THE
NATURAL HEALING
COOKBOOK

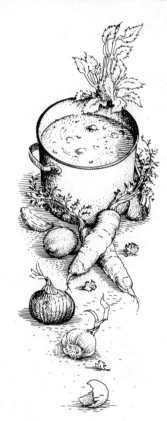

THE NATURAL HEALING COOKBOOK

Over 450 Delicious Ways
To Get Better and Stay Healthy

by

Mark Bricklin

Executive Editor, Prevention® *Magazine*

and

Sharon Claessens

Design

John F. Carafoli

Layout

Jerry O'Brien

Illustrations

Heather Preston

Pat Dypold

Darlene Schneck

Hayward Blake

RODALE PRESS
Emmaus, Pa.

Printed in the United States of America on recycled paper, containing a high percentage of de-inked fiber.

Library of Congress Cataloging in Publication Data

Bricklin, Mark.
The natural healing cookbook.

Includes indexes.
1. Diet therapy. 2. Cookery for the sick.
3. Nutrition. I. Claessens, Sharon, joint author.
II. Title.
RM216.B844   641.5'631   80–29170
ISBN 0-87857-338-0 hardcover
ISBN 0-87857-358-5 hardcover deluxe

		8	10	9	7			*hardcover*
4	6	8	10	9	7	5	3	*hardcover deluxe*

Table of Contents

Notice

The information in this book is meant to complement the advice and guidance of your physician, not replace it. If you are under the care of a physician, you should by all means discuss any major change in your diet with him or her. That is especially important if you are diabetic and taking insulin, because the recipes in this book have a very powerful health effect on the body, and may well make it necessary for you to reduce your insulin dosage.

Because this is a book, and not some kind of medical consultation, keep in mind that the information presented here may not apply in your particular case, because of food allergy, medication, or other individual differences. Whenever a question arises, discuss it with your physician.

Acknowledgments

We gratefully acknowledge the assistance and inspiration of many people at Rodale Press. Our recipes were tested by Anita Hirsch and others at the Rodale Test Kitchen. The researchers and fact-checkers were Carol Baldwin (Chief), Tom Wolff, Carol Munson, Carol Matthews, Eileen Mazer, Susan Rosenkrantz and Marian Wolbers, who also worked on the copy editing. Writers whose work we consulted and often used to help fill in our work include John Feltman, William Gottlieb, Carl Sherman, Jane Kinderlehrer, Sharon Faelten, John Yates, Linda Shaw and Jeanne-Nell Gover. Typing was done by Carol Petrakovich, Brenda Peluso, Barbara Hill and Pat Hasik. Library assistance was given by Shirley Keck and Liz Wolbach. Copy editing was done by Dolores Plikaitis. Emrika Padus helped edit the book, Karen Schell helped in the design; Henry DeWeerd and Robert Rodale gave us inspiration. We are also grateful to the many scientists and physicians who talked to us, and who patiently double-checked our work for accuracy. Then there are Barbara and Mat, who gave us encouragement, energy and more.

Getting It All Together

MORE THAN A COOKBOOK

This is not just a collection of good-tasting recipes, but a new way of eating that you can *live* with—and live longer.

Because this book may be quite different from other cookbooks you have read, we'd like to take a few minutes to orient you to its approach.

Health Improvement Is Paramount

First and foremost, *The Natural Healing Cookbook* offers you a way of eating which we believe to be optimally healthful for most people. From individual ingredients to cooking methods, right down to condiments, *everything* has been selected and designed to promote health and well-being. The idea is not simply to avoid what is bad, but to maximize what is good, what is strengthening and healing.

The great majority of recipes can be used with benefit by almost all readers. That's because many of the most common chronic illnesses in this country—such as heart and circulatory disease, high blood pressure and bowel problems—seem to respond well to the same overall dietary approach. They may also be prevented from occurring, or progressing, in large degree, by the same approach. In that sense, what we have assembled here is a vast menu of meals that heal.

In addition, there are special recipes and dietary programs for helping specific problems, such as overweight, insomnia, hearing problems, convalescence and others. In many instances, people interested in these recipes could also benefit greatly from recipes designed to promote overall health.

If you want to, you may think of these recipes, and the whole approach described here, as the new *cuisine sante*—the cuisine of health.

Scientific Basis

Our choice of ingredients and preparation methods in this book is based on extensive research in the fields of clinical nutrition, food science and experimental medicine. It is not based on any special system or belief to which we are committed at all costs. Adherence to such special systems often leads to exaggerated claims of benefits on the one hand and curt dismissal of different approaches on the other. We have tried to be as open-minded as possible, accepting scientific findings on their merits, and using them in the spirit of pragmatism and common sense.

A Cookbook To Live With

These recipes aren't meant to be prepared once a month, or whenever the fancy strikes you, as is the case with most other cookbooks. Rather, they are designed to be a way of eating, from morning to bedtime, every day, as long as you feel they are appropriate for you. Not only recipes, but overall dietary strategies are given.

A Practical Approach

If we expect you to use this cookbook as an everyday guide for better eating, we have to offer something practical—*very* practical. So we've put great emphasis on making sure that you can genuinely *use* it, really reap its benefits, trust it and enjoy it, like a good friend.

Specifically, that means, among other things, that the recipes must taste good. You can be sure that there are many dishes we tried that didn't make print. Recipes had to have real character, and please the people we served them to. Many of the dishes were offered and received very well at Sunday night suppers, dinner parties, buffets and picnics. After we were satisfied, our test kitchen prepared each recipe according to our directions, served it to several groups of taste-testers and let us know the results, as well as suggestions for improvements or clarification of the cooking procedures. All that doesn't mean we can guarantee each recipe to be positively delicious to everyone, but at least it increases the chances you'll be quite pleased with how your meal turns out.

Another facet of food enjoyment is appearance, and these recipes are, we feel, very attractive. They don't need fancy tableware or capes of cream sauce to make them look that way, either.

Food should also be filling—*satisfying*—especially if you're trying to control your food budget, and maybe your waistline at the same time. These recipes fill the bill nicely, we think. The variety of food tastes, zesty herbs and spices, and plenty of natural fiber take care of that. And the meals you'll be enjoying are so low in fats and sugars that there's very little danger of taking in too many calories as you satisfy your appetite.

Another practical aspect is that these recipes are quite flexible. We often give tips for substituting what you happen to have around the kitchen.

No Exotic Ingredients

Nothing is more maddening to a cook than to find a great-sounding recipe that calls for hard-to-find ingredients—the kind of thing you almost never keep in your pantry or refrigerator. In some cases, you might not even know where you could buy them—or how to pronounce them if you did! There are no exotic ingredients in *The Natural Healing Cookbook*—no black Chinese mushrooms, no European saffron, no pompano, no quail or venison, no green peppercorns or papayas—and certainly no candied orange peels or *kirschwasser*. We did all of our shopping at typical large supermarkets and several small—*very* small—health food stores. Occasionally we visited ethnic groceries to buy something like fresh ricotta cheese, or a farmers' market to get fresher vegetables, but never to seek out exotic items.

But we go even further. Before we even get to the recipes, we give you a list of ingredients that will be used over and over again and suggest that you always keep some on hand. These ingredients, which can easily be kept in the kitchen, will enable you to always find a very wide selection of recipes—hundreds, actually—that can be made perfectly with those ingredients alone.

No Fancy Equipment

To make these recipes, you will not be required to purchase any expensive or elaborate equipment—no food processors, convection ovens, deluxe juicers or grain grinders. But we'll tell you what you *do* need to make your work easier and more efficient.

Economical

If the spiral of higher and higher food prices is pinching your budget and torturing your sense of kitchen economy, these recipes will ease the pain. You won't find a recipe that sounds good and then grimace when you realize it entails buying budget-busters like veal and lobster. (In the course of writing this book, we were so impressed with the drop in our food budgets that we thought of renaming it *The Save-Money-and-Live-to-Enjoy-It Cookbook!*)

How is that possible? Here's a clue: the latest government figures show that of the total price of a loaf of bread, only about *four cents* goes to farmers who produce the actual food. The rest goes to middlemen and retailers. To a large extent, we teach *you* how to become the middleman. The money you *do* spend will all go for good nutrition and fresh flavor, not processing and fancy labels.

And here's something else: How would you like to go for weeks without ever throwing away a single thing from your refrigerator because it went bad? Imagine how pleasant it is to be able to look into your refrigerator and never see anything except fresh, attractive food—no wilted heads of lettuce, no pieces of fruit covered with large brown spots, no shriveled pieces of dry meat. Both of us made that wonderful discovery independently, and it wasn't because we were trying to pinch pennies. Rather, it was the natural result of the new culinary system we were following, a system that encourages versatility and the creative use of leftovers.

Creative But Simple

We don't stint on giving clear instructions on how to prepare our recipes. And the techniques we use are quite simple. Anyone familiar with a kitchen should have no trouble understanding our directions. At the same time, we frequently give tips for variations. The idea is not to make each dish come out so that it looks and tastes exactly like some famous chef made it, but to have it come out plain *terrific.*

Because natural food lends itself to a kind of casual, free-wheeling approach, you can mix and match ingredients as the season—or your taste buds—may dictate. And because our food is generally low in calories and fat, you can enjoy eating *more* of it, too—feeding your appetite in royal style while catering to your health.

TOOLING UP

Cooking for better health does not mean turning your kitchen upside down and investing in lots of new equipment. In fact, your kitchen is probably adequate right now for the preparation of most recipes in this book.

Rather than investing in specialized equipment, remember that it is possible to improvise. For example, rather than purchase a special steamer for vegetables, put your metal colander to double duty. Place enough water in a large kettle so that the water level is just below the colander, place the colander in the kettle, add food when the water is boiling, cover, and steam. Or, set a square cooling rack atop an electric skillet, bring water to a boil in the skillet, and place the food to be steamed on the rack. Cover with the lid, and you're set.

A double boiler can be fashioned from two pans, one just a bit larger than the other, or a stainless steel mixing bowl set inside a pot. Place water in the larger pan, set the smaller pan over the boiling water, and proceed.

If you don't already have them, here are a few items that can simplify meal preparation:

blender	muffin tins
garlic press	bread pans
cooling racks	pie pans
sieve	heavy cast-iron pans
grater, with fine, medium, and large holes	stainless steel pans
sharp knives	pressure cooker
mechanical grater	wooden spoons
nutmeg grater	eggbeater
	wire whisk

A blender is handy for making soups and sauces, although it is quite possible to do without one. A blender can also be used to grind nuts, and even to make peanut butter.

A mechanical grater can simplify grating chores. Carrots, nuts and cheese can be grated in a small, hand-held model. Consider a food mill, too, for making soups and purees. Purees can also be made by pressing foods through a sieve with the back of a wooden spoon.

A sharp knife, or set of knives, is essential in preparing vegetables and meats. Keep a sharpening tool handy and use it frequently.

Our muffin recipes are based on muffin cups which hold one-quarter cup of batter. Bread recipes are based on pans measuring 8½ × 4½ inches.

Cast-iron pans are useful, easy to clean, and impart a certain amount of iron to foods. A small cast-iron pan is perfect for toasting sunflower or sesame seeds atop the stove on the occasions they are called for. Alternately, these can be toasted in a moderate oven or broiled until golden.

Some prefer a pressure cooker for beans and grains as it greatly shortens cooking time. Beans can foam, however, clogging the steam vent. An alternative method we recommend is cooking beans in the oven while baking other dishes. This is safe, easy and economical.

Stainless steel pans are a good investment because they are less likely than aluminum to react with foods. To cash in on efficient heat conduction—but at the same time protect yourself from food reactions—choose aluminum-clad stainless steel or lined copper pans.

STOCKING UP

By keeping certain staples on hand, you'll be able to prepare a wide variety of healthful meals from our book. Here is what we suggest keeping in your pantry and refrigerator.

Whole grains: whole wheat flour, whole wheat pastry flour, rolled oats, brown rice, whole grain cornmeal, soy flour, buckwheat flour, rye flour, millet, whole grain pastas.

Beans, nuts and seeds: kidney, lima, pinto, soy or other beans; lentils and dried peas; peanuts, almonds, walnuts, cashews; natural peanut butter; sesame (hulled), sunflower and pumpkin seeds.

Vegetables: carrots, green and sweet red (bell) peppers, spinach, potatoes, broccoli, cabbage, brussels sprouts, cauliflower; also, yellow onions, scallions, garlic.

Cheeses: low-fat cottage cheese, ricotta cheese, Parmesan cheese (used for flavoring), Swiss or Jarlsburg, and *Yogurt Cream Cheese* (see *Index*).

Fruits: bananas, grapefruit, oranges, apples, lemons, assorted dried fruits (prunes, dates, apricots, raisins, currants).

Herbs: dried basil, thyme, marjoram, sage, rosemary, tarragon, dill, oregano, bay leaves, mint, celery seeds, caraway seeds, ground cumin, coriander, chili powder, mustard powder, paprika, cayenne pepper, fresh parsley (flat-leaf or curly-leaf), dried hot red pepper flakes.

Spices: allspice, cardamom, curry, ground and whole cloves, nutmeg, mace, cinnamon, turmeric, ground ginger, fresh ginger root.

Flavorings: cider and white vinegar, tamari, kelp powder, lemon juice, *Vanilla Extract* (see *Index*), tomato paste, Dijon-style mustard, carob powder.

Oils: sunflower, safflower, corn, soy, olive.

Miscellaneous: wheat germ, bran, gluten flour, active dry yeast, agar-agar flakes, baking soda, *Baking Powder* (see below for recipe without aluminum compounds).

Note that any ingredient, such as rice, vegetables or fish, is raw unless otherwise specified. Herbs are dried, unless "fresh" is listed. Spices are ground, not whole.

Getting Acquainted

When you are stocking up, you will want to choose the most healthful varieties of each food. The following notes will help explain the form and function of these ingredients.

Agar-agar: This is a vegetable gelatin made from sea algae. Available in health food stores and Oriental food shops.

Baking powder: Most brands of baking powder on the market are undesirable because they contain aluminum salts. There is evidence that ingested aluminum accumulates in the brain and could, over time, cause memory loss and brain deterioration. Baking powder without aluminum salts is available at health food stores. Do not exceed the recommended amount of baking powder used in our recipes, because excess alkalinity plus heat destroys thiamine, a B vitamin. And be aware that one teaspoon of our baking powder contains 225 milligrams of sodium, slightly over one-tenth of the amount found in one teaspoon of table salt.

Here is a simple recipe for making your own baking powder:

Baking Powder

Makes ¼ cup (60 ml)
1 tablespoon (15 ml) baking soda
2 tablespoons (30 ml) cream of tartar
2 tablespoons (30 ml) arrowroot

Mix the ingredients together in a small bowl with a wooden spoon. Crush any lumps. Store in a tightly covered jar in a cool, dry place.

Baking soda: Again, baking soda affects the alkalinity of the batter, and thiamine, sensitive to heat in an alkaline environment, can be lost. If the entire range of B vitamins, which whole wheat flour provides, is to be part of your diet, do not depend heavily on chemically leavened baked goods. Try the many delicious and easy yeast-raised breads included here. Baking soda contains 1,123 milligrams of sodium per teaspoon, over half that contained in the same amount of salt.

Baking yeast: Often cheaper purchased in bulk, one tablespoon is equal to the small packets available commercially. Active dry yeast is available in health food stores; if you prefer compressed yeast, try a bakery. Keep it dry and tightly covered, stored in a cool place. Yeast is usually dissolved in warm water before combining with flour. About 100 degrees F., or lukewarm, is sufficient to activate the yeast without killing it by too high temperature. A little honey in a recipe encourages the little yeasts to feed. As they multiply, the yeasts release carbon dioxide, which creates bubbles and makes the dough rise. A warm (between 80 to 85 degrees F.), draft-free spot is best for rising. If you are uncertain about the viability of your yeast, place a teaspoon of honey in the warm water when dissolving it. If the yeast does not bubble up, chances are it is no longer "active" and you will have to discard it.

Bran: We usually use wheat bran, the hull of the wheat berry, which is discarded in the making of white flour. Inexpensive and valuable as a source of fiber, bran is available in supermarkets and health food stores. Do not use commercial breakfast cereal bran, which often contains sugar and other additives. Store in a cool, dry place.

Brewer's yeast: This nonleavening yeast is an excellent source of B vitamins, and is high in protein. It can be added to bread, baked goods, cereals, pancakes, soups, sauces and many other foods. Available in health food stores. Store in a cool, dry place.

Buckwheat: Roasted buckwheat groats are called kasha. This product resembles a grain, but is related, instead, to rhubarb. Buckwheat has over twice the iron of brown rice. Buy it hulled at health food stores. Store in a cool, dry place.

Buckwheat flour: Buy the whole, dark flour, made from unfumigated buckwheat, available at health food stores. Store, tightly wrapped against moisture, in the refrigerator.

Bulgur: Parboiled, dried and cracked wheat, bulgur is a good substitute for brown rice or potatoes. Try it as a quick-cooking cereal for breakfast. Available in health food stores. Store in a cool, dry place.

Buttermilk: Contrary to what the name implies, this cultured milk is low in calories and butterfat, and provides a tasty, tangy beverage. The acid content makes buttermilk useful in baking as it will interact with baking soda and also tenderizes yeast breads. Contains somewhat more sodium than regular milk. Sold at supermarkets, it should be stored in the refrigerator.

Carob powder: Made from ground carob pods (also called St. John's bread), carob resembles chocolate in taste. But here the similarity ends. In terms of healthy eating, carob has several advantages over chocolate or cocoa.

1. Carob is naturally sweet, so there is no need to rely heavily on concentrated sweeteners to mask bitterness, as is the case with chocolate.
2. Carob is high in fiber and low in fat, with one-tenth the amount of fat found in chocolate.
3. Carob contains approximately four times the calcium of cocoa or chocolate.
4. Chocolate contains oxalic acid, which actually inhibits the absorption of calcium.
5. Chocolate contains caffeine, which is addictive, and theobromine, a related stimulant.
6. Carob, a legume, does not cause the allergies that chocolate can incite.

Carob powder is found in health food stores. Store tightly covered in a cool, dry place.

Cheese: Unprocessed cheese should be chosen, such as Swiss or cottage cheese. Avoid products labeled "processed cheese" or "cheese food." Note labeling on cottage cheese containers and choose those with only natural ingredients. Some are available without salt. Cheese can be purchased at supermarkets, specialty shops and health food stores. Keep cheese wrapped and refrigerated.

Corn tortillas and tacos: These are made with very simple ingredients—whole grain cornmeal, water and lime. But they are extremely difficult to make yourself unless you have exactly the right kind of cornmeal and equipment. We have found it very convenient to buy them at the supermarket. Most brands have no preservatives and many have no salt. Tortillas are usually kept in the dairy case or freezer section. They are great for making sandwiches when you don't want to eat two whole slices of bread along with the filling. You just wrap the filling up in one thin tortilla which has been heated in the oven. Or heat up a crisp taco shell and stuff with filling.

Cornmeal: Choose stone-ground, whole grain cornmeal. Buy the cornmeal freshly ground and store in the refrigerator. Available in health food stores.

Crumbs: Recipes may call for soft or dry bread crumbs. For soft crumbs, use fresh whole grain bread and separate crumbs lightly with a fork while holding the bread in place on a cutting board. Soft crumbs can also be made by crumbling fresh bread by hand. To measure, pile the fresh crumbs lightly in a cup. Use them immediately. For dry crumbs, use very dry, stale whole grain bread. To remove any moisture, place bread slices on a baking sheet and place in a 200-degree F. oven just until dry. Do not let the bread darken; this will affect the taste. Crumbs can be made by placing broken slices in a blender and processing in short bursts at high speed. A rotary hand grater can be used for small amounts. Dry crumbs can be placed in a tightly covered container and frozen.

Dried fruits: Buy fruits that are naturally dried, without preservatives. These fruits may look darker and seem tougher than the artificially softened fruits. To soften, just cover with boiling water and allow to stand up to 24 hours, or until tender. Available at health food stores. Store in a cool, dry place.

Dried legumes: Buy these in supermarkets and health food stores. Dried beans, peas and peanuts, available for pennies a pound, provide a real protein bargain, along with valuable vitamins and minerals. Combine them with whole grains, nuts, seeds or dairy products for balanced, nourishing protein that comes accompanied by fiber. Store in a cool, dry and dark place.

Cooking Beans and Other Legumes

There are two basic methods of preparing beans and other legumes for cooking. One is to wash the beans, drain, then place with enough water to cover in a container for several hours or overnight. Use sufficient water to accommodate the beans as they expand.

The second method is to wash the beans, drain, then place in a pan with enough water to generously cover. Bring to a boil, reduce heat and simmer for one or two minutes. Remove from the heat, cover, and let stand one hour.

These two soaking methods will greatly reduce cooking time. To reduce flatulence, the soaking water can be discarded, and the beans cooked in fresh water. This will result in the loss of some nutrients, but may make the beans acceptable to some who would not otherwise enjoy them.

Lentils and split peas need not be soaked before cooking.

To cook beans, place in a pan with water to cover, bring to a boil and simmer gently until beans are tender. Cooking times for beans will vary from about one-and-a-half hours for lima, kidney and small white beans such as navy beans to about three hours for chick-peas, azuki and soybeans. Most dried beans will double in bulk after cooking.

An alternate method of cooking beans is to place the soaked beans with water to cover in an ovenproof casserole dish. Cover and bake at about 350 degrees F. until tender. Place soybeans in an oversized container, such as a roasting pan covered with foil, as soybeans tend to foam as they cook. A container of beans can be prepared in the oven along with other baked goods, saving energy.

Flours: Buy whole grain flours with their vitamins, minerals, fats and trace elements intact. Stir lightly before measuring, or sift and then stir in the bran that is left behind. Grind grains yourself, if possible (there are several manual and electric grinders on the market), or get them as freshly ground as possible. Soy flour is a protein-enhancing addition to whole wheat flour. Substitute two tablespoons of soy flour for an equal amount of whole wheat flour per cup. Store in moistureproof containers in the refrigerator.

Fruit juices: Purchase unsweetened, unstrained, and fresh juices, if possible. (Make your own orange juice, with pulp; nothing fresher!) Fresh apple cider is preferable to strained and overprocessed apple juice, which may contain added sugar. Juices are available at fruit stands, farmers' markets, supermarkets or health food stores. Store in the refrigerator.

Herbs: Grow them fresh, or buy them fresh or dried. Since none of our recipes call for salt, herbs are an important way of highlighting the natural flavor of foods. Crush dried herbs between the fingers before adding; this enhances their ability to impart flavor. Popular herbs are: basil, parsley, thyme, oregano, tarragon, dill, bay leaf, caraway, coriander, cumin, horseradish, marjoram, sage, mint, chives, cayenne pepper, chili, rosemary, sage and savory. Herbs can be purchased at the supermarket, health food stores, specialty shops or farmers' markets. Store tightly covered in a cool, dry and dark place. Fresh herbs can be frozen for later use.

Honey: Buy honey raw and unfiltered in supermarkets, farmers' markets and at health food stores. Honey is used in place of white sugar. But it is still a potent sweetener (64 calories per tablespoon), and should be used very sparingly. Store in a cool, dry place—but not in the refrigerator where it may crystallize.

Lecithin: Occurring naturally in soybeans, lecithin is composed of two B vitamins and oil. It is sold in health food stores in both an oil and granular form. Soybean lecithin, used in the granular form, has been shown to have an effect in reducing cholesterol. Lecithin oil, mixed half and half with a vegetable oil, is perfect for lightly oiling baking pans and casserole dishes. A thin layer prevents sticking and adds no taste to baked goods. Mix and keep on hand on a pantry shelf.

Meat and poultry: These should be purchased fresh, preferably from animals raised organically, that is, without hormones or unnecessary chemicals. These are available from local farmers, health food stores or companies that specialize in such meat products. Keep refrigerated or frozen until ready to use.

Milk: Skim or buttermilk, both low in fat and calories, is preferred. Available in supermarkets or dairy stores, it should be stored in the refrigerator.

Molasses: Molasses, especially blackstrap, is rich in minerals. Here you'll find a storehouse of iron, calcium and potassium, and even some essential chromium. Molasses keeps breads and cakes moist longer. Medium, unsulfured molasses can be substituted for honey in most recipes without an appreciable difference in taste. Store in a cool, dry place.

Nuts: Choose unsalted, fresh nuts. Cashews must be cooked before eating as they are toxic raw. Although high in calories (they are used sparingly here), nuts are a valuable source of protein, vitamins and minerals. The best way to store nuts is in their shells in a cool, dark, dry place. If nuts have been shelled, refrigerate or freeze, tightly covered.

Oats: Rolled oats are made from hulled groats, steamed and rolled flat. Steel-cut oats are passed through special cutting machines to convert groats to uniform granules. Oats have the highest protein content of all the cereals, and the highest quality protein. Available in supermarkets and health food stores. Store in a cool, dry place.

Oils: Use corn, safflower, sunflower or soy oil for cooking or salad dressings.

Sesame oil has a distinctive flavor, and is used sparingly for that reason. Olive oil is used only occasionally, for its special flavor, because it is not as high in polyunsaturates as the other oils. Avoid cottonseed oil, which is higher than most vegetable oils in saturated fat. Coconut oil is extremely high in saturated fat. We never use it. Note that ingredients listed as "vegetable oil" on product labels might in reality be cottonseed or coconut oil. Store in a cool, dry, dark place if oil is purchased in small quantities and use quickly. Otherwise, refrigeration is best. Olive oil, which begins to solidify under refrigeration, can be left to stand at room temperature until liquid before using. When oils turn rancid (with an "off" taste and odor), they must be discarded.

Pastry flour: While whole wheat bread flour is made from hard winter wheat, pastry flour is made from soft spring wheat. It contains little or no gluten, which gives dough its "stretchy" quality, so is unsatisfactory for yeast breads. For quick breads, pie crusts and cakes, however, it provides the flaky, crumbly texture desired. Store in the refrigerator in a moistureproof container.

Peanut butter: Buy peanut butter made from whole peanuts, without sugar, salt or stabilizers added. If the peanut butter separates, just stir—you'll be avoiding the hydrogenated fats that are added for smoothness to other brands. Try making peanut butter in your blender, adding up to one tablespoon of corn or soy oil per cup of peanuts to get the proper consistency. Use walnuts, almonds and toasted cashews to make a variety of nut butters, or try raw sunflower seeds. Peanut butter made from whole peanuts, including the germ, should be kept in the refrigerator. Natural peanut butter can be purchased at some supermarkets and at health food stores.

Rice: Brown rice, because it is far higher in fiber and nutrients than polished white rice, is the rice to buy. Long or short grain rice is available in health food stores. Short grain may be used more commonly in puddings, desserts, stuffings or other dishes, while long grain, which separates more easily after cooking, is commonly used plain, as a side dish. Try both and see which you prefer. Supermarkets often carry the long grain rice. Store in a cool, dry and dark place.

Cooking Brown Rice

Wash rice and drain. Place in a saucepan with two-and-one-quarter cups of water for each cup of rice and bring to a boil. Reduce heat, cover and slowly simmer for about 35 minutes, or until the water is absorbed and the rice is tender.

To save time, cook two to three cups of rice at a time. Cool the unused portion and refrigerate or freeze for later use.

Seafood: To determine freshness of whole fish, see that the eyes are shining and bulging, and the gills are reddish. If you can, touch the fish to see if the flesh is firm and the scales are firmly attached. Fresh fish does not have a strong, offensive odor. With frozen fish, choose packages that are solidly frozen, without tears in the package. Never refreeze fish that has been frozen, or that you suspect may have been frozen. Use any unfrozen fish within a day or two, storing it in the refrigerator over ice, carefully wrapped.

Be careful not to overcook fish. When the fish turns from translucent to opaque, it is done. Fish that is too "flaky" after cooking, and has no moisture remaining, is overdone. Frozen fish will require about double the cooking time for fresh fish. With canned salmon, break up the soft bones with some of the flesh for added calcium. In our recipes the crushed bones are undetectable.

Seeds: High in vitamins and minerals, seeds are one of the best snack and cooking ingredients available. Seeds even complement some of the proteins in nuts and grains, proving their meal-worthiness. Seeds are best bought at a health food store, where they are available untreated and in bulk. Buy seeds raw and unsalted, the sunflower and sesame seeds hulled. Seeds can be stored in a cool, dry place, or tightly covered in the refrigerator.

Sesame tahini: Tahini is made of ground hulled sesame seeds. An oily paste, it is used in some Middle Eastern dishes. Tahini can be used in sandwich spreads, salad dressings, dips and baked goods. It is available in health food stores and some ethnic food shops. Store in a cool, dry place, or in the refrigerator if it is not used frequently.

Soy flakes: These are toasted soybeans rolled into flakes. Soy flakes can be eaten without additional cooking, mixed with dry cereals or with seeds and nuts. Available in health food stores. Store in a dry place.

Sprouts: Most important is to use seeds, beans or grains that have not been fumigated or treated with pesticides or fungicides, as are seeds meant for planting. Buy seeds meant for human consumption in health food stores. Sprouting greatly increases vitamin content, and sprouts are especially high in vitamin C. Using one-quarter cup of most beans or seeds will yield about one pint of sprouts. Try alfalfa, mustard, radish and sunflower seeds, mung beans, lentils, chick-peas, soybeans, and wheat or other grains. Store sprouts in a moistureproof container in the refrigerator.

How to Make Sprouts

Sprouts are best made in a wide-mouth glass jar anywhere from one quart to one gallon in capacity. The important thing is to make sure that the mouth is wide. If you are using a large jar, you will also need a piece of cheesecloth and a rubber band, to be fixed over the mouth of the jar during rinsing operations.

The amount of seeds that you will put in the jar will vary with how large it is and how many sprouts you need. If you are using a gallon jug, and making sprouts for four people, for instance, you might want to use about one-half cup of seeds. The amount also depends on the *kind* of seed to be sprouted. Alfalfa sprouts increase tremendously in size, while the larger seeds, like lentils and soybeans, increase relatively little. You will soon get the hang of judging amounts. A good mixture is equal parts of alfalfa and lentils sprouted together.

Begin by putting the seeds in the jar and covering them with water. Let them sit overnight or an equivalent amount of time, and then pour off the water and rinse the seeds very well. With your cheesecloth tied over the mouth of the jar, shake the seeds vigorously so that the only water remaining in the jar is the water clinging to the seeds. Then shake the seeds again so they are distributed as widely as possible and lay the jar on its side on your kitchen counter. Make sure there is something in front of it so it doesn't roll off the counter! Many people seem to think that seeds should be sprouted in a dark place, but that only encourages the growth of mold. Seeds will sprout very well in full light and you can have fun watching them develop. The most important thing is to rinse your sprouts very well about three or four times a day, making sure that they get plenty of fresh water and are then completely drained. Don't worry if you have to work during the day. Rinse them first thing in the morning, as soon as you come home from work, once during the evening, and one more time just before you go to bed. During the last day or two of sprouting, we like to put the jar in full sunlight. Alfalfa sprouts, especially, will turn a beautiful green, develop valuable chlorophyll, and improve their texture and taste if they get some good sunlight. After about three or four days, your sprouts will be ready. Alfalfa sprouts are best harvested when the sprout is about two inches long, but the larger the seed, the less the sprout has to grow before harvesting time. Sunflower seeds and soybeans, for example, may have sprouts only about a quarter of an inch or so long when they are ready. If you let them get *too* long, they won't be tender and sweet. While some people say they have trouble making sprouts, we've found that you can get perfect results every time if you make sure that you don't put too many seeds in a jar, that they aren't lying in water, and that they get plenty of fresh air and light. When your sprouts are ready, put them in a transparent storage bag, and store in the refrigerator. Sprouts will generally retain their crispness and good taste for four or five days. When one batch is done, start another so that you never run out.

Tamari: This oriental-style soy sauce is made from fermented soybeans, sometimes with wheat added. Use tamari that has been naturally fermented, unlike some commercial brands, which are produced by chemical means. Available in some oriental food shops (where it may be labeled ''soy sauce'') and in health food stores. Use sparingly because of high sodium content. Store on the shelf.

Vanilla: Use either the vanilla bean or a pure extract. (See *Index* for recipe for making extract without alcohol.) Vanilla beans are available at some supermarkets and at health food stores. Store in a cool, dry and dark place.

Vegetables: The best option is to organically grow your own, if possible, so you are certain to get fresh, wholesome produce without chemicals. If that is impossible, try to find a small-scale local farmer who grows produce organically. Visit a farmers' market and ask how the vegetables are grown. Many health food stores carry organic produce. Be sure vegetables are firm, fresh and with good color. The following are most frequently called for in our recipes: broccoli, cabbage, brussels sprouts, cauliflower, carrots, green and red sweet peppers, spinach, potatoes, onions, leeks, scallions, garlic, leafy salad greens, sweet potatoes and squash. Try fresh lemon juice rather than salt to spark salads and cooked vegetable dishes.

Wheat germ: The nutritional ''heart'' of the wheat, the germ is rich in protein,

B vitamins, vitamin E, potassium and zinc. Wheat germ should be stored tightly covered or wrapped in the refrigerator or, if not used regularly, in the freezer. Toasting destroys some of the food value, but prolongs storage time.

Yogurt: Yogurt is easily made at home, which makes it inexpensive as well as healthful and nutritious. To make, heat one quart of skim milk to just under the boiling point in a stainless steel or enameled pan (small bubbles will appear around the edges of the liquid in the pan). Set aside to cool. When the milk is lukewarm, stir in about one-half cup of store-bought yogurt (yogurt with *Lactobacillus acidophilus* is preferred as these beneficial bacteria establish themselves most easily in the bowels). Cover the pan, place in a warm spot—either a gas oven with pilot light, sunny window, or counter-top in a kitchen warmed by baking—and allow to rest, undisturbed, for eight hours or longer, until it thickens. Do not move the pan, or the yogurt may not set. Store yogurt in the refrigerator.

Miscellaneous: Kelp powder, made from seaweed, is used in some recipes, though with moderation because of its high sodium content. Kelp is, however, also rich in potassium, and contains iodine, a mineral that regulates the thyroid gland. Kelp also contains calcium, iron, zinc and phosphorus. Cracked wheat, which is cut wheat grains, is good for morning cooked cereal or mixing into breads. Gluten flour adds extra body to some whole wheat doughs. Eggs are used only occasionally in our recipes because of the high-cholesterol content of the yolks. For barley, buy the whole grain, hulled, not "pearled" barley. Store in cool, dry place. Herbal teas are a more healthful hot or cold beverage than caffeine-laced teas and coffee. Maple syrup is occasionally used for sweetening.

PROMINENT AMONG THE MISSING

Throughout this book, you will get clues as to why we never use certain foods or ingredients and use others sparingly. Right now, though, we'd like to gather them all together for a look at the whole unhealthful lot.

First, here are the foods and ingredients we *never* use.

Salt is almost 40 percent sodium, which we believe to be a major contributing cause of high blood pressure. Besides not using salt in cooking, we avoid any prepackaged foods that contain added salt (such as olives, pickles and anchovies).

Sugar is among the missing for more reasons than we have time to count here. Just briefly, sugar contains nothing but calories; tends to deplete the important B vitamin, thiamine; can lead to or aggravate both hypoglycemia and diabetes; works synergistically with salt to promote high blood pressure; promotes tooth decay when eaten with sticky foods; and, although few people realize it, has been shown to actually depress the body's immune response, and so lowers our resistance to disease. Brown sugar is marginally better than white, but is still far from being a healthful food. Foods and condiments that contain large amounts of added sugar, such as jams, jellies and ketchup (which is 30 percent sugar) are also excluded.

Coffee, needless to say, is not used as a beverage. But we've also nixed its use for flavoring desserts, because we feel if you're trying to get coffee out of your life, there's no sense keeping some around just for a very occasional dessert. As for decaffeinated coffee, it's true that most of the caffeine has been taken out, but it still contains chlorogenic acid, which is capable of causing its own mischief, such as heartburn. And the chemicals used in the decaffeination process are suspected of being potential cancer agents.

Chocolate not only contains caffeine, but because it is bitter, is almost always prepared with copious amounts of sugar. Probably the worst thing about chocolate is that it is usually used in foods that are basically unhealthful, such as cakes, candies and pies —so hard to resist.

Butter is practically pure fat—and dairy fat at that, which some health researchers consider to be especially unhealthful. It's also loaded with calories, a single tablespoon delivering about 100 of the little buggers. Cooking without butter is both healthier and easier than most people imagine.

Cream, sour cream, and **cream cheese** are, along with butter, the fattiest dairy products and we do not use them at all.

Mayonnaise, which is basically an amalgam of fat and oil, and contains cholesterol-rich egg yolks, is probably one of the most unhealthful of all condiments.

Coconut sounds like a wonderful natural food, but by some quirk of nature, coconuts are positively loaded with fat, and scientists who study atherosclerosis report that the fastest way to give an experimental animal a good case of bad circulation is to feed it coconut oil. Since the coconut meat contains ample amounts of the oil, we do not use even small amounts of shredded coconut.

Wine, brandy, beer and other alcoholic beverages are frequently used in sauces prepared by cooks following low-fat diet principles, but we have not permitted ourselves this easy luxury. Although much of the alcohol in these beverages may evaporate during cooking, we don't want you to keep them around the house just for occasional use in the kitchen. Over-consumption of alcohol is such an enormous health problem that we feel it's not right to encourage its use in any form.

White flour has become for many the very symbol of overly processed, devitalized foods, and for good reason. Even when it is called "enriched," it's actually impoverished, because only a few of the vitamins and minerals that are depleted are put back, and in the case of iron, it's put back in a form that is almost totally unusable by human beings. And of course, nearly all the fiber is gone, too.

Pepper, although few people realize it, is now considered to be a "mild co-carcinogen," which means it can act together with other more powerful substances to promote the development of cancer. Although this effect is not an especially powerful one, the regular use of pepper has no place in a diet designed for health. That goes for black *and* white pepper.

Granola. We're banning *granola?* Yes, and we didn't even have to think twice about it. Whether you make it at home or buy it from the supermarket shelf, almost everyone understands granola to be a mixture of grains and seeds to which generous amounts of honey and oil have been added before roasting. Some recipes (or brands) call for brown sugar as well as honey. And if you buy granola that lists "vegetable oil" as an ingredient, chances are it's coconut oil which, as we mentioned before, is probably the worst oil of all for your heart. Now, we wouldn't get that upset if a little bit of honey or vegetable oil was being added to something extremely low in fat, but nuts, seeds and grains are already quite rich in oil, while the dried fruits normally added to granola, like raisins, are high in natural sugar. What we offer in our book instead of granola are a variety of muesli recipes, which give you all the taste, crunchiness and natural energy of nuts, seeds and grains, but without the entirely unnecessary extra oil and extra sugar, which turn a high-energy breakfast into candy-in-a-bowl.

So much for the absolute no-no's. Now let's do a quick review of those foods that we use either very rarely and/or in very small amounts.

Whole milk is used only for a few special applications where it seems to be needed. Ordinarily, we use skim milk exclusively, or buttermilk, which is also low in fat but which has more sodium in it. If you're new to the health food game, we suggest using either low-fat milk, which is a compromise between whole milk and skim milk, or keeping two quarts of milk in the refrigerator—one whole and one skim, and combining them in different proportions as the use dictates.

Cheese, because of its high saturated fat, salt and cholesterol content, is used only in small amounts, never more than about one ounce per person in the case of firm cheeses, but more if the cheese is less dense. And usually, we use a low-fat or low-salt cheese, such as ricotta or cottage cheese. Occasionally, we'll sprinkle on some cheddar or Parmesan for flavoring, but in general we stay away from the hard cheeses.

Honey and **maple syrup** have largely undeserved reputations as health foods. While they are a little better than plain sugar, the difference is not worth getting excited about. We use both very sparingly. On occasion, we also use some blackstrap molasses, which is loaded with sugar, but also loaded with minerals. Medium unsulfured molasses, though ordinarily not thought of as a health food, is in fact much more nutritious per calorie than honey.

Mustard contains a substantial amount of salt and so should not be used regularly or liberally. However, for certain technical uses such as in making our wonderful *Tofu Mayonnaise* (see *Index*), a little bit of Dijon-style mustard goes a long way.

Tamari, which is similar to soy sauce, is high in salt, but some of our recipes call for a small amount—never more than half a teaspoon per person. That has 133 milligrams of sodium—about as much as a cup of skim milk. We have made this slight compromise because a small amount of tamari can make rice and vegetables much more palatable. However, if you are on a low-sodium diet or concerned about your blood pressure, skip this flavoring entirely.

Red meat is used in only a handful of recipes, and even then often with large amounts of high-fiber foods, which tend to balance out the fattiness of the meat. But we do feel that some meat, particularly liver, but also, occasionally, lean hamburger, may be advisable for people on the mend or who for other reasons may be trying to build up their iron, zinc or protein status. In general, though, there is now widespread agreement that eating less red meat, particularly beef, is a good way to help prevent a wide number of health problems, ranging from heart disease to osteoporosis.

COOKING TERMS DEFINED

Bake: To cook with dry heat in an oven. Turn on the oven to the required heat some 5 to 10 minutes before the food is inserted. Do not crowd pans together or place pans directly over other pans set on a lower shelf. If it is necessary to use two shelves while baking, stagger the pans to provide for good heat circulation. Leave at least two inches of space between pans, and between pans and the side of the oven. Baking times may vary according to the type of pan used (bright pans reflect heat; dark pans absorb heat) and the temperature of the ingredients when they are placed in the oven. It is generally recommended that oven temperatures for breads baked in glass be set 25 degrees F. lower than for those baked in aluminum. (Our bread recipes are based on the use of metal pans; pie recipes are based on glass pie plates.) Yeast breads should sound hollow when tapped, indicating they are baked through. Other baked goods can be tested by touching lightly in the center; if it springs back, it is done. Also, if a toothpick inserted in the center comes out clean, baking is completed. A mixture of half liquid lecithin and half corn or soy oil is most effective for lightly oiling bread pans, baking sheets or muffin cups.

Baste: To spoon a liquid or marinade over food while cooking or marinating in order to add flavor or to prevent the food from drying out.

Beat: To mix rapidly and vigorously with a regular motion that lifts the mixture over and over in order to incorporate air into the mixture. In beating egg whites, be certain to have the whites at room temperature. Utensils must be clean and dry, and no amount of egg yolk must slip into the whites. When whites are shiny and stand in peaks, they are properly beaten.

Boil: To cook food in liquid at 212 degrees F. A liquid at the boil has many bubbles of steam rising and breaking on the surface. As a general rule, root vegetables should be placed in cold water and brought to the boil, while vegetables growing aboveground should be placed in water that is already boiling. In both cases, heat is reduced and vegetables are simmered until done.

Boil down: To reduce or condense a liquid by rapid boiling.

Broil: To cook by direct radiant heat.

Chop: To cut into small pieces with a knife or other sharp tool.

Cube: To cut into square pieces.

Dice: To cut into small, square pieces.

Dredge: To sprinkle or coat with flour.

Dry: To place in a warm oven until the moisture has evaporated, as with bread for making dry crumbs.

Fold in: To gently add an ingredient, such as beaten egg whites, with a careful motion to preserve the air bubbles in the mixture. Often a spatula is used; the tool is pushed down on one side of the mixture and brought up the opposite side, lifting the ingredients and "folding" them together.

Garnish: To add a decoration.

Grate: To rub a food over a grater. Graters, which shave a thin layer from foods, have a range of sizes. Very tiny openings are effective for grating orange and lemon rinds to a fine powderlike consistency. For carrots and other vegetables, coarsely grate (see "Shred") with larger crescent-shaped openings.

Knead: To work dough with the hands until the dough is smooth. Kneading should be done on a floured surface to prevent sticking. In bread making, this process distributes yeast cells throughout the dough and develops the gluten of the flour, which holds the gases from the yeast cells in place, allowing the bread to rise. Kneading also develops the gluten (the "stretchy" part of the wheat) in other doughs, such as pasta or pizza doughs. To knead, flatten the dough slightly, then fold the farthest edge toward the front, and press down and away with the heels of the hands. The work surface should be low enough to allow "leaning into" the dough. Turn the dough and repeat the process. If dough sticks, a little more flour can be dusted on the work surface. Too much flour, however, will change the basic proportion of the recipe. When kneading is complete, the dough should be satiny smooth and not too stiff.

Marinate: To cover with a liquid in order to flavor or tenderize food. Because of their acid content, marinades and the foods they flavor should be placed in a glass, enameled or stainless steel container. Refrigerate any food that is to be marinated for more than one hour.

Mince: To cut or chop extremely fine.

Parboil: To boil until partially cooked.

Pare: To remove the outside covering of a food with a knife.

Peel: To remove the skin of a fruit or vegetable.

Puree: To press food through a sieve, or to place in a blender and process until food is of a thick liquid or paste consistency.

Roast: To cook meats with dry heat, usually in an oven.

Scald: To heat milk just below the boiling point. Small bubbles will appear along the edges of the liquid in the pan.

Shred: To cut into very thin strips, as for cabbage, or to pass over crescent-shaped holes of a grater, as for carrots.

Simmer: To cook in a liquid that is heated just to the point where bubbles come gently to the surface. The liquid is about 185 degrees F.

Steam: To use a moist cooking technique in which food is placed over, not in, boiling water, so that it is surrounded by steam.

Steam-stir: To cook in an open pan in just a few drops or spoonfuls of water or other liquid to prevent scorching. The liquid replaces the oil generally used in sauteing or panfrying. The food, chopped or minced, is stirred until tender.

Stir: To mix ingredients with a circular motion in order to combine them or to obtain a uniform consistency.

Toast: To brown food with dry heat.

Whip: To beat rapidly to incorporate air into an ingredient or mixture, usually with a whisk, hand beater or electric mixer.

Tuning In to the Taste of Health

(Please read before tying on your apron)

When some people hear that we use no butter, no salt, no cream, no sugar, no mayonnaise and scarcely any honey in our recipes, they can hardly believe that human beings can survive on such a diet. When we assure them they not only live, but live *longer,* they ask: "But what's the use of living if you can't enjoy your food?" Our answer is this: You can live longer and *love* it!

First, every recipe appearing in this book has not only satisfied our individual palates, but has been tested by another cook who served it to an average of half-a-dozen people and asked them to literally score what they ate. Only those recipes with the highest scores are included in this book. But beyond this testing process and its statistics, there is another dimension to taste which is extremely important to all of us who are trying to eat more healthfully.

Probably the most fundamental fact about taste differences is that people tend to like what they are accustomed to. There are exceptions, naturally, but that is the rule. People all over the world are presumably born with the same taste buds, but we generally enjoy only those foods and methods of serving we've become accustomed to. There is nothing intrinsic about a cheeseburger or raw fish or cassava root or ripe cheese that make them acceptable only to certain cultures. It's simply a question of habituation. When we are exposed to a food often enough, we usually get to like it. It's as simple as that.

The same thing is true on an individual basis. As children, we liked those foods that we were served or that our elders thought we would like—corn flakes, cookies and probably Cokes, too. But some of us managed to get enough exposure to other kinds of foods as we grew older and learned to change our tastes. Our early fondness for chocolate milk and Coke gave way, perhaps, to a love of coffee and beer. And from coffee and beer to whiskey and wine. Perhaps from a sweet wine to dry wine. From dry wine to spring water.

For many of us, habit is not something that's set in concrete, but a constantly changing process of discovery and education. For some reason, we're not content to just stand pat with the same familiar tastes. Although trying different things may be somewhat disconcerting, confusing, and on occasion even slightly disagreeable, we do it because it seems important to keep developing.

But maybe the driving force behind our changes in taste has something more to it than the sheer love of adventure and change. If you think back to when you first tried coffee, chances are you didn't like it very much. But it was the grown-up thing to do and you probably felt that it *must* taste terrific in order for all those grown-ups to be drinking it. So you kept at it, kept waiting for that terrific taste to emerge until one day, almost without your knowing it, there it was. You may have gone through the same process with many other foods and condiments, such as mustard, hot peppers, alcohol, and perhaps even more exotic items like strong, aged cheeses or fiery Mexican foods.

If you think back for a moment on your journey to various levels of taste, it should become clear that the taste of food—assuming it's wholesome and nutritious—is to a much greater extent in the mind of the diner than the substance of the food. And in order for that good taste to get into your mind, you have to permit your taste buds to become accustomed to it. Which brings us now to one extremely practical point: although the food and recipes in this book are supremely healthful, don't expect all your eating habits and tastes to change instantaneously. *Because our preferences grow from habit, the logical course of action is to gradually allow our taste buds to learn to like what we know we should be eating.*

Make no mistake about it. Most of our recipes will taste very good to you from the word go. Some of them are fabulous, our taste-testers told us. But certain other recipes are going to surprise you somewhat when you take your first mouthful. If at that point you simply shake your head and say "Sorry, that's not for me!" you will be doing yourself an enormous disservice.

You must understand that the reaction our taste buds have to food that is prepared in a way new to us (without salt, for instance) is *not* a reflection of whether that food is good-tasting or not. All we are reacting to is the *newness.* Give yourself a chance to get past that first moment of confusion, of novelty. *Don't make the mistake of interpreting it as a judgment or evaluation of the food.* We're not saying this in a preaching or apologetic kind of way, because we've gone through it ourselves. We know that very frequently, by the time you get to the second or third or maybe even the fifth or sixth mouthful, the good natural taste of the food begins to come through. What you're doing is giving yourself the same chance to enjoy perfectly healthy food that you gave yourself to enjoy coffee, brandy, and the many other unhealthful food and drinks that tasted weird, awful or (in the case of certain whiskeys) practically poisonous when you first sampled them.

Now, after you have taken a few mouthfuls of food, it's possible that you will still be put off by its newness. If we're talking about a dish to which you would ordinarily be adding some salt or sugar or butter, you can at this point use a little bit of creative imagination. In other words, cheat. It's far better to use a little salt or a little honey in the beginning while your taste buds are in training, than to attempt to finish the dish in its "pure" form and wind up feeling disappointed and deprived. Our recipes are, after all, healthful in many ways—not just because they don't contain salt or sugar or butter. So if you find yourself adding a light sprinkle of salt, for instance, don't feel you aren't getting any of the health benefit of that recipe. You're getting lots of vitamins and minerals, and perhaps a lot of fiber and many healing factors for various parts of the body as well. As days go by, simply use *less* salt or sugar or butter or whatever you have been adding. You may look upon the form in which our recipes are given here as the "advanced" version, suitable for people whose taste buds have been through a reeducation process.

That process happens to be one of the more fascinating things we have experienced ourselves in recent years. We are sure you will find it fascinating too. Probably the first realization that something new is happening to you will come when, perhaps after one or two weeks of following our recipes, you are served some soup in a restaurant, and find it tastes oversalted. Meanwhile, you will be discovering a whole new rainbow of tastes in vegetables whose uniqueness hasn't been extinguished with salt and sugar. After a month or so, you may begin wondering why in the world *anyone* would put salt on vegetables.

With other foods, it may take more time to get used to the salt-free taste. Our guess is that bread will be among the last foods to become acceptable without salt. But just continue to use less, over a period of weeks, until you decide it's time to go all the way and leave it out completely. We've been eating bread that way for many months, of course, and we can honestly say that we no more miss the presence of salt in our bread than we would pepper. Follow the same general plan with sugar, gradually cutting down until you no longer feel it's necessary. As for butter, a pat or two here and there while you are adjusting to your new eating habits is perfectly okay. Slowly, but only slowly, replace butter with lemon juice, herbs or even small amounts of fruit juice. Remember, what we're trying to do is reeducate the taste buds, not stun them. The transition period may take a few weeks or even a few months. No matter. *The important thing is the years of healthier life ahead of you.*

During the transition period, don't for a moment imagine that you're depriving yourself of some wonderful pleasure by gradually eliminating salt, sugar and added fats. What those unhealthful additives do, more often than not, is to mask what's really unique about each food. There are plenty of really good foods and herbs that can give you that creamy or piquant taste when you need it. If anyone is deprived, it's the person who can't eat anything unless it's drenched with sugar, salt or fat. By eating natural foods, you're connecting with all the variety and subtlety and pizzazz of the real thing.

What makes the growth process so much easier, of course, is the knowledge that every mouthful you eat is a step on the road to better health. With that kind of motivation, you'll discover that your tastes are a lot less ingrained than you imagined!

Understanding the Symbols We Use in This Book

Each chapter of our book goes into considerable detail about the kinds of foods believed healing or protective in relation to specific health problems. Recipes that feature such foods follow the textual part of each chapter. But there are many more recipes considered beneficial for each problem besides those included in that chapter. These additional recipes can be found throughout the book and are easily identified by means of symbols. To match the symbols with the health problems, consult either the Table of Contents or the *Index of Recipes according to Problem.*

The appearance of a symbol next to a recipe means that one or more beneficial factors—as described in the chapter dealing with that problem—are found in that recipe. In some cases, the symbol indicates the recipe is very low in a food element, such as salt or fat, which may aggravate a certain condition. In other cases, the symbol reflects the presence of one or more positive healing elements.

As we point out elsewhere in our book, people under medical care should consult their doctor before making any dramatic changes in their diet. Also, understand that neither we nor anyone else are in a position to offer individual assurances that eating in a certain manner is going to result in a specific benefit. When we put various symbols of healing next to a recipe, what we are saying is that the best information available to us suggests that the food is likely to be helpful. In other words, the symbols are informational, not prescriptive. Although this information represents the combined work of many editorial researchers and hundreds of health professionals, the question of specific benefit to the individual can only be answered by you and your physician. The two of you may also find that our symbols make it much easier to translate medical advice about a dietary change (like low salt) into actual meals that you can prepare and enjoy.

Recipe ingredients appearing in italic type are recipes themselves, and they may be located by referring to the *General Index.*

Chapter 1

A Healthier Heart Can Begin Today

The evening news would have us believe that our lives are endangered because of earthquakes, hurricanes, revolutions, nuclear accidents and terrorism. But in fact, the chances of any one of those disasters affecting you directly are extremely slim. If the television were to show you what was most likely to do *you* in as you lie in your bed tonight, it would show you a picture of your own heart, ticking away politely in your own chest.

An unsettling thought—that we are each carrying a potential assassin within us. But that is not the news we want to leave you with in this chapter. Rather, we want you to understand that—quite unlike all the disasters that TV thrusts at us like characters in a Punch-and-Judy show—there is something we can *do* about that most real, most personal of all dangers that threaten us. We can, in a word, rehabilitate that potential assassin and turn him into what nature intended him to be—our best and closest friend.

Mind you, diet is not the only way to make friends with your heart. Not smoking and getting a reasonable amount of exercise are both of great importance. Too much stress, the kind that turns your nerves into a kind of clenched fist inside your chest, is also something that can be changed with a little effort, although you may need professional help. Here, we're concentrating on just one aspect of a healthy heart, but one that we can all use to our advantage, regardless of age, family history, or personality type.

The dietary approach to a healthier heart which is agreed upon by more experts than any other is a reduction of fat in the diet. Specifically, a reduction in *saturated* fat, which occurs mostly in animal-source food such as beef, and a fatlike substance that we all know about called *cholesterol*. Working together, many heart researchers believe, saturated fat and cholesterol encourage deposits of fatty material on the lining of our arteries, creating a condition known as atherosclerosis (or arteriosclerosis). As this buildup of fat and other materials increases, blood flow is slowly squeezed off, creating a situation where even a fairly small blood clot which happens to be floating along can cause a disastrous blockage of circulation. Atherosclerotic heart disease is by far the most common form of heart disease and the variety we are talking about here. It is also the major underlying cause of strokes. Other forms of heart disease, such as inherited faults with valves, may involve diet only very marginally.

If you rank the major nations of the world according to the incidence of heart disease, and rank them once again for the average intake of cholesterol, it becomes obvious that the more cholesterol and saturated fat that is eaten, the higher the rate of heart disease. Now, there are certainly other factors in the diet related to heart disease, but none of them impress epidemiologists quite to the extent that the cholesterol association does. Yet, curiously, when you try to apply the cholesterol link to individuals inside the borders of any one country, it doesn't work very well. The fact that John eats more cholesterol in his diet than Bill, who in turn eats more cholesterol in his diet than Jack, doesn't necessarily mean that their blood levels of cholesterol are going to be arranged in the same descending order, or that they will develop symptoms of heart disease accordingly. Some people have interpreted this to mean that cholesterol in the diet really doesn't matter very much, if at all. But it does. Here, we think, is the most practical and realistic way to look at the importance of cholesterol and fat in the diet.

THE ROLE OF CHOLESTEROL AND SATURATED FAT

Think of cholesterol and saturated fat as laying down a kind of basic foundation for the development of atherosclerosis. When there is a lot of them in a diet, there is a large foundation. But where they are scarce, the foundation is small. Now, given a particular foundation, what will be built on it is largely a result of individual characteristics. Heredity is certainly one. Some people, we all know, have an exaggerated tendency to develop deposits of cholesterol, while others seem to enjoy a kind of natural protection. Smoking habits are another big factor. So is blood pressure. Exercise. Personality type. Stress level. Calorie intake. And then a whole host of dietary factors, such as vitamins, minerals and fiber. So what we have is a situation in which the foundation of a disease process is usually laid by cholesterol and saturated fat, while further construction of the disease state (atherosclerosis) is largely an expression of individual tendencies and vulnerabilities. No wonder we see so many cases of people eating a very similar diet who differ dramatically in their health. You might compare it to a situation where two people earn the same basic salary, yet one is rich and the other poor because of differences in thrift, investments, gambling habits and so on. We wouldn't assume from such a case that income is meaningless, because it's quite clear that—*on the average* —you're better off having a high income than a low income. It's the same story with diet and your heart. The overwhelming *trend* is for people who eat a fat-rich diet to have a lot of fat in their bloodstream, and for these same people to suffer more heart attacks, strokes, thrombosis and other expressions of atherosclerosis. Ancel Keys, Ph.D., of the University of Minnesota's School of Public Health, points out that in an occasional case

Heart Disease:
As American as Apple Pie?

one medium apple

fat:	1.3 grams
calories:	123
sodium:	1 milligram
total fiber:	6.8 grams
vitamin C:	8 milligrams
potassium:	233 milligrams

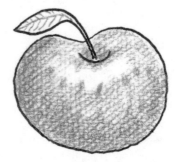

Once we have some idea how different foods and food elements affect the circulatory system, it's easy to see why heart disease is our number one killer —and how to get yourself off its hit list. Consider the transformation of the apple into apple pie. Every harmful dietary element has been greatly increased; every protective element decreased. *Fat has gone up over 900 percent, calories by 145 percent. Sodium, which in excess can lead to high blood pressure, a major heart risk factor, has increased almost 200 fold! Meanwhile, protective fiber has dropped 82 percent; vitamin C, 88 percent; and potassium 60 percent. When you begin eating more natural foods, this health arithmetic does a flip-flop and* you come out on top!

one slice apple pie
(⅛ of pie)

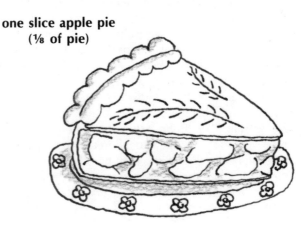

fat:	13.1 grams
calories:	302
sodium:	355 milligrams
total fiber:	1.2 grams
vitamin C:	1 milligram
potassium:	94 milligrams

of sudden death, the autopsy reveals relatively clean coronary arteries and no other findings to explain the death. "But such cases are rare indeed," he declares, going on to cite several studies showing that in most cases of sudden coronary deaths, extensive atherosclerotic damage had laid the groundwork for catastrophe (*Acta Medica Scandinavica,* vol. 207, no. 3, 1980).

Because it is difficult if not altogether impossible to control the diets of large numbers of people, ironclad proof of this hypothesis is hard to come by. But World War II made unwilling experimental subjects out of millions of Europeans who suddenly found their food supply drastically changed. Finland, Norway and Sweden all experienced extreme shortages of foods rich in animal fats, particularly butter, whole milk and meat. Whole grains, potatoes, fresh vegetables and fish filled the gap. Interestingly, the result was a very sharp drop in deaths from heart attack and other circulatory problems. However, within a few years after the end of the war, when the fat-rich diet had once again become the norm, the heart attack rates went right back to where they were before.

Now, it's easy to suppose that the drop in heart attacks could have been related to social changes, not diet. But consider the case of Denmark. Denmark, like the other Scandinavian countries, was occupied during the war, but its production of food was not seriously disturbed. In fact, Denmark had previously imported large amounts of soybeans and fish oil with which to manufacture margarine, but during the war, butter was substituted for margarine. So consumption of saturated fat remained high all through the war—as did deaths from heart attacks. In the United States, it was much the same story. No diet change, no heart change.

All this may sound a little remote, dealing as it does with trends rather than specific events. But if it's a close-up look at what fat does to you that you want, we can turn to a classic study carried out more than a quarter of a century ago by Peter P. Kuo, M.D., and Claude R. Joyner, Jr., M.D., of the University of Pennsylvania. Selecting 14 patients who had all been diagnosed as having angina pectoris (episodes of severe pain in the chest caused by insufficient blood reaching the heart), the doctors gave each a fatty meal consisting of nothing but cocoa-flavored heavy cream. The amount of butter fat was adjusted for the weight of each person, but it worked out so that a 150-pound man was receiving about 3 ounces of butter fat, roughly equal to the amount of fat in 10 ounces of cheddar cheese. Following the ingestion of the cream, each person remained at rest, not being permitted to smoke or eat anything else. Meanwhile, numerous tests were taken of the blood, and the patients' condition observed. Within three to five hours after drinking the cream, 6 of the 14 patients developed attacks of angina which were "identical" with those they had suffered in the past when they overexerted themselves. What's more, the actual onset of the angina attack corresponded perfectly with the absorption of the fat into their bloodstreams, coming precisely at the moment when fat levels reached their peaks. Interestingly, it was discovered that the younger patients experienced peak fat levels (and anginal attacks) about three hours after eating, while the older patients suffered their attacks an average of about five hours after fat ingestion.

At the time this test was conducted, it was widely believed that attacks of angina following a meal were a result of an increase in cardiac work or pressure on the coronary arteries from a distended stomach. Since the meal eaten, however, was of very small volume, it seems clear that the real trigger of the angina was nothing but fat clogging up the body's blood vessels. This study, by the way, may also give us an understanding of why many acute coronary episodes occur during sleep, rather than at a moment of unusual effort. If a heavy, fat-rich meal is eaten at 7:00 or 8:00 P.M., for instance, the worst danger in an older person would come about five hours later, or about 12:00 to 1:00 A.M. It's even been suggested by other doctors that because blood flow is very slow during sleep, the sudden onslaught of fat may have more of a clogging effect than it would during a period of activity. That in turn leads to the suggestion that people who are prone to circulatory ailments should avoid eating heavy meals for six hours or so before going to bed.

We mentioned before that saturated fat and cholesterol, over a period of years, tend to create deposits inside the arteries and constrict circulation. But as the University of Pennsylvania study showed, fat can also have an acute effect on circulation. The excess fat in the bloodstream can coat red blood cells, causing them to clump together, and get jammed in capillaries as they try to bring oxygen to the tissues. The chances of a major blood clot are also much greater at such times.

Our recipes, you will not be surprised to learn, are generally very low in fat of all kinds, but particularly saturated fat and cholesterol. Butter, for instance, which is just about pure fat and has virtually no nutritional value except for a small amount of vitamin A, is excluded altogether. We often think of lard as being the worst kind of fat, but there is actually more saturated fat in butter than in lard. And there's more saturated fat in just two pats of butter than in a whole cup of spaghetti, meatballs, sauce and a sprinkling of cheese. Cream cheese is another no-no: a single ounce has more saturated fat than three-quarters of a pound of white meat chicken, while at the same time, it's very low in calcium and protein—which are the major nutritional reasons for eating cheese at all. Cream, sour cream and mayonnaise are likewise very high in saturated fat and are excluded. Only a very few recipes in our book call for beef, and none of those marked with the symbol of the heart contain beef. That's because beef—even the very leanest you can buy—has more than twice as much total fat as white meat chicken and more than three times as much saturated fat. Whole milk, because of its fat and cholesterol, is used only very rarely in our book and not at all for any heart recipes. The general rule for the heart is to avoid dairy fats, red meat, and foods such as pies and cakes which are frequently baked with butter or lard. We rarely call for eggs in our recipes in the heart section and precious few anywhere in the book. Eggs, although nutritious, contain very high levels of cholesterol and, if you have reason to be seriously concerned about your circulatory system, you're better off not eating them.

Two Looks at One Ounce of Fat

To get the same amount of fat in the Big Mac (31.4 grams or a little more than an ounce), you'd have to eat the entire "sandwich" of more natural foods on the right, consisting of half-a-pound of broiled chicken (skinned), one halibut fillet, a whole head of Bibb lettuce, one onion, six scallops, a cup of cooked kidney beans, a cup of brown rice, one pound of green beans, one sweet potato, an ear of corn, a cup of raisins, an orange, two red beets, four asparagus spears, half-a-pound of green peas in their pods, a cup of popcorn, a cup of cooked spaghetti and two slices of whole wheat bread. And don't think there's anything all that unusual about the Big Mac—compared to other common processed foods. Two hot dogs have just as much fat; so do a couple of Danish. You can see that while nature made it very difficult for us to get too much fat in our diets, we have outsmarted her—and ourselves at the same time.

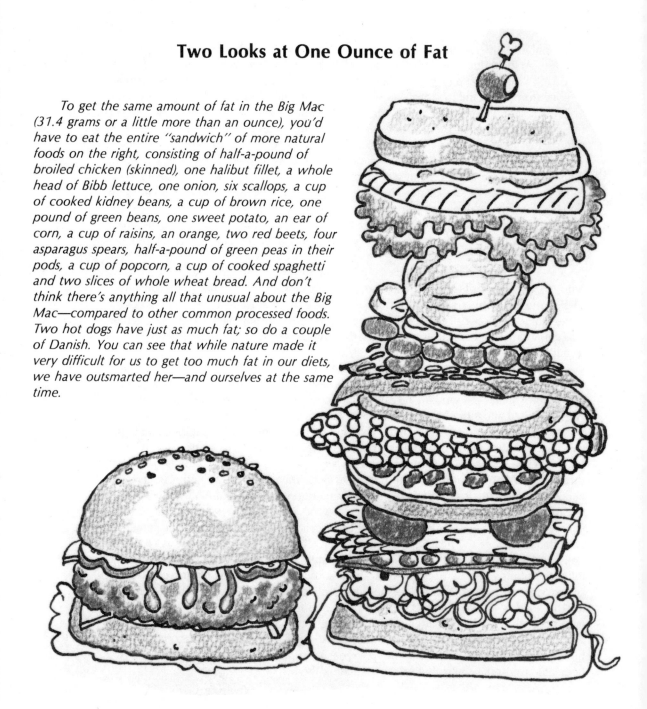

Vegetable products contain no cholesterol at all, and most have very little saturated fat, with the exception of avocados and coconuts. Coconuts, particularly, are bad news: in animal experiments, coconut oil produces atherosclerosis more efficiently than any other kind of fat. Even the meat of the coconut is very high in fat and for that reason we don't use even small amounts of shredded coconut in any of our recipes. Incidentally, when the label of a packaged food says it contains "vegetable oil," it's likely to be coconut oil.

OILS THAT EASE THE CIRCULATION

While we do not recommend eating very large amounts of *any* kind of fat or oil, substituting polyunsaturated oils for most of the saturated oils you typically eat seems to be a very wise move. In Finland, long-term patients at one mental hospital were given the normal Finnish diet, which is very high in such saturated fat sources as eggs and milk products. In another hospital, much of the saturated fat was replaced with polyunsaturated fat. After six years, the diets were switched. Researchers found that when patients received the experimental diet, their blood cholesterol dropped sharply. More to the point, the rate of deaths from coronary heart disease in the hospital on the experimental diet fell to *half* the rate at the other institution (*Circulation,* January, 1979).

Other studies have suggested that the substitution of polyunsaturated for saturated fats can reduce the tendency of the blood to form thrombi, or tiny blood clots, that may initiate heart attacks and strokes. In whole foods, polyunsaturated oils are found in many grains, seeds and nuts, as well as fish. For cooking purposes, sunflower, safflower, corn and soy oil are good sources of polyunsaturates.

While everyone has heard a lot about polyunsaturates, there is one particular kind that is currently the focus of intense interest by scientists studying the link between diet and heart disease. It's found—of all places—in fish oil.

Interest was sparked in the relationship of fish oil to cardiovascular disease, thanks to obscure tribes of Greenland Eskimos. Those tribes eat a high-fat, high-cholesterol diet—just the kind that, as we have seen, ought to promote atherosclerosis. Yet, atherosclerosis and its attendant evils, stroke and heart disease, are rare among Eskimos. How could that be?

The answer comes from Danish scientists, who were intrigued by the fact that both Danes and Eskimos ate a high-fat diet, but only the Danes seemed to suffer for it. Noting that the main source of fat in the Eskimo diet is fish, they studied the fatty acids in those animals and soon found that fish fats are unique: they contain an unusually high amount of omega-3 fatty acids, one of the two main classes of polyunsaturated fats. But much more exciting, they discovered that these omega-3 fatty acids reduced the production of a substance in the blood that causes blood platelets to stick together, leading sometimes to blocked arteries and eventual stroke or heart attack. It seemed to be a case of one kind of fat—the omega-3 fatty acids—neutralizing the bad effects of other fats (*Lancet,* July 15, 1978).

"Unfortunately, the average North American diet seldom contains foods rich in these omega-3 fatty acids," William Harris, Ph.D., Research Fellow in nutrition at the University of Oregon Health Sciences Center, told us. "Virtually no omega-3 fatty acids are found in beef, chicken or any food other than fish. The average American diet consists of 40 percent fat, but it's mostly saturated fat. That creates an imbalance of the 'bad' kind of fatty acids which may then be converted by cellular metabolism into substances that set the stage for stroke and heart attack."

Would normal Americans who changed to an Eskimo-type diet derive the same benefits? Dr. Harris and two colleagues set out to test the effect of fish oil on the risk factors of heart disease in a study subsequently presented to a major meeting of experimental biologists in 1980.

"Our study was designed to answer two questions," Dr. Harris explains. "First, does fish oil in a diet reduce levels of blood fats, such as cholesterol and triglycerides, and thus conceivably help to prevent heart disease? Second, does dietary fish oil make blood platelets less sticky and thus reduce the tendency to form blood clots?" (High levels of cholesterol or triglycerides are possible warning signs of coronary trouble.)

They recruited 10 volunteers (5 men, 5 women) whom they placed on two different diets. For one month, the 10 ate a typical American diet, high in fat but including vegetables and fruit. Then tests were done to determine their blood chemistry. The next month the volunteers were switched to the second diet, identical to the first except that all fat came from salmon meat and salmon oil. Blood chemistry tests were performed again and the results compared with those of the first diet.

"After a month on the salmon diet, the average blood cholesterol levels went down 17 percent, which is a moderate decrease. But triglyceride levels dropped 40 percent, which is exciting. There is something unique about the effect of fish oil on triglyceride metabolism. Polyunsaturated vegetable oils will lower cholesterol levels too, but they don't do much to triglyceride levels," Dr. Harris said.

Of course, high blood cholesterol and triglyceride levels are not the only risk factors for atherosclerosis. The stickiness of the blood platelets (the smallest formed elements in the blood) may also play a role in the development of heart disease. The more adhesive the platelets, and the more of them there are in the blood, the greater the likelihood of dangerous clotting. The salmon reduced the stickiness of the platelets and their numbers as well. The researchers found that with the salmon diet, platelet counts actually dropped 40 percent, from 350,000 per cubic millimeter of blood to 212,000. "Both values are within the normal range. Whether the platelets were being destroyed faster or being made more slowly is not known," Dr. Harris said. The time it takes to stop bleeding is another indicator of the tendency of the blood to form clots. While it's obviously not good for the blood to clot too little, for the person prone to heart disease it *is* good for it to clot slightly less than normal. Normal bleeding time for those on a control diet was 7.5 minutes. On the salmon diet, bleeding time averaged 10 minutes. "That is not dangerously long," Dr. Harris told us.

What is the practical significance of all this? "Although we certainly cannot say that fish oil in the diet will prevent heart disease," Dr. Harris suggested, "we can say that it does act against preconditions for heart disease by lowering cholesterol and triglyceride levels and improving platelet function. I think the most promising application of this research would be to isolate the active components in the salmon diet, which are probably omega-3 fatty acids, and to concentrate them into capsule form. Until that happens, people at high risk of developing cardiovascular disease might benefit from increasing their consumption of fish rich in oil."

Another study by a team of researchers at the University of Michigan Medical School at Ann Arbor, shows that fish oil may also prevent or lessen the severity of brain stroke. Working with laboratory animals, they determined that those supplemented with fish oil suffered less brain damage when a stroke was artificially induced. They hypothesized that the fish oil kept open the small, collateral blood vessels that can take on the work of the main ones when they are blocked, and maintain the brain's blood supply (*Prostaglandins and Medicine,* November, 1979).

At this writing, we don't know of any large institution that has carried out a major study of the effect of fish oils on cardiovascular health over a period of years. However, some years ago, Averly M. Nelson, M.D., of Seattle, Washington, decided that a diet high in seafoods might benefit heart patients. He conducted a study of 80 coronary patients eating such a high-seafood diet and 126 patients eating the usual diet. Results? Patients on the seafood diet lived almost twice as long as the other patients, he reported. The older the patients, he noted, the more they seemed to need such a diet. In the 56 to 70 age group, 32 percent of those on the special diet remained alive throughout the years of the study, compared to only 5 percent of the others (*Geriatrics,* December, 1972).

Where do you get omega-3 fatty acids? Salmon, tuna, trout, mackerel, shad and bass are all rich in these valuable oils. Since tuna is extremely difficult to buy in its fresh state, it is one of the few foods that we don't hesitate to buy in cans.

We do buy it packed in water instead of oil, though. The oil that is added is usually soy oil, so you aren't losing any of the omega-3 fatty acids by dispensing with the extra calories.

At this point, a brief reminder: as we said in the front of this book in our Notice, if you are under medical treatment for any condition, such as heart disease, by all means check with your physician before going on any major diet change. If you are taking blood thinners, your dose of medication may need to be adjusted as your new diet naturally changes your clotting tendency. And in fact, as you will soon see, there are foods other than fish oils which naturally reduce the tendency of your blood to clot. If you have not been eating them, and begin abruptly, the combined effect of diet plus medication could lead to serious problems. The ideal situation would be to reduce the amount of medication, if possible, under your doctor's guidance. However, none of the doctors and researchers who have studied this question feel there is any danger to people who are not on blood thinners. Many people, after all, not only eat a good deal of fish on a regular basis, but also take supplements of cod liver oil, which contain large amounts of omega-3 fatty acids.

WHY ONION AND GARLIC HELP THE HEART

Two other common foods which have a similar protective effect against blood fats and clotting are onion and garlic. This is not medieval herbalism we're talking about, either, but the voice of modern science. *Nutrition Reviews,* one of the most conservative of all scientific nutrition journals, reported in their issue of February, 1976, that onions can reduce cholesterol levels after a fatty meal, and perform the job equally well if eaten raw, boiled or even fried. Onions have also been shown to slightly increase the breakdown of fibrin, a substance necessary for blood clotting. As we said before, if blood didn't clot, we would be in big trouble, but most Westerners have the opposite problem —too much fibrin and too much clotting, which can create blocked blood vessels. Onions, reported *Nutrition Reviews,* reduce fibrin just enough to prevent an unneeded clot, but pose no danger whatsoever.

At Queen Elizabeth College in London, investigators gave nine healthy volunteers three different test breakfasts. One was a low-calorie, low-fat meal, which included grapefruit, corn flakes, skim milk, bread and marmalade. Another was a hearty breakfast, high in calories and in saturated fats—cream, bacon, sausage, bread, butter and fruit. For the third test meal, the experimenters added about two-and-a-half ounces of fried onions to the heavy repast.

"The rate of platelet aggregation was significantly greater after the fat meal, compared with the control," they reported. "But when onion was included in the fat meal, the results were not significantly different from the control values." In other words, a high-fat meal increased the dangerous aggregation of platelets—but the onions neutralized the effect (*Lancet,* January 8, 1977).

In India, a team of researchers led by Dr. G. S. Sainani of the B.J. Medical College in Poona analyzed blood samples from three groups of people with slightly different dietary habits. All three groups ate a primarily or entirely vegetarian diet. But the first group spiced their meals with a good deal of onion and heavy amounts of garlic —about two to three cloves daily. The second group never touched onion or garlic, while the third preferred only small amounts of the pungent vegetables.

Among those who shunned onion and garlic, Dr. Sainani found, there were consistently higher blood levels of cholesterol and triglycerides than among the herb eaters. Interestingly, they also had higher levels of low-density lipoproteins (LDL)—that fraction of cholesterol associated with an increased risk of heart disease. Finally, the people who ate a lot of onion and garlic had even healthier levels of blood fats than those who ate just a little (*Indian Journal of Medical Research,* May, 1979).

Now, you might be wondering if these fascinating effects were due entirely to onion and not to the garlic as well. But other tests show that garlic, like onion, really works when it gets into our systems.

Dr. Arun Bordia, of the R.N.T. Medical College in Udaipur, India, found that when he added small amounts of garlic oil to blood samples, platelet aggregation was slowed down considerably. When the garlic oil was added before a chemical used to cause aggregation, it kept the platelet clumps from forming. When the garlic was added after the platelets had begun to aggregate, it seemed to reverse the process. Dr. Bordia found a similar result when he put volunteers on a diet that included a little bit less than an ounce of garlic oil daily. After five days, there was a marked reduction in platelet aggregation, suggesting that eating garlic is a natural way to help reduce the stickiness of platelets (*Atherosclerosis,* August, 1978).

According to another experiment of Dr. Bordia's, garlic may help dissolve clots that have begun to form by increasing the blood's fibrinolytic activity—its ability to dissolve the chemical fibrin, which makes clots thick and strong. Dr. Bordia gave 10 healthy adults hefty doses of garlic oil for three months, testing their blood regularly. He found a gradual rise in fibrinolytic activity. Three months of garlic, in fact, more than doubled this clot-dissolving ability. When garlic was discontinued, fibrinolysis gradually dropped back to its original level. A high level of fibrinolytic activity is especially important for people who have had heart attacks—to prevent recurrences. Dr. Bordia gave garlic to one group that had suffered myocardial infarction more than a year before; he started another group on garlic within 24 hours after their heart attacks. Here, too, garlic led to a swift, significant rise in fibrinolytic activity—"within a few hours," Dr. Bordia said. For those patients in the crucial recovery period after their heart attack, 10 days of garlic therapy led to a 63 percent increase in fibrinolysis. After 20 days, clot-dissolving activity had nearly doubled.

There are drugs, of course, that can do the same thing—reduce the tendency of blood to clot. But those must be watched closely, to avoid side effects such as excessive bleeding. "In our studies," Dr. Bordia noted, "administration of as much as 60 grams of crude garlic (the equivalent of some 20 cloves) daily for three months has led neither to side effects nor to a bleeding tendency. As such this herbal remedy seems to be clinically acceptable and safe."

Don't be put off by that mention of 20 cloves of garlic. Nowhere near that amount is necessary to achieve a real benefit. Dr. R. C. Jain of the University of Benghazi Faculty of Medicine in Libya reported that a little more than a sixth of an ounce (about one or two cloves, depending on size) of crushed garlic bulbs daily reduced both cholesterol and triglyceride levels in six healthy men after three weeks (*American Journal of Clinical Nutrition,* September, 1977). Meanwhile, the fibrinolytic activity of the men's blood rose significantly. Dr. Jain suggests that people with high cholesterol and triglyceride readings eat garlic "as a vegetable in daily meals" to help keep their blood fat levels under control.

Garlic, like onion, retains its cholesterol-fighting potency even when cooked. In one scientific test, two ounces of garlic cloves which had been boiled for 30 minutes were still able to hold cholesterol levels in check even after volunteer subjects ate a quarter pound of butter spread on four slices of bread!

Needless to say, we use plenty of onion and garlic in our recipes. If you find the taste a bit too pungent, try baking (or boiling) your garlic before using it. That makes the taste much milder, but apparently does not weaken its health potency.

SOYBEANS ARE SOMETHING SPECIAL

Of course, you can't live on onions and garlic even if the only one smelling your breath is your pet dog who has a head cold. But soybeans—that's another story. Exceptionally high in protein for a legume (the bean family), and rich in minerals, soybeans can be a dietary staple and yet have an extraordinary ability to police cholesterol. "The hypocholesterolemic [cholesterol-lowering] effect of soybean was remarkable; it was achieved within a few weeks and was probably superior to that expected even from months' treatment with a low-lipid [low-fat] diet." Those words come from C. F. Sirtori and five colleagues associated with leading medical research centers in Milan, Italy. The "remarkable" reduction in cholesterol achieved was 14 percent after two weeks and fully 21 percent just after three weeks. The patients involved all had quite high levels of cholesterol (over 300) when all the animal protein in their diet was replaced with textured soybean protein. In one test, the average cholesterol levels went from 335 down to 258; in other tests, they dropped from 313 to 254. And this came *after* these patients had tried to get their cholesterol down—without success—by eating a diet very low in fat. Furthermore, when a good wallop of cholesterol was added to the soybean regimen, it had virtually no impact on the cholesterol-lowering effect of the program. Finally, the Italian doctors noted that the drop in cholesterol was accompanied by an equally sharp drop in undesirable LDL levels (*Journal of the American Oil Chemists' Society,* July, 1976).

What the Italian doctors actually fed their patients was a textured soybean protein product, which they used in preparing a variety of typical Italian dishes. We prefer to use real soybeans rather than the isolated protein because of the lower cost, absence of additives which are sometimes used in textured soybean products, and the fiber in the soybeans. However, we do frequently use tofu, which is fairly similar to what the Italian researchers used, being essentially a kind of nondairy "cheese" made from soybean curd. By itself, tofu has little or no taste (unless you make it yourself at home and eat it fresh). But tofu has the quality of taking on the taste of almost anything it is marinated or cooked with, and is especially good when mixed with spicy or savory foods, such as wok-steamed vegetables with garlic and other herbs.

When you eat whole soybeans, you get the bonus of lecithin, a fatlike substance which has been shown in many tests to favorably effect elevated blood fat levels. Some of our recipes call for granulated lecithin, which is a very concentrated form.

FIBER FIGHTS FOR YOUR LIFE

You have probably heard the exciting news from medical researchers about the importance of food fiber in preventing and healing certain problems of the digestive tract (which we'll get to in a later chapter). But you may not know that fiber also plays an important role in protecting the heart. Food fiber is not all the same, though, and scientists are still busily engaged trying to sort out which fibers do which jobs. But we already know enough to say with some confidence that if your diet includes ample amounts of whole grains and whole grain products—which we use plentifully in our recipes—you are on the right track. Consider the following evidence:

A United States government scientist reported in 1978 that hard red spring wheat and corn bran (part of the whole kernel) work to increase the percentage of high-density lipoproteins (HDL)—the fraction of cholesterol now believed to protect the heart, probably by helping to remove other fractions of cholesterol from the blood before they can build up on artery walls. As a bonus, the wheat caused a decrease in LDL—which is also considered good—and a 17 percent decrease in total cholesterol, another good sign. Juan Munoz, M.D., formerly with the Human Nutrition Laboratory in the U.S. Department of Agriculture, also said that wheat and corn, as well as a number of other sources of fiber, reduced triglycerides, another form of blood fats, by about 15 percent.

One medical scientist has reported finding actual improvement in the clinical signs of heart disease in patients taking supplementary fiber. Renzo Romanelli, M.D., professor of Gerontology and Geriatrics at the University of Pisa in Italy, reported to a conference of the International College of Surgeons in the United States in 1978 that a number of patients taking wheat bran daily enjoyed a reduction in the number of angina attacks. In 5 patients over 70 years of age, Dr. Romanelli said, tests showed improvement in cardiac efficiency, and EKG signs of lack of oxygen in the heart muscle were diminished. In 14 patients between 72 and 94 years of age, he added, there was complete disappearance of a particular type of circulatory inefficiency which commonly occurs during straining at stool. The professor explained that with a low-fiber diet, which often results in constipation and the need to strain, high pressures can build up in the area of the colon and reduce the output of the heart. Bran stops this cycle from occurring. Fiber, this specialist in the health problems of aging told the assembled surgeons, is so important that its inclusion in the daily diet should be considered an important part of preventive medicine.

The same thought is apparently shared by several English physicians writing in the *British Medical Journal* (November 19, 1977). Dr. J. N. Morris and colleagues suggested that lack of fiber in the diet may well be a major cause of coronary thrombosis, a blood clot that blocks the flow of oxygen to the heart. In another communication to the same journal, Dr. A. D. Robertson argues that the reason Scotland has seven times as much coronary thrombosis as it did before World War II is lack of fiber. "Prewar," Dr. Robertson says, "the common Scottish breakfast included porridge made from coarse meal, soaked overnight. The main meal frequently included homemade soup, thick with a good supply of vegetables and pulses [peas and beans]. Now it is flakes (if that) and creamed tin soup. . . ." (December 17, 1977).

Other British doctors have put the fiber thesis to a harsh test. "Over the past four years, I've operated on over 1,500 patients, and not one of them has suffered any postoperative blood clotting," English surgeon Dr. Maurice Frohn told us in an interview. According to the consultant surgeon at London's Bethnal Green Hospital, anesthesia induces a type of temporary paralysis. The body becomes limp; breathing is taxed and the blood becomes stagnant, inviting the formation of blood clots. "To avoid dangerous clots after an operation, there must be a good flow of blood through the veins," he explains. "Many of my colleagues in the profession use a drug called heparin to keep the blood flowing. But I prefer to use the natural method by feeding my patients with dosages of bran. Bran keeps the bowels moving—which is imperative after surgery," he insists. "Otherwise the colon becomes overweighted and causes extreme pressure on the leg veins. This often leads to clotting and deep vein thrombosis."

Another English surgeon, Dr. Conrad Latto of the Royal Berkshire Hospital in Reading, has had similar results with feeding bran to the surgical patients. "In the past four years," he told us, "I have operated on many cases of high-risk thrombosis. In each case I've insisted that the patient be given an adequate diet of bran both before and after surgery. In all that time, I've had only one difficult case. That was in someone who had deep vein thrombosis, but wouldn't take his bran."

Dr. Latto has seen dramatic proof of fiber's benefits in other medical institutions. Once, when he was in Kashmir, India, he visited a 700-bed hospital responsible for treating an enormous number of people and was told that in 14 years, there had only been a single case of death from embolism—the obstruction of a vein by a clot. "I have seen postoperative patients in Kashmir sitting up in bed in their customary cross-legged position within hours of surgery," he relates. "By Western medical standards, that should have created blood clots in the legs. But in their case, it did not."

Perhaps we should point out that the citizens of India and other Asian and African countries where deep vein thrombosis is almost unknown do not take bran supplements. Some may not eat any wheat at all. But they do eat plentiful amounts of fiber from other sources, such as rice and various kinds of beans. Since our recipes include large amounts of a variety of high-fiber foods, we do not make extensive use of bran in our recipes. However, if you feel the need to get your fiber from sources other than whole foods, you can certainly turn to a couple of tablespoons of bran a day, taken with plentiful fluids. Recently, some very promising experimental work has been done with oat bran, and should that become available commercially, it would make an excellent supplement.

Pectin, a form of fiber found abundantly in apples, but also in the white rind of oranges, is another natural substance that can help lower cholesterol. A review by A. Stewart Truswell, M.D., of Queen Elizabeth College, London University, England, points out that there are at least seven reports in medical literature on pectin and its effect on plasma cholesterol and "all found significant reduction of plasma cholesterol." (*Nutrition Reviews,* March, 1977). For this reason, many of our recipes for breakfast cereal mixes suggest slicing an apple over the whole grains to increase the anticholesterol potency. Homemade applesauce mixed with a little fruit and spread over bran muffins or whole wheat pancakes is another obvious—and tasty—possibility. Good crisp whole apples also make excellent snacks and desserts.

In many of our recipes, you will see directions for topping various dishes with alfalfa sprouts. That's done not just for the sake of appearance and taste—which are both important—but also because alfalfa, like apples, is a cholesterol fighter. That has been proven both in animals and human beings. Most of the experiments done have used unrealistically large amounts of alfalfa, so we can't tell exactly to what extent a big handful of alfalfa sprouts is going to help, but, as they say, it can't hurt. Also in the "can't hurt" category are eggplant and yogurt. There is experimental evidence suggesting that both may help to reduce cholesterol. The interesting thing about yogurt is that even when it's made from whole milk, which contains saturated fat and cholesterol, it *lowers* serum cholesterol when fermented into yogurt. There is still some controversy about whether the cholesterol-lowering effect of yogurt is due to the bacteria, the calcium, or something in the milk itself, but there is no question that yogurt is a good addition to the diet. We often use it as a substitute for mayonnaise and other fatty dressings or sauces.

HELP FROM BREWER'S YEAST

Another familiar "health food" that does good things for your circulatory system is brewer's yeast. Rebecca Riales, Ph.D., a nutritionist, told us that her interest in brewer's yeast began because it is a naturally rich source of chromium, a trace element which has important influence on normalizing blood sugar and insulin levels. She reasoned that since insulin has important roles in connection with fat metabolism (in addition to sugar metabolism), perhaps something that improves the efficiency of insulin might have beneficial effects on blood fats, too — especially on HDL, which, as we've explained, appears to actually protect against heart disease. Her first step was to give a daily dose of brewer's yeast to her physician-husband. She was astonished when his HDL levels took a tremendous upward bound. "You can imagine my excitement!" she relates. "So I enlisted the cooperation of eight physician friends. Believe me, I couldn't have found a more skeptical group, but with a little persuasion they agreed to take yeast for me for six weeks." After six weeks of taking two teaspoons of yeast a day, all but one of the seven subjects completing the study (one dropped out) showed increased HDL levels. In fact, HDL cholesterol levels rose an average of 17.6 percent. In one person it increased by almost 38 percent. "Another significant finding for my little yeast study," Dr. Riales says, "was that as HDL cholesterol levels rose, total fat in the blood decreased by 10 percent. This just happens to be in perfect harmony with the studies in the literature which suggest that HDL removes fats from the body."

VITAMINS AND MINERALS HELP, TOO

So far, we haven't said much about vitamins. But they, too, can help your circulatory system. The vitamin C in your food or supplements, for instance, may be doing your circulatory system at least as big a favor as it is your immunity. Experiments carried out at the Oak Ridge National Laboratory in Tennessee showed that animals fed extra vitamin C along with a high-cholesterol diet had 60 percent less plaque on the walls of their arteries than those that received no supplements. And the plaque in the untreated animals contained more than twice as much cholesterol as the plaque in the vitamin C group (*International Journal for Vitamin and Nutrition Research,* vol. 46, no. 3, 1976). Further, experimental research carried out by biochemist Anthony Verlangieri, Ph.D., suggests that vitamin C actually protects the *lining* of the arteries, by helping to prevent rough spots believed to serve as snags for fats and other materials in the bloodstream. Because human beings cannot be autopsied at will to see how their arteries are doing, human evidence of this plaque-fighting ability of vitamin C remains to be established. But researchers in the studies we've mentioned here have told us that it makes sense to get plenty of vitamin C in your diet in hopes of helping to keep your arteries clean. Good sources of vitamin C are citrus fruits, melons, broccoli, brussels sprouts, cabbage, green and red sweet peppers, strawberries and dark green leafy vegetables. These foods are all low in calories and high in nutrients other than vitamin C, so it's easy to fit them into an overall good diet plan.

Vitamins E and B_6 (pyridoxine) have also been reported to be a potential help to the circulatory system. Preliminary tests with vitamin E show that 600 international units a day significantly raises the desirable HDL fraction of cholesterol. Vitamin B_6 apparently is another natural protection against abnormal platelet aggregation, which can lead to deadly blood clots. However, work with these vitamins so far has been done only with supplements in amounts much larger than would ordinarily exist in a diet, or with blood samples in test tubes. We can't say, then, exactly what effect they might have when eaten in whole food form. Peanuts and wheat germ are good sources of both vitamin E *and* vitamin B$_6$. B$_6$ is also found abundantly in bananas, brewer's yeast, chicken, brown rice, salmon, sunflower seeds, whole grains and liver. Vitamin E is found in almonds, and foods rich in polyunsaturated oils, such as sunflower seeds, and the oil of soybeans, safflower, corn and sesame seeds.

When it comes to the minerals, the ones that have received the most attention are magnesium, potassium and the trace element selenium. Magnesium, particularly, seems to be crucial in maintaining the heart muscle in a state of relaxed and rhythmic functioning. A fascinating study by Carl J. Johnson, M.D., of the University of Colorado School of Medicine, and colleagues suggests that "more emphasis must be placed on the importance of magnesium in the diet" (*American Journal of Clinical Nutrition,* May, 1979). Dr. Johnson's team found that there were unusually low concentrations of both magnesium *and* potassium in the heart tissues of men dying suddenly from heart attacks. Of course, it's possible that following any kind of sudden death, there could be a tendency for these minerals to leave the heart, but their studies revealed that this marked shortage of minerals in the heart does not occur in men dying a sudden death from causes other than heart attacks. What's more, they found that the four lowest potassium values were obtained for the four men who had a history of angina. And three of these four also had the lowest magnesium levels in their heart muscles. The possibility that this would occur from mere chance, they point out, is exceedingly remote.

Fortunately, both magnesium and potassium occur in goodly amounts in foods which a health-minded person would be eating for *other* reasons as well. Good sources of magnesium, for instance, include nuts, tofu, wheat germ, soybeans, blackstrap molasses, potatoes, whole grains and beans. Potassium is found in nearly all garden vegetables, such as broccoli, carrots, spinach and tomatoes, as well as apples, bananas, chicken, oranges, potatoes, raisins, salmon, sunflower seeds, tuna and wheat germ. *Notice, by the way, how so many of the vitamins, minerals, oils and other substances good for your heart are found in the same foods. These are precisely the foods that we try to use most frequently in our recipes.*

The trace mineral selenium has not received much medical attention until the last few years, when more and more evidence began to pile up that it may have an important protective effect on the heart. In America, the work has been done mostly with laboratory animals, but in China, scientists reported at an international conference in 1980 that supplements of selenium seem to be wiping out a virtual epidemic of a certain type of heart disease affecting young people, and which is rampant in areas of that country where the soil is very low in selenium. In the United States, most wheat is grown in the Midwest, where the soil content of selenium is naturally high, so whole wheat products are a good source. Fish, other whole grains, along with mushrooms, beans, garlic and liver are also rich in selenium.

Finally, we should say something about recent reports from Europe that the moderate use of alcohol, particularly wine, seems to be associated with a lower incidence of heart attacks. Most of the experts we talked to were extremely cautious about interpreting this, warning that anyone who increases his intake of alcohol because of such reports would probably be doing himself a lot more harm than good. For one thing, while drinking alcohol does—as grandpop's family physician may have told him—dilate the arteries somewhat, it does not and cannot dilate arteries that are narrowed and clogged by atherosclerosis. As Howard S. Friedman, M.D., chief of cardiology at the Brooklyn Hospital told us, while alcohol dilates healthy vessels, a narrowed or obstructed vessel already is dilated as much as possible. "The narrowed vessel cannot take any more blood, so the blood is redistributed away from that area to the good areas of the heart. This might be considered a 'coronary steal,' endangering the ailing part of the heart," he says. Four shots of hard liquor or four beers taken very quickly could create this same effect in people with heart failure or coronary artery disease. "Those people should limit their use of alcohol," he warns. "If used at all, alcohol should be used with moderation."

Another word of caution on alcohol comes from Finland. A study of the case histories of 76 patients at the University of Helsinki found that even occasional intoxication seems to increase the risk of strokes in young adults (*Lancet,* December 2, 1978). Scientists in the university's department of neurology had noticed that strokes in young patients were often preceded by drinking bouts. They decided to take a look at the medical records on file for all stroke patients under the age of 40. They found that drunkenness preceding strokes was two to three times as common in men, and three to four times as common in women, as the general rate of intoxication in Finns of the same ages and sex. Fifteen of the 76 patients were stricken within 24 hours of a drinking spree, and 2 suffered strokes while they were still drunk. Over half the cases were reported on a weekend, when drinking in Finland is heaviest.

As you can see from all of the above, the story of nutrition and the heart is still unfolding. Yet, from all that's been done so far, it's easy to see that as far as the heart is concerned, to a large extent we are carving our destinies with our knives and forks. We can also see that, despite all the different factors involved, foods that are generally good for the heart are the grains, vegetables and fruits of the earth and the fish of the sea. The foods that are bad for the heart are those that come from intensive agricultural and food processing techniques, which have made available to us large amounts of artificially fattened beef, fat-added products like sausages and cold cuts, and the products of the dairy industry. You may be thinking "what's so unnatural about dairy foods?"— but remember that the keeping of cows for their milk is a relatively recent invention of civilization. And how "natural" can it be for human beings to drink milk designed to nourish calves?

Looked at in such a light, you can say that the recipes and the dietary approach we present in this book are simply a return to a more natural way of eating. Dining on ham and eggs, hot dogs, steaks, ice cream and cake may be the *typical* way of eating, but it's *not* natural—unless you think heart disease is natural! If you believe a *healthy* heart is natural . . . *bon appetit!*

BREAKFASTS

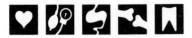

Dutch Muesli

This is based on a formula developed by Dutch chemist Dr. Jacobus Rinse. He ate it every morning with some vitamin E and C and claimed his angina cleared up.

Makes four cups (1 l)
- 1 cup (250 ml) bran
- 1 cup (250 ml) rolled oats
- 1 cup (250 ml) wheat germ
- ¾ cup (175 ml) soy flakes
- ¼ cup (60 ml) lecithin granules
- ¼ cup (60 ml) sunflower seeds
- 1 tablespoon (15 ml) sesame seeds
- 1 tablespoon (15 ml) brewer's yeast
- 1 teaspoon (5 ml) bone meal (optional)

Mix ingredients in a large bowl and store in covered jar. Soy flakes can be broken up in blender before adding, if desired. Serve over chopped apples with milk or yogurt. Raisins, sliced bananas and chopped nuts are other tasty additions.

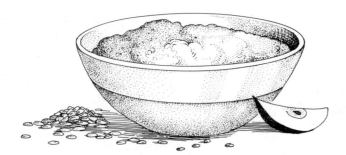

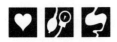

Apple Chunk Porridge

Makes two servings
- 1 unpeeled apple, finely diced
- 1¼ cups (300 ml) water
- ⅓ cup (80 ml) rolled oats
- ¼ cup (60 ml) *Dutch Muesli*

Place apple in a medium saucepan, add water, bring to a boil and then reduce heat and simmer about two minutes. Add oats and muesli and cook until creamy. Serve with milk or apple juice.

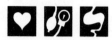

Raisins 'n' Spice Oatmeal

Makes two servings
1½ cups (375 ml) water
⅔ cup (150 ml) rolled oats
3 tablespoons (45 ml) raisins
½ teaspoon (2 ml) cinnamon
⅛ teaspoon (0.5 ml) cloves
   pinch coriander
1 teaspoon (5 ml) honey

Bring water to a boil in a medium saucepan, and stir in oats, raisins and spices. Reduce heat and simmer, stirring, about three to six minutes, until mixture is thickened and creamy. Remove from the heat. Cover, and let stand for five minutes, if desired, for a thicker consistency.

Stir in honey before serving oatmeal plain or with skim milk.

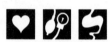

Porridge-Fruit Melange

Makes two servings
1 unpeeled apple, coarsely
   chopped
½ banana
½ teaspoon (2 ml) finely grated
   lemon rind
¼ cup (60 ml) yogurt
⅔ cup (150 ml) rolled oats
1½ cups (375 ml) water

Place apple with banana and lemon rind in a blender and process on low speed until smooth.

Place the fruit sauce in a medium saucepan with the yogurt, oats and water. Bring to a boil, then reduce heat and simmer 5 to 10 minutes, until oats are creamy.

Note: Serve hot with skim milk or orange juice, or stir in additional yogurt and a little honey to taste.

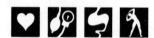

Bulgur Breakfast

Makes two servings
¾ cup (175 ml) bulgur
1½ cups (375 ml) water
1 unpeeled apple, chopped
¼ cup (60 ml) raisins
   dash cinnamon

Place ingredients in a saucepan and bring to a boil over medium heat. Cover, reduce heat and simmer mixture for 15 minutes, stirring occasionally.

Serve hot with skim milk or as is.

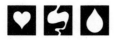

Apple-Raisin Cracked Wheat Cereal

Makes four to six servings
1 cup (250 ml) cracked wheat
4 cups (1 l) water
¾ teaspoon (4 ml) cinnamon
½ cup (125 ml) raisins
1 unpeeled tart apple, cubed
2 tablespoons (30 ml) sunflower
    seeds
2 tablespoons (30 ml) sesame
    seeds

Try eating this hot cereal plain, to best enjoy its hearty flavor.

To shorten cooking time, soak the cracked wheat in the water overnight. Combine the wheat, water, cinnamon, raisins and cubed apple in a heavy-bottom saucepan, and bring to a boil. Reduce heat and simmer until the wheat is soft, between 10 and 30 minutes. Stir in the sunflower and sesame seeds and serve.

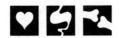

Molasses Pancakes

Makes two servings
1 cup (250 ml) whole
    wheat flour
¼ cup (60 ml) bran
1 tablespoon (15 ml)
    lecithin granules
1 teaspoon (5 ml) baking
    soda
1½–1¾ cups (375–425 ml)
    buttermilk
1 tablespoon (15 ml)
    medium unsulfured
    molasses
2 egg whites, beaten

Place the dry ingredients in a large bowl, breaking up any lumps and stirring until combined. Add the buttermilk (more or less, depending on the thickness desired), the molasses and egg whites. Cook on a lightly oiled, hot skillet.

Pancakes can be served with fresh fruit.

Wheat-Oatmeal Dollar Pancakes

Makes two servings
1 cup (250 ml) rolled oats
2 tablespoons (30 ml) bran
2 tablespoons (30 ml) wheat
    germ
½ teaspoon (2 ml) baking soda
⅔ cup (150 ml) buttermilk

Dollar-size little pancakes are filling when served with chopped fresh fruit topping.

In a medium bowl, combine the oats, bran, wheat germ, soda and buttermilk. Allow to stand for a couple of minutes, until the oats have absorbed most of the milk. Shape into eight small patties and bake in a hot, lightly oiled skillet, turning when browned. Serve hot.

SOUPS

French-Style Onion Soup

Makes two servings
1 tablespoon (15 ml) corn oil
1 large Spanish onion, thinly
　　sliced
1 clove garlic, crushed
2 cups (500 ml) *Chicken Stock*
2 teaspoons (10 ml) tamari
½ teaspoon (2 ml) blackstrap
　　molasses
1 bay leaf
2 thin slices whole wheat bread
1 teaspoon (5 ml) grated
　　Parmesan cheese

With good Chicken Stock *as its basis, this soup wins well-earned praise.*

Place oil in skillet, add the onions and saute. Add a tablespoon (15 ml) of water, if needed, to keep onions from sticking to bottom of the pan. When onions are slightly tender, and beginning to get translucent, add garlic, stock, tamari, molasses and bay leaf. Simmer for 30 to 45 minutes. Remove bay leaf. Place in two ovenproof serving dishes. Top each with a thin slice of whole wheat bread sprinkled with Parmesan cheese. Place under a broiler until cheese begins to melt.

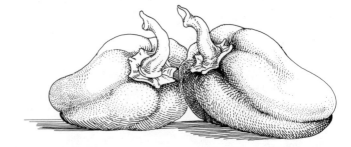

Green Pepper Soup

Makes four servings
1 teaspoon (5 ml) sesame oil
3 cups (750 ml) chopped green
　　peppers
1 cup (250 ml) chopped onions
1 tablespoon (15 ml) whole
　　wheat flour
½ teaspoon (2 ml) marjoram,
　　crumbled
1 cup (250 ml) buttermilk

Place oil in a heated skillet and add 2½ cups (625 ml) of the green peppers, and the onions. Saute until the onions are translucent, adding a few drops of water if necessary to prevent scorching. Place the remaining green peppers in a blender and add two-thirds of the cooked pepper and onion mix.

Add flour, marjoram and buttermilk to blender and process on medium speed until smooth. Return blended mixture to the skillet, stir to combine with remaining pepper and onion mixture, and bring to a boil, stirring, until the soup thickens. Serve hot.

Note: This can also be served cold with a dollop of yogurt and mint garnish.

Makes four to six servings

½ cup (125 ml) finely chopped
    mushrooms
 1 teaspoon (5 ml) corn oil
 1 clove garlic, crushed
 1 cup (250 ml) finely chopped
    tomatoes
¾ cup (175 ml) finely chopped
    green or sweet red
    peppers
½ cup (125 ml) finely chopped
    onions
½ cup (125 ml) finely chopped
    celery
½ cup (125 ml) finely chopped
    cucumbers
 1 teaspoon (5 ml) minced
    chives
 2 teaspoons (10 ml) minced
    fresh parsley
¼ cup (60 ml) *Tarragon
    Vinegar*
¼ cup soft whole grain bread
    crumbs
1½ cups (375 ml) tomato juice
    or ¼ cup (60 ml)
    tomato paste and 1¼
    cups (300 ml) water

Gazpacho

Saute mushrooms in the oil in a small skillet, adding just a few drops of water if necessary to prevent sticking. Combine with the remaining ingredients in a large bowl and chill thoroughly before serving. Makes about one quart (1 l).

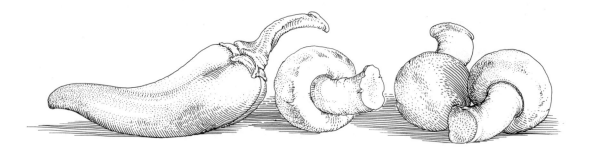

SALADS

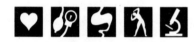

Tuna Tabbouleh

Makes six servings
½ cup (125 ml) bulgur
½ cup (125 ml) water
¼ cup (60 ml) lemon juice
2–3 medium tomatoes, seeded
    and chopped
5 scallions, chopped
1½ cups (375 ml) minced fresh
    parsley
¼ cup (60 ml) minced fresh
    mint
6½ ounces (184 g)
    water-packed tuna,
    drained
1 tablespoon (15 ml) corn oil
    curly endive or escarole
    leaves

Soak the bulgur in the water and lemon juice for about 30 minutes. Add remaining ingredients and toss until thoroughly combined. Makes about four cups (1 l). Serve as a luncheon dish atop a bed of curly endive or escarole.

Simply Super Bean Salad

Makes two servings
2 cups (500 ml) broccoli florets,
    lightly steamed
1 cup (250 ml) cooked small
    white beans with cooking
    liquid
1 medium red onion, thinly
    sliced
1 tablespoon (15 ml) oil

Every ingredient here is working for your health—and somehow they all manage to harmonize beautifully for your taste buds as well.

Toss ingredients together and let sit for 30 minutes or more before serving, if possible.

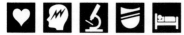

Tuna-Rice Salad

Makes four servings
- 1 cup (250 ml) long grain brown rice
- 2 cups (500 ml) whey (see *Index, Yogurt Cream Cheese*)
- 1 small green pepper, finely chopped
- 1 carrot, shredded
- 6½ ounces (184 g) water-packed tuna, drained
- 1 tablespoon (15 ml) minced fresh parsley

Cook rice, substituting whey for water. This will give the rice a lemony tartness, a fine background for the tuna salad. While rice is still warm, combine it in a bowl with green pepper, carrot, tuna and parsley. Chill before serving.

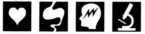

Sunday Night Rice and Lentil Salad

Makes four servings
- ¼ cup (60 ml) *Black Magic Sauce*
- 1 teaspoon (5 ml) sunflower oil
- 1½ cups (375 ml) cooked brown rice
- ½ cup (125 ml) shredded carrots
- ½ cup (125 ml) roughly chopped savoy cabbage
- ¼ cup (60 ml) chopped scallions
- 2 tablespoons (30 ml) grated Parmesan cheese
- ½ cup (125 ml) roughly chopped endive
- ½ cup (125 ml) sprouted lentils

Pour half of *Black Magic Sauce* and all of oil into wok or skillet and turn heat to high. When liquid begins to steam, add rice, carrots, cabbage and scallions. Stir briskly until the food becomes hot, which will take one or two minutes. Add more sauce as required. Sprinkle in Parmesan cheese and toss in endive. Continue stirring briskly for another 15 seconds, then add sprouted lentils and any remaining liquid. Stir for another 30 seconds or until food is hot and serve immediately.

Note: As a main dish, this salad serves two and is well complemented by a dessert of yogurt and fresh fruit.

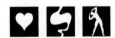

Macaroni Salad

Makes four servings
1 cup (250 ml) whole wheat
    macaroni
½ cup (125 ml) peas
2 stalks celery, chopped
¼ green pepper, chopped
1 tablespoon (15 ml) *Tarragon
    Vinegar*
2 tablespoons (30 ml) sunflower
    oil
2 tablespoons (30 ml) tomato
    paste
1 teaspoon (5 ml) basil
½ teaspoon (2 ml) oregano
½ teaspoon (2 ml) marjoram

Bring a large saucepan half-filled with water to a boil and add the macaroni. Return to a boil, and cook only until the pasta is still firm to the bite, about four to five minutes. Drain.

In a smaller pan, bring a small amount of water to a boil and add the peas. Simmer until crisp-tender, about one to two minutes.

In a serving bowl, combine celery and pepper with macaroni and peas. Blend vinegar, oil, tomato paste and seasonings and pour over macaroni salad. Toss to combine. Chill before serving.

Tarragon Vinegar

Makes two cups (500 ml)
2 cups (500 ml) white vinegar
3-inch (8 cm) fresh tarragon
    sprig
1 clove garlic, halved

Place ingredients in a small saucepan and heat, but do not boil. Remove garlic clove. Place sprig of tarragon and vinegar in a sterile jar or the bottle in which vinegar was purchased.

Note: Tarragon is easy to grow in your herb garden and can be purchased at certain produce markets in season.

Chopped Tomato Salad

Makes four servings
2 large, ripe tomatoes
4 scallions or ½ small onion
½ green pepper
½ medium cucumber
1 stalk celery
3 tablespoons (45 ml) lemon
    juice
    lettuce leaves

Chop all vegetables. Sprinkle with lemon juice and chill thoroughly before serving on lettuce leaves.

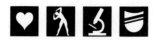

Green Bean Salad

Makes three servings
2 cups (500 ml) sliced green
   beans
½ sweet red pepper, chopped
1 stalk celery, thinly sliced
2 scallions, finely chopped
1 cup (250 ml) alfalfa sprouts
Creamy Garlic Dressing
lettuce leaves

Combine the beans, pepper, celery, scallions and sprouts. Toss with enough dressing to coat. Chill and serve on lettuce leaves.

Creamy Garlic Dressing

*Makes about 1½ cups
(375 ml)*
¼ cup (60 ml) mild vinegar
1 teaspoon (5 ml) Dijon-style
   mustard
½ cup (125 ml) sunflower oil
1 clove garlic
1 cup (250 ml) yogurt

Combine vinegar and mustard in a blender on low speed, and slowly add oil.

Add garlic and yogurt. Store in a covered jar in refrigerator.

Lemon Vinaigrette Dressing

Makes ¾ cup (175 ml)
¼ cup (60 ml) lemon juice
½ teaspoon (2 ml) Dijon-style
   mustard
½ cup (125 ml) soy or
   sunflower oil
¼ teaspoon (1 ml) grated lemon
   rind

This dressing is nice for fruit salad combinations.

In a blender, combine lemon juice and mustard on low speed, slowly adding the oil, until mixture is thick. Place in glass jar, add lemon rind, and shake. Store unused portion in the refrigerator.

Celery Dressing

Makes 1¼ cups (300 ml)
1 stalk celery
6 ounces (170 g) tofu
2 tablespoons (30 ml) mild
    vinegar
1 teaspoon (5 ml) Dijon-style
    mustard
1 scallion or ½ small onion

Place ingredients in a blender and process on slow, then medium speed, until smooth. This can be used on salads or, for a twist, try serving on baked potatoes.

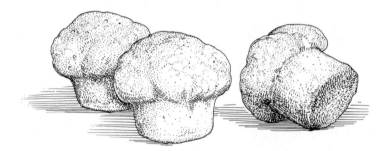

BREADS

Buttermilk-Bran Muffins

Makes one dozen
1½ cups (375 ml) whole wheat
    pastry flour
2½ cups (625 ml) bran
2 teaspoons (10 ml) *Baking
    Powder*
1 egg
1½ cups (375 ml) buttermilk
⅓ cup (80 ml) maple syrup
1 tablespoon (15 ml) sesame
    tahini

For all their fiber, these muffins are surprisingly light and tasty. Try them for breakfast with applesauce.

Combine flour, bran and *Baking Powder* in a large bowl. Beat egg in a separate bowl, and add the buttermilk, syrup and tahini, beating to mix. Add wet ingredients to flour mixture and stir just until combined. Some lumps can remain. Divide mixture between 12 lightly oiled muffin cups. Bake in a preheated 400° F. (200° C.) oven for 20 minutes, until golden.

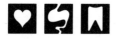

Crunchy Fruit Muffins

Makes one dozen

1½ cups (375 ml) whole wheat
   pastry flour
2½ teaspoons (12 ml) *Baking
   Powder*
 ½ cup (125 ml) wheat germ
 ½ cup (125 ml) bran
 ½ cup (125 ml) sunflower
   seeds
 ¼ cup (60 ml) sesame seeds
 1 cup (250 ml) fruit
 ¾ cup (175 ml) buttermilk or
   yogurt
 2 eggs, beaten
 ¼ cup (60 ml) honey

These muffins are sure favorites, and a great way to use up extra fruit.

Combine dry ingredients in a large mixing bowl. For fresh fruit, you might try peaches, plums, apples, pears or berries. Chop fruit, if necessary, and combine with buttermilk, eggs and honey in a medium bowl. Combine wet and dry ingredients, stirring lightly just until combined. Some lumps can remain. Divide batter between 12 lightly oiled muffin cups. Bake in a preheated 400° F. (200° C.) oven for 20 to 25 minutes, or until golden brown.

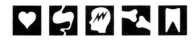

Strawberry Muffins

Makes one dozen

 1 cup (250 ml) whole wheat
   flour
 ½ cup (125 ml) bran
 2 tablespoons (30 ml) wheat
   germ
 1 tablespoon (15 ml) lecithin
   granules
 1 teaspoon (5 ml) bone meal
 1 tablespoon (15 ml) brewer's
   yeast
 1 teaspoon (5 ml) baking soda
 1 egg, beaten
 1 tablespoon (15 ml) safflower
   oil
 3 tablespoons (45 ml) honey
 ½ cup (125 ml) buttermilk or
   yogurt
 1 cup (250 ml) strawberries
 2 apples

Combine dry ingredients in a large mixing bowl. In another bowl, combine egg, oil, honey and buttermilk. Process strawberries and apples in a blender on medium speed until pureed. Add to egg mixture. Mix thoroughly and then add to dry ingredients. Combine with light strokes of the fork, just until moistened. Place in a lightly oiled muffin pan and bake at 350° F. (175° C.) for 30 minutes. Serve with additional blended strawberries and apples, if desired, instead of jam.

MAIN DISHES

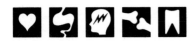

Sharon's Best Pizza

Makes four 10-inch (25-cm) pizzas

Sauce:
- 1 tablespoon (15 ml) corn oil
- 1 cup (250 ml) finely chopped onions
- 1 tablespoon (15 ml) minced garlic
- 6–8 large, ripe tomatoes, or 4 cups (1 l) Italian plum tomatoes with juice
- ⅔ cup (150 ml) tomato paste
- 1 tablespoon (15 ml) oregano, crumbled
- 2 teaspoons (10 ml) basil, crumbled
- 1 bay leaf
- 1 teaspoon (5 ml) blackstrap molasses

Dough:
- 2 tablespoons (30 ml) active dry yeast
- 1¼ cups (300 ml) lukewarm water
- ½ teaspoon (2 ml) honey
- 2½ cups (625 ml) whole wheat flour
- 1 cup (250 ml) gluten flour
- 2 tablespoons (30 ml) sesame tahini or corn oil
- whole grain cornmeal

In a three or four quart (3 or 4 l) enamel or stainless steel saucepan, heat oil and cook onions over moderate heat, stirring, for seven or eight minutes. When they are soft, add garlic; continue stirring one or two minutes. Add the remaining ingredients, bring to a boil, then reduce heat and simmer one hour, stirring occasionally. Remove bay leaf. For a smoother sauce, puree tomato sauce in a food mill or blender. Makes about 3½ cups (875 ml).

In a small bowl, sprinkle yeast over ¼ cup (60 ml) lukewarm water into which the honey has been stirred. Let mixture stand until yeast is dissolved, about two or three minutes. Stir yeast mixture and place in a warm spot until the yeast bubbles up and the mixture doubles in volume, about three to five minutes. If the yeast does not bubble, discard and use fresh yeast.

Place whole wheat and gluten flours into a large bowl. Make a "well" in the center of the flour and into this pour the yeast mixture and remaining cup of lukewarm water. Add tahini or oil, and begin mixing the dough with a wooden spoon or your fingers. When it begins to grow elastic, gather the dough into a ball and turn out onto a floured board. Knead the dough for about 15 minutes, until it is smooth and shiny. Dust the dough lightly with flour and place in a large, clean bowl, covered with a plate or lid. Place in a warm, draft-free place to rise about double in bulk, about 1½ hours. (In a pinch for time, pizzas can be made without allowing the dough to rise, with acceptable results.)

Preheat oven to 500° F. (260° C.). Punch the dough down and divide into four equal pieces. Knead each piece on the floured board for a minute or two. Then flatten the piece into a round about an inch (2.5 cm) thick. Grasp the circle in your hands and stretch the dough by pulling your hands apart gently, rotating the dough to get an even circle. When the dough is about 7 or 8 inches (18 or 20 cm) across, place on the floured board and roll with a rolling pin, sprinkling with flour to prevent sticking to board or roller. If dough sticks to the board, gently lift it up and dust board with flour. When dough is about 10 inches (25 cm) across, flute the edge to make a small rim, which will help to contain the pizza sauce.

Sprinkle a baking sheet with cornmeal and carefully lift dough onto sheet. To make pizza, pour ¾ cup (175 ml) of tomato sauce on dough, and spread evenly with the back of a spoon. Repeat for remaining pizzas.

Topping:

1½ cups (375 ml) shredded mozzarella or Swiss cheese

3 tablespoons (45 ml) grated Parmesan cheese

chopped garlic

sliced tomatoes

thinly sliced onions

cooked spinach

flaked tuna

chopped green or sweet red peppers

sliced mushrooms

crumbled tofu

Sprinkle each pizza with shredded cheese and dust with grated Parmesan. Garnish with your choice of additional toppings.

Bake on lowest shelf of a 500° F. (260° C.) oven for 8 to 10 minutes, until crust is golden. Cut and serve. Pizzas may be frozen before baking, in which case they must be thawed or baking time adjusted to allow for defrosting.

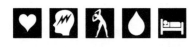

Makes two servings

1 whole chicken breast, skinned
   and boned
6 tablespoons (90 ml) orange
   juice
1 cup (250 ml) chopped
   mushrooms
½ cup (125 ml) chopped green
   peppers
¼ cup (60 ml) chopped
   scallions
1 clove garlic, crushed
½ cup (125 ml) freshly shelled
   peas
½ cup (125 ml) chopped
   tomatoes
1 teaspoon (5 ml) lemon juice
1 teaspoon (5 ml) tamari
2 teaspoons (10 ml) curry

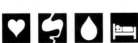

Makes six to eight servings

3 yellow onions, chopped
2 green peppers, chopped
1 teaspoon (5 ml) corn oil
3 cups (750 ml) cooked fava
   or kidney beans
3½ cups (875 ml) tomato puree
6 cloves garlic, minced
2 tablespoons (30 ml) chili powder
2 teaspoons (10 ml) cumin powder
1 teaspoon (5 ml) cumin seed
1 teaspoon (5 ml) tamari
1 tablespoon (15 ml)
   blackstrap molasses
1 teaspoon (5 ml) basil
1 teaspoon (5 ml) oregano
½ teaspoon (2 ml) marjoram
½ teaspoon (2 ml) thyme

Curried Chicken and Peas

Low-fat flavor is the theme of this savory dish.

Cut chicken into small, thin strips. Put two tablespoons (30 ml) of the orange juice into a hot skillet or wok. When hot, add mushrooms and cook over medium-high heat for about five minutes. Add green peppers, scallions and garlic and cook for three minutes. Finally, add the peas and tomatoes and cook for one minute. Now pour contents of wok or skillet into another pan. Pour the lemon juice, the remaining orange juice, and the tamari into the original wok or skillet and turn the heat up to high. When steaming, add the chicken and curry. Stir vigorously. If necessary, pour some liquid from the vegetables into the chicken. The chicken will be done very quickly, in two to three minutes. Be careful not to overcook. The only reliable way to see if the chicken is done is to fork out the thickest piece and slice it. The center should be pale white, but not pink. Taste it to make sure. When just *barely* done, add the vegetables to the chicken, stir vigorously for about 20 seconds, or until you are sure the vegetables are the proper temperature, and serve. Rice makes a good side dish.

Chili Non Carne

In a large pot, saute onions and peppers in oil, adding a few drops of water, if necessary, to prevent sticking. Stir in beans and remaining ingredients and bring to a boil. Reduce heat and simmer, stirring occasionally, for 30 to 45 minutes. Serve with whole wheat bread, corn bread, on tortillas or as a taco filling. Makes six to seven cups (1.5 to 1.75 l).

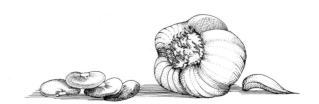

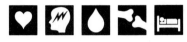

Skillet Turkey Dinner

Makes two servings
1 small onion, chopped
½ sweet red pepper, chopped
1 tablespoon (15 ml) corn oil
1½ tablespoons (25 ml) whole
    wheat flour
1 teaspoon (5 ml) basil
1 cup (250 ml) skim milk
1 cup (250 ml) cooked, cubed
    turkey breast
1 teaspoon (5 ml) tamari
1 teaspoon (5 ml) minced
    fresh parsley

In a skillet, saute the onion and pepper in the corn oil until tender. Stir in flour and basil, and cook over low heat for a couple of minutes. Stir in the skim milk slowly, to prevent lumping.

Add turkey meat, tamari and parsley and simmer until thickened. Serve *Skillet Turkey Dinner* hot over whole wheat noodles, brown rice or whole grain toast.

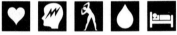

Boston Scrod and Vegetables

Makes two servings
10 ounces (280 g) Boston scrod
1 teaspoon (5 ml) sunflower oil
1 teaspoon (5 ml) tamari
1 clove garlic, crushed
6 mushrooms
2 scallions
1 medium tomato
2 tablespoons (30 ml) lemon
    juice
2 tablespoons (30 ml) orange
    juice

A classic, yet so-easy dinner that always pleases.

Slice fish into six pieces and marinate in the oil, tamari and garlic for 30 minutes. Chop vegetables into very small pieces. Place fish on foil under broiler. Begin steam-stirring the mushrooms and scallions in the lemon and orange juice. After about 5 minutes, add tomato and continue stirring. Adjust the heat if necessary to avoid overcooking. In about 10 minutes from the time you put the fish under the broiler, both the vegetables and the fish should be done. Spoon the vegetables over the fish and serve while hot. A perfect marriage of tastes.

Variation: Substitute haddock or cod for Boston scrod.

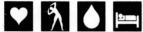

Makes two servings
1 pound (450 g) haddock fillets
1 onion, finely chopped
⅓ cup (80 ml) minced fresh
   parsley
1 clove garlic, crushed
2 tablespoons (30 ml) *Tarragon
   Vinegar*
½ teaspoon (2 ml) thyme
3 large tomatoes, chopped

Portuguese Poached Fish

Color and flavor abound in this easy entree.

Place the fish in a heavy pan or electric skillet and cover with remaining ingredients. When mixture has come to a boil, simmer, covered, for 10 minutes. Carefully remove fish fillets from the vegetable sauce and place on a serving platter. Keep the fish warm by covering with foil while you boil down the sauce. Turn up heat under the vegetables and boil quickly to reduce mixture by half. Pour the sauce over the fish and serve.

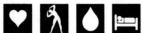

Makes four servings
1 pound (450 g) haddock
   fillets
¼ cup (60 ml) finely chopped
   celery
½ cup (125 ml) finely chopped
   onions
½ cup (125 ml) shredded
   zucchini
1 teaspoon (5 ml) corn oil
1 cup (250 ml) soft whole
   grain bread crumbs
¼ teaspoon (1 ml) tarragon
⅛ teaspoon (0.5 ml) rosemary
1 tablespoon minced flat-leaf
   parsley
1–2 large tomatoes, thinly sliced

Baked Fillet of Haddock

Place haddock fillets in a shallow baking dish. Combine celery, onions and zucchini in a skillet with the oil and saute until slightly tender, adding a few drops of water, if necessary, to prevent scorching. Sitr in bread crumbs and herbs, including parsley. Spread bread crumb mixture over the fish in the casserole dish. Place thin slices of tomato to cover the bread crumb mixture. Bake in a 375° F. (190° C.) preheated oven for 35 to 40 minutes.

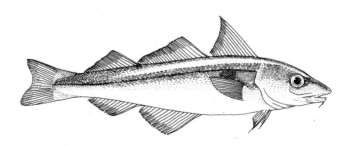

Haddock Souffle

Makes four servings
1½ tablespoons (25 ml)
safflower oil
1½ tablespoons (25 ml) whole
wheat flour
1 cup (250 ml) skim milk
1 cup (250 ml) cooked, flaked
haddock
⅓ cup (80 ml) finely chopped
carrots
1 tablespoon (15 ml) minced
fresh parsley
freshly grated nutmeg
4 egg whites

Heat oil in a heavy skillet, and add the flour. Stir until combined, and continue stirring over medium heat one or two minutes. Add milk gradually, stirring after each addition, to prevent lumps. Set aside to cool.

Stir haddock (flounder, tuna or other soft fish can be substituted), carrots, parsley and nutmeg to taste into the cream sauce.

Beat egg whites by hand with an eggbeater, or on low to medium speed with a hand mixer until the whites are stiff but not dry. Stir ½ cup (125 ml) of the beaten egg whites into the cream sauce, then gently fold in the remaining whites.

Turn mixture into a lightly oiled 1¾-quart (1.75-l) souffle dish. Bake in a preheated 325° F. (165° C.) oven until firm, about 35 to 40 minutes. Serve immediately, either plain or with a tomato sauce.

  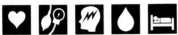

Haddock with Mushroom and Bulgur Stuffing

Makes four servings
¼ cup (60 ml) finely chopped
onions
½ cup (125 ml) finely chopped
sweet red peppers
2 teaspoons (10 ml) sunflower
oil
2½ cups (625 ml) sliced
mushrooms (about ½
pound [225 g])
½ cup (125 ml) bulgur
1 cup (250 ml) *Chicken Stock*
or *Vegetable Stock*
½ teaspoon (2 ml) basil
1 pound (450 g) haddock
fillets
1 tablespoon (15 ml) chopped
fresh parsley (garnish)

Fish with a meat-hearty kind of flavor.

Steam-stir the onions and peppers in the oil, adding a little water, if needed, to prevent scorching. When the onions are translucent, add the mushrooms and cook until water evaporates and mushrooms are tender.

Add bulgur, stock and basil. Cook covered on low heat for 10 minutes. Stir. Place fish fillets on bulgur dressing, cover, and cook an additional 10 minutes, until fish is opaque and cooked through.

Serve hot, garnished with fresh parsley.

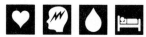

Makes two servings

Salad:

¼ cup (60 ml) unpeeled diced apples

¼ cup (60 ml) seedless grapes, quartered

¼ cup (60 ml) walnuts, chopped

6½ ounces (184 g) water-packed tuna, drained

½ cup (125 ml) cooked navy beans

spinach or lettuce leaves

Dressing:

1 cup (250 ml) yogurt

2 tablespoons (30 ml) sesame tahini

3 tablespoons (45 ml) tomato paste

Rosy Tuna Salad

Combine apples, grapes, nuts, tuna and beans in a medium bowl. Stir together dressing ingredients in a small bowl, and toss salad with enough dressing to moisten. Serve on spinach or lettuce leaves.

Note: Use leftover dressing on cooked vegetables or tossed salad. It is also good on lightly steamed vegetables, served chilled as a salad.

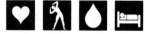

Makes four servings

1 cup (250 ml) finely chopped green peppers

2 cups (500 ml) unpeeled diced apples

6½ ounces (184 g) unsalted water-packed tuna, drained

2 teaspoons (10 ml) sesame seeds, toasted

½ cup (125 ml) raisins

½ cup (125 ml) *Tofu Mayonnaise*

lettuce or spinach leaves

Tuna-Apple Salad

Here's a super-fast combo that balances the protein and good oils of tuna with the crunch and sweetness of vegetables and fruit.

Combine the first five ingredients in a medium mixing bowl. Toss with *Tofu Mayonnaise*. Makes about four cups (1 l).

Serve on lettuce or spinach leaves as a luncheon main course.

Variation: For a sweeter salad, substitute a dressing made of two tablespoons (30 ml) apple juice, one tablespoon (15 ml) sesame tahini and one tablespoon (15 ml) yogurt for the *Tofu Mayonnaise*.

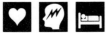

Makes three servings
2 medium onions, chopped
4 cloves garlic, minced
1 tomato, chopped
⅔ cup (150 ml) tomato
     paste
6½ ounces (184 g) unsalted
     water-packed tuna
2 cups (500 ml) water
2 teaspoons (10 ml) basil
1 teaspoon (5 ml) oregano
2 tablespoons (30 ml)
     minced fresh parsley
¼–½ teaspoon (1–2 ml) dried
     hot red pepper flakes
2 tablespoons (30 ml)
     lemon juice
grated Parmesan cheese
     (garnish)

Hot Tuna Sauce

Steam-stir onions in a small amount of water until they are translucent and slightly tender. Add remaining ingredients, including the water from the tuna. Bring to a boil and simmer over medium heat for about 20 minutes. Serve over whole wheat spaghetti or pasta and sprinkle lightly with grated Parmesan cheese.

Makes six servings
6 green peppers
½ tablespoon (7 ml) soy oil
1 medium onion, finely
     chopped
3 cloves garlic, minced
1½ cups (375 ml) chopped
     tomatoes
2½ cups (625 ml) sliced
     mushrooms (about ½
     pound [225 g])
2 tablespoons (30 ml) fresh
     basil
1 tablespoon (15 ml) tamari
1½ cups (375 ml) cooked
     brown rice
Lentil-Tomato Sauce

Stuffed Peppers

Remove the tops and seeds from green peppers. Set aside. In a large skillet, heat oil and add onion. Stir, adding a few drops of water if necessary to prevent sticking, until onions are translucent. Add garlic and tomatoes, stirring until tomato pieces begin to lose their shape. Add mushrooms, basil and tamari. Cook until mushrooms are tender. Stir in rice and heat through. Place stuffing in the peppers, and arrange peppers in a colander. Place colander in a large kettle with one to two inches (2.5 to 5 cm) of water in the bottom and steam the stuffed peppers until tender, about 20 minutes. Serve immediately with *Lentil-Tomato Sauce* spooned over top, or pass the sauce separately.

Note: The steamed, stuffed peppers can also be placed in a casserole dish, covered with tomato sauce and a sprinkling of grated Parmesan cheese and held in a warm oven until served.

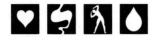

Chili Beans

Makes six servings
4 cups (1 1) cooked kidney
    beans
2½ cups (625 ml) liquid from
    cooking kidney beans
    (or add enough
    Vegetable Stock to
    make 2½ cups
    [625 ml])
⅔ cup (150 ml) tomato paste
2 tablespoons (30 ml) chili
    powder
1 teaspoon (5 ml) cumin
    powder
1 teaspoon (5 ml) tamari
2 teaspoons (10 ml) blackstrap
    molasses
½ teaspoon (2 ml) dried hot
    red pepper flakes

Combine ingredients in a large skillet or saucepan. Simmer 10 to 15 minutes to develop flavor. Makes about five cups (1.25 l).

Chili beans can be served over corn bread, or baked under a layer of *Corn Pone.*

Variation: Steam-stir one green pepper, seeded and chopped, in a little water until crisp-tender. Add remaining ingredients and cook as above.

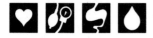

Oven-Baked Lentils

Makes 2½ cups (625 ml)
1 cup (250 ml) dried lentils
3 cups (750 ml) water
1 onion, chopped

This is a handy way to have cooked lentils on hand. Plan to make the lentils when the oven is heated for other baking—a good way to conserve time and fuel!

Wash the lentils and place them in an ovenproof casserole dish with the water and onion. Place in a 350° F. (175° C.) oven and bake one hour. Drain before using in recipes calling for cooked beans or lentils.

Note: Cooked lentils can be used to enrich soups, can be added to tomato sauces for pasta or, seasoned with chili and cumin powders, can be used in a tomato sauce for tortillas. Try a chili-flavored lentil sauce with *Corn Pone.*

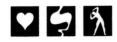

Soy-Bulgur Casserole

A hearty protein fare lightly spiced with chili flavor.

Makes six servings
1½ cups (375 ml) bulgur
3 cups (750 ml) water
1½ cups (375 ml) cooked
　　soybeans
4–5 scallions
⅔ cup (150 ml) tomato paste
1 cup (250 ml) *Chicken Stock*
½ green or sweet red pepper,
　　chopped
¼ cup (60 ml) minced fresh
　　parsley
1 tablespoon (15 ml) brewer's
　　yeast
1 tablespoon (15 ml) tamari
1 tablespoon (15 ml) chili
　　powder
2 teaspoons (10 ml) cumin
　　powder
½ teaspoon (2 ml) oregano

Place the bulgur in the water in a large saucepan; bring to a boil, reduce heat and simmer 15 minutes. Meanwhile, in a blender, place ½ cup (125 ml) of cooked soybeans with two scallions, tomato paste and stock. Process on medium speed until smooth.

Place blended mixture in a large mixing bowl. Chop remaining scallions and add to blended mixture along with remaining ingredients, including bulgur when it is cooked. Turn into a lightly oiled casserole dish and bake in a 350° F. (175° C.) oven for 45 minutes.

Corn Casserole

Makes four servings
1 onion, chopped
1 sweet red pepper cut in long,
　　thin slices
1 tablespoon (15 ml) corn oil
1 teaspoon (5 ml) tamari
4 cups (1 l) fresh or frozen corn
6 ounces (170 g) tofu
1 egg, beaten

In a heavy skillet, saute onion and pepper in oil until nearly tender. Add tamari and corn kernels and cover, turning off heat. Mash tofu or process in a blender on low speed until smooth. Combine tofu with the egg in a medium casserole dish, and add corn mixture, stirring to combine ingredients. Bake in a 400° F. (200° C.) oven for 25 minutes. Serve hot.

SIDE DISHES

Green Beans Provencale

Makes four servings
4 cups (1 l) sliced green beans
3 large shallots, minced
1½ teaspoons (7 ml) sunflower
    oil
1 clove garlic, minced
3 medium tomatoes, chopped
    dash cayenne pepper
    dash freshly grated nutmeg

Our taste panel said this was one of the very best vegetable dishes.

Steam green beans just until crisp-tender. Rinse in cold water, or place in ice water, to stop cooking.

Meanwhile, in a skillet, saute shallots in oil for a minute or two, add garlic, and continue to stir until shallots turn translucent. Do not brown. Add a few drops of water if necessary to prevent scorching. Add tomatoes and continue to simmer, stirring occasionally, until mixture is reduced by one-third. Add green beans to tomato mixture, a faint dusting of cayenne and nutmeg, and stir to combine. Serve hot.

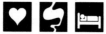

Molasses Baked Soybeans

Makes eight servings
2 cups (500 ml) dried soybeans
1 small onion, chopped
½ green or sweet red pepper,
    chopped
2 tablespoons (30 ml) soy oil
⅔ cup (150 ml) tomato paste
2 tablespoons (30 ml)
    blackstrap molasses
1 tablespoon (15 ml) honey
1 tablespoon (15 ml) tamari
¼ teaspoon (1 ml) oregano
2 cups (500 ml) liquid from
    cooking soybeans (or
    add enough *Vegetable
    Stock* to make 2 cups
    [500 ml])

One of the tastiest ways to eat soybeans we've ever discovered.

Soak soybeans overnight. Cook atop the stove or in the oven until tender (see Index "Cooking Beans").

Saute onion and pepper in oil in a medium skillet until tender. Combine all ingredients in a large mixing bowl and transfer to a covered casserole dish. Bake, covered, for one hour in a preheated 350° F. (175° C.) oven. Remove the cover, and bake 45 minutes longer, stirring occasionally.

Variation: For a more traditional "baked beans" dish, substitute dried lima beans for the soybeans. Proceed as above.

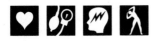

Red Rice

Rice takes on a different hue prepared this Middle Eastern way.

Makes four servings
1 small onion, finely chopped
1 tablespoon (15 ml) soy oil
2 cloves garlic, crushed
1 cup (250 ml) brown rice
1 cup (250 ml) stewed
    tomatoes or tomato
    puree
1½ cups (375 ml) *Chicken
    Stock* or *Vegetable
    Stock*

Place the onion in a large saucepan with the oil and stir over medium heat until the onion is translucent. Add the garlic and the rice, and stir 1 or 2 minutes over the heat. Add the remaining ingredients and bring to a boil. Reduce the heat and simmer until the rice is tender and the liquid has been absorbed, about 25 to 35 minutes.

Scalloped Eggplant

Makes four servings
1 medium eggplant
2 tablespoons (30 ml) chopped
    parsley
1 small onion, finely chopped
1 cup (250 ml) soft whole grain
    bread crumbs
½ teaspoon (2 ml) oregano,
    crumbled
½ teaspoon (2 ml) basil,
    crumbled
¼ teaspoon (1 ml) kelp powder
½ cup (125 ml) buttermilk

Dice eggplant and simmer until tender in boiling water to cover in a medium saucepan. Drain well in a colander and sprinkle with parsley. In a small skillet, steam-stir onion in a small amount of water until translucent. Do not brown. In a mixing bowl, combine onion with bread crumbs, herbs and kelp.

Preheat oven to 350° F. (175° C.). Lightly oil a baking dish and place a layer of eggplant in the bottom. Top with a layer of crumb mixture. Repeat until eggplant and crumbs are used up, ending with a topping of crumbs. Pour buttermilk over casserole and bake, uncovered, for 30 minutes.

Note: To prevent discoloration, eggplant should be cooked in glass, enamel, pottery or stainless steel.

Fiesta Corn

Makes four servings
¼ cup (60 ml) chopped
   green peppers
½ small onion, chopped
½ stalk celery, chopped
1½–2 cups (375–500 ml) fresh
   or frozen corn
dash cayenne pepper

Steam-stir green peppers, onion and celery in a little water until onion is translucent. Add corn and stir a few minutes more, until corn is tender. Add a dash of cayenne. Serve hot.

Variation: For *Corn Creole,* add one cup (250 ml) drained, canned, or peeled and seeded fresh garden tomatoes to sauteed onion, celery and peppers. Simmer two or three minutes before adding corn. Continue to simmer until corn is cooked through.

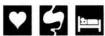

Creamy Succotash

Makes four servings
½ onion, finely chopped
1 teaspoon (5 ml) corn oil
1 cup (250 ml) fresh or frozen
   corn
1 cup (250 ml) fresh or frozen
   lima beans
½ teaspoon (2 ml) brewer's
   yeast
2–3 tablespoons (30–45 ml)
   yogurt

In a medium saucepan, saute onion in the oil until translucent. Add the corn and lima beans and stir occasionally until tender. Add a few spoonfuls of water, if necessary, to prevent scorching. When tender, sprinkle with brewer's yeast, remove from heat, and add enough yogurt to make a creamy sauce. Serve hot.

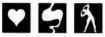

Sweet and Sour Cabbage

Makes two servings
3 cups (150 ml) shredded red
   cabbage
1 onion, chopped
2 tablespoons (30 ml) cider
   vinegar
1 unpeeled tart apple, chopped
1 bay leaf
1 teaspoon (5 ml) honey
1 teaspoon (5 ml) caraway seeds
   (optional)

Prepare cabbage and set aside. In a large skillet, steam-stir onion over medium heat with just a few drops of water to prevent scorching. When onion is soft, add vinegar, apple, bay leaf, cabbage, honey and caraway seeds, if desired. Cover and cook over medium heat, stirring occasionally, for 15 to 20 minutes, until cabbage is just tender. Add a few drops of water, if necessary, to prevent sticking. Remove bay leaf before serving.

Steam-Stirred Red Onions

Makes four servings
2 large red onions
1 teaspoon (5 ml) tamari
½ teaspoon (2 ml) medium
    unsulfured molasses

Peel the onions and cut in half lengthwise. Cut into thin slices. Place the onions in a heavy-bottom pan over medium heat, and add a few spoonfuls of water. Stir in tamari and molasses.

Steam and stir onions, covering occasionally, until tender. Serve as is, as a side dish, or add thin slices of calf liver and steam just until the liver is pink and the juices run clear.

Baked Onions in Their Jackets

Makes two servings
2 large yellow onions

A delicious and easy dish which is a nice addition to a complete oven-baked meal—with baked potatoes and a casserole, for example.

Bake onions in their skins in a preheated 350° F. (175° C.) oven 30 to 40 minutes, until tender. Let each person cut open the juicy onion on his or her own plate.

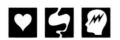

Baked Stuffed Onions

Makes four servings
4 medium Spanish onions
½ cup (125 ml) cooked brown
    rice
½ cup (125 ml) cooked lentils
¼ cup (60 ml) chopped celery
½ cup (125 ml) *Good Gravy*
1 tablespoon (15 ml) minced
    fresh parsley
1 tablespoon (15 ml) walnuts,
    chopped
1 teaspoon (5 ml) tarragon
½ teaspoon (2 ml) coriander

Bake onions in their skins in a preheated 350° F. (175° C.) oven for 25 to 30 minutes. Cut off tops, and scoop out most of the insides, leaving two or three layers of onion and skin. Take a thin slice off the bottom (root end) of the onion, being careful not to cut into the cavity, so that the onion will stand upright.

Chop the centers of the onions and combine with the remaining ingredients in a medium bowl. Stuff onion shells, and place in the oven for an additional 25 to 30 minutes, until onions are tender.

Mushroom Stuffing

Makes three cups (750 ml)
1 teaspoon (5 ml) corn oil
1 small onion, chopped
3½ cups (875 ml) chopped
   mushrooms (about ¾
   pound [340 g])
2 teaspoons (10 ml) tamari
1 cup (250 ml) soft whole
   grain bread crumbs
¼ cup (60 ml) chopped fresh
   parsley
¼ cup (60 ml) wheat germ
1 teaspoon (5 ml) basil
¼ teaspoon (1 ml) marjoram
¼ teaspoon (1 ml) thyme
1 teaspoon (5 ml) brewer's
   yeast
dash freshly grated nutmeg

Delicious with boned chicken breasts or fish fillets.

Heat oil in a heavy skillet, and add the onion and mushrooms. Saute until the mushrooms have released their liquid and the excess liquid has evaporated, about 10 to 15 minutes. Add the tamari, bread crumbs, parsley, wheat germ, herbs, brewer's yeast and nutmeg. Toss together and remove from heat.

Onion-Apple Stuffing

Makes four servings
4 cups (1 l) water
2 cups (500 ml) chopped
   onions
1 cup (250 ml) dry whole grain
   bread crumbs
1 cup (250 ml) soft whole grain
   bread cubes, crumbled
1 unpeeled tart apple, chopped
1 egg, beaten
2 teaspoons (10 ml) tamari
1 teaspoon (5 ml) basil
¼ teaspoon (1 ml) thyme

Bring water to a boil. Place onions in boiling water and simmer 10 minutes. Drain, saving water for later use.

Mix the cooked onions with the bread crumbs and crumbled fresh bread, apple, egg and seasonings.

Recipe can be used for stuffing turkey breast or chicken breasts before roasting, or bake separately. Place in an 8 × 8-inch (20 × 20-cm) casserole, cover with aluminum foil and bake in a preheated 350° F. (175° C.) oven about 45 minutes, until apples are tender.

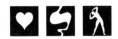

Makes four servings
3 cups (750 ml) cubed turnips
2 cups (500 ml) peeled,
    cubed celery root
    (celeriac)
2 teaspoons (10 ml) *Baked Garlic*
2–4 tablespoons (30–60 ml)
    yogurt, warmed

Autumn Vegetable Puree

This vegetable dish is more work than most, but is tasty and unusual.

Boil turnips and celery root until quite tender. Rub cooked vegetables and garlic through a sieve or use a food mill. Stir in warmed yogurt to taste. Serve hot.

MISCELLANEOUS

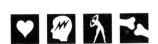

Makes 1½ cups (375 ml)
¾ cup (175 ml) tofu
2 tablespoons (30 ml) mild
    vinegar
1 teaspoon (5 ml) Dijon-style
    mustard
½ teaspoon (2 ml) tamari
1 tablespoon (15 ml) sunflower
    oil

Tofu Mayonnaise

You'll be astonished at how much like real mayo this tastes. It may even taste better. Yet it has 90 percent less fat and calories and zero cholesterol!

Combine first four ingredients in a blender and begin blending at lowest speed. When tofu is creamy, blend on higher speed and slowly pour oil into the mixture. Continue blending until thoroughly combined.

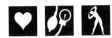

Makes 2½ cups (625 ml)
1 cup (250 ml) chopped onions
4 cloves garlic, minced
1 tablespoon (15 ml) corn oil
2 cups (500 ml) Italian plum
    tomatoes with juice

Thick Onion-Tomato Sauce

Delicious on pizza, over lasagna or polenta, or with the addition of cooked beans or lentils, as a pasta sauce.

Saute onion and garlic in oil in a skillet until the onion begins to become transparent. Chop tomatoes and add with the juice to the onion mixture. Simmer for 30 minutes.

Raw Marinated Mushrooms

Makes five cups (1.25 l)

5 cups (1.25 l) mushrooms
(about 1 pound [450 g])
6 tablespoons (90 ml) sunflower
oil
3 tablespoons (45 ml) lemon
juice
1 tablespoon (15 ml) tomato
paste
1 clove garlic, sliced
1 teaspoon (5 ml) thyme,
crushed

Use these as a garnish on salads.

Brush dirt from mushrooms. (A fingernail brush kept in the kitchen for such chores is handy.) Cut off stems, saving these for another use. Leave small mushroom caps whole; cut medium mushrooms in half, large mushrooms in quarters.

Combine oil, lemon juice, tomato paste, garlic and thyme in a large bowl. Toss with mushrooms until they are well coated. Chill for one to two hours before serving.

Basic Tomato Sauce

Makes one quart (1 l)

1 large onion, chopped
2 green or sweet red peppers,
chopped
1 cup (250 ml) sliced
mushrooms
2 cloves garlic, crushed
4 cups (1 l) tomato juice
2 teaspoons (10 ml) oregano
1 teaspoon (5 ml) basil
½ teaspoon (2 ml) thyme

Serve over whole wheat pasta, with vegetables or chicken.

Steam-stir vegetables and garlic in a large pan in a few spoonfuls of water, stirring frequently. When vegetables are tender, add the tomato juice and herbs. Bring to a boil, then cover, reduce heat and simmer for 30 to 45 minutes.

Hot Taco Sauce

Makes 3 ½ cups (875 ml)

1½ cups (375 ml) light green
hot peppers, finely
chopped
1 onion, finely chopped
2 cups (500 ml) chopped
tomatoes with juice

Serve with tortillas, tacos, or other Mexican-style favorites.

Place hot peppers and onion in a skillet and steam-stir with a few drops of water for 4 to 5 minutes. Add tomatoes with their juice to the peppers and onion. Cook over medium heat about 5 to 10 minutes. The longer the peppers are cooked, the milder in taste they will be; however, the mixture will also lose flavor, so it should not be cooked too long.

Stockpot Tomato Sauce

Makes two quarts (2 l)
2 onions, chopped
1 green pepper, finely
    chopped
6 cloves garlic, minced
1 tablespoon (15 ml) oil
1–2 stalks celery with leaves,
    finely chopped
1 beet, shredded
1 zucchini, shredded
3 carrots, shredded
5–6 scallions, chopped
1 cup (250 ml) chopped fresh
    parsley
6 cups (1.5 l) water
1¼ cups (300 ml) tomato paste
½ cup (125 ml) fresh basil or
    2 tablespoons (30 ml)
    dried basil
other garden herbs to taste
1 tablespoon (15 ml) paprika
3 bay leaves
1½ tablespoons (25 ml) tamari
2 tablespoons (30 ml)
    blackstrap molasses
1 teaspoon (5 ml) *Tarragon
    Vinegar* or red wine
    vinegar

In a stockpot or kettle, saute onions, pepper and garlic in the oil until onions are transparent, adding a little water if necessary to prevent scorching. Combine remaining ingredients and simmer for 30 to 45 minutes. Remove bay leaves. To make a smoother sauce, puree some of the sauce in a blender, and return to pot.

Some can be frozen for later use.

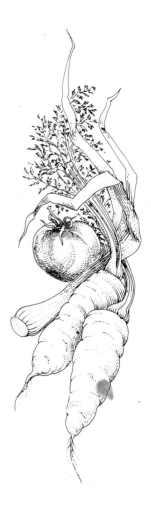

Black Magic Sauce

Makes one cup (250 ml)
10 tablespoons (150 ml) water (a little more than ½ cup)
2 tablespoons (30 ml) lemon juice
2 tablespoons (30 ml) orange juice
2 teaspoons (10 ml) tamari
1 teaspoon (5 ml) blackstrap molasses
1 teaspoon (5 ml) vinegar
4 cloves garlic, crushed
½ teaspoon (2 ml) bay leaves, cracked
¼ teaspoon (1 ml) dillweed
¼ teaspoon (1 ml) oregano

A slightly fruity, slightly savory sauce we often use in place of oil when making steam-stir dishes in a skillet or wok.

Mix all ingredients together and use as stock in preparing steam-stir dishes. Usually, about ¼ cup (60 ml) of the mixture is used per serving.

Tamari, which is similar to soy sauce, contains about 265 milligrams of sodium per teaspoon (5 ml). So each person would be getting about 135 milligrams of sodium. Ordinarily, *Black Magic Sauce* is used no more than a few times a week. However, it should not be used by anyone on a *salt-free* diet prescribed by a physician.

Feel free to experiment with the ingredients in *Black Magic Sauce.* The version given has a pleasantly sweet, slightly orangy flavor. You may want to add more orange juice, cut it out altogether, reduce the amount of tamari or add other herbs, such as coriander.

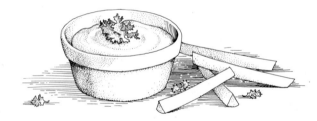

Soybean Tahini Dip

Makes 1¾ cups (425 ml)
1 cup (250 ml) cooked soybeans
¼ cup (60 ml) sesame tahini
2 tablespoons (30 ml) sesame seeds
½ cup (125 ml) lemon juice
3 tablespoons (45 ml) water
6 cloves garlic
2 teaspoons (10 ml) tamari
paprika
parsley sprigs

Like its Middle Eastern counterpart, Hummus Tahini, Soybean Tahini Dip *is a popular party dip with* Pita Bread *or a successful sandwich spread for the lunch set.*

Place the ingredients, except paprika and parsley, in a blender and process on low speed until smooth. Chill. Serve with *Pita Bread.*

Variation: For sandwiches, spread some *Soybean Tahini Dip* inside halved pitas. Fill "pocket" with chopped tomatoes, sprouts, lettuce and chopped scallions.

Hummus Tahini

Makes 2 ½ cups (625 ml)
2 cups (500 ml) cooked
    chick-peas
1 clove garlic
⅓ cup (80 ml) lemon juice
¼ cup (60 ml) sesame tahini

We love hummus as a dip for raw vegetables.

Place the chick-peas with the remaining ingredients in a blender. Process on low speed until smooth, stopping the blender when necessary to scrape down the sides of the container with a spatula. Serve as a dip with whole wheat *Pita Bread,* or raw vegetables.

White Lightning Cheese Dip

Makes one cup (250 ml)
¾ cup (175 ml) cottage cheese
2 teaspoons (10 ml) fresh
    parsley
¼ cup (60 ml) yogurt
2 cloves garlic
1 teaspoon (5 ml) sesame tahini

For a milder version, reduce garlic to one clove. For a hotter version, increase garlic to three cloves and serve with a "chaser" of ice water.

Place ingredients in a blender and process on low speed until smooth. Chill before serving to blend flavors. Serve with raw vegetables such as cauliflower florets, carrot sticks, celery, Jerusalem artichoke slices, cucumbers, green beans or zucchini sticks. Or, serve at room temperature as a garnish for cooked broccoli or brown rice.

Eggplant Dip

Makes 1 ½ cups (375 ml)
1 large eggplant
½ cup (125 ml) yogurt
1 clove garlic
1 teaspoon (5 ml) tamari
1 tablespoon (15 ml) soy oil
    dash cayenne pepper
1 tablespoon (15 ml) fresh
    parsley

Traditionally, the eggplant can be charred by thrusting it through with a sword, and holding it over an open campfire. If you don't want to dirty the sword, place eggplant under a broiler or in a 450° F. (230° C.) oven until the skin of the eggplant is charred and the eggplant is very soft. This will take 30 to 45 minutes.

Place eggplant in a glass or ceramic bowl and remove pulp from the skin with a wooden spoon. Place cooked eggplant pulp in a couple of layers of cheesecloth or linen kitchen towel and squeeze liquid out, until eggplant is dry. Place eggplant with remaining ingredients in blender and process on medium speed until thoroughly combined. Chill and serve with *Pita Bread.*

Baked Garlic

2 heads garlic (whole garlics,
with about 16 cloves
each)

Baking tames the pungent taste of garlic.

Place the garlic heads in a baking ramekin or ovenproof custard cup, and place in a 350° F. (175° C.) oven. Remove from oven in 30 to 45 minutes, when the garlic is soft.

Squeeze each clove of garlic toward its root end and press out the softened garlic clove. *Baked Garlic* can be used as a spread or stirred into soups, stews or sauces where a hint of garlic is desired without pungency.

Herbed Garlic Spread

Makes ¼ cup (60 ml)
2 tablespoons (30 ml) *Baked
Garlic*
2 tablespoons (30 ml) yogurt
1 teaspoon (5 ml) minced fresh
parsley
¼ teaspoon (1 ml) tamari
¼ teaspoon (1 ml) marjoram
⅛ teaspoon (0.5 ml) thyme
⅛ teaspoon (0.5 ml) basil

This spread can be served on bagels, whole wheat crackers or sandwiches.

Combine ingredients with a wooden spoon in a small bowl until blended.

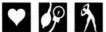

Garlic Broth

Makes five cups (1.25 l)
1 head garlic (whole garlic with
about 16 cloves)
6 cups (1.5 l) water
1 onion
2 whole cloves
1 tablespoon (15 ml) fresh
parsley
½ bay leaf
1 carrot, sliced

A versatile and surprisingly mild-tasting way to eat more garlic.

Peel garlic cloves. Cut garlic cloves in half and place in the water in a large saucepan. Add the onion, which has been stuck with the whole cloves, and remaining ingredients. Bring to a boil and simmer for 30 to 45 minutes. Strain, crushing garlic cloves through a sieve to release flavor.

Through long simmering, the pungent qualities of the garlic give way to a subtleness that will help flavor many soups and sauces. As it is handy to have broth around for many cooking purposes, the broth can be doubled and most of it frozen for future use. Divide among small containers so that broth can be defrosted quickly and easily.

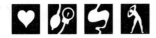

One-Minute Cinnamon Applesauce

Makes 1½ cups (375 ml)
2 medium unpeeled tart apples,
    coarsely chopped
cinnamon

The name says it all: quick, tasty and no cooking.

Place apples in a blender with a little cinnamon, to taste, and process on low speed until rather smooth. Stop blender and scrape down the sides of the container as you go.

Note: For a thinner applesauce, add ¼ to ½ cup (60 to 125 ml) of apple cider to the apples before processing.

Strawberry Applesauce

Makes two cups (500 ml)
1 cup (250 ml) strawberries
2 unpeeled apples, chopped

Try this delicious variation for pancakes or slathered on whole grain bread or muffins.

Blend together on low speed until smooth. It's that simple, and surprisingly delicious. Also saves using syrup and butter (practically pure sugar and fat).

Cinnamon-Apple Snack

Makes one serving
1 tablespoon (15 ml) lemon
    juice
1 unpeeled tart apple, sliced
dash cinnamon

How to make a good snack last twice as long.

Squeeze fresh lemon juice over the apple slices and dust with a bit of cinnamon. That's all there is to it! The lemon juice brings out the natural sweetness of the apple.

Spiced Pear Spread with Pineapple

Makes one cup (250 ml)
2 medium pears, chopped
½ cup (125 ml) chopped fresh
   pineapple
¼ cup (60 ml) pitted dates
¼ teaspoon (1 ml) cinnamon
⅛ teaspoon (0.5 ml) ginger
   dash cloves

Substitute this spread for butter or sugar-laden jams. Incredibly delicious on whole grain toast!

Combine ingredients in a blender and process on low speed until smooth. Stop blender and scrape down the sides of the container as necessary.

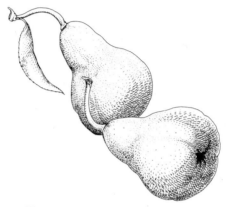

Vanilla Extract

Makes ¼ cup (60 ml)
1 vanilla bean
¼ cup (60 ml) boiling water
1 tablespoon (15 ml) honey
1 tablespoon (15 ml) sunflower
   or soy oil
1 teaspoon (5 ml) liquid lecithin

A familiar, natural flavoring, without the alcohol of commercial varieties.

Cut the vanilla bean into small pieces and place in a small bowl. Pour the boiling water over the bean pieces, cover, and allow the mixture to steep overnight. Place the mixture in a blender and process on medium speed until bean pieces are pulverized. Strain the mixture through cheesecloth, then return the liquid to the blender.

Add the honey, oil and lecithin and blend on medium speed until thoroughly combined. Pour the extract into a small bottle, cap tightly and store in the refrigerator. Shake well before using. Measure the same amount as for any commercial vanilla extract.

DESSERT

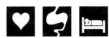

Banana Pound Cake

Makes one loaf
1 cup (250 ml) whole wheat
    flour
1½ cups (375 ml) barley flour
1½ teaspoons (7 ml) *Baking
    Powder*
½ teaspoon (2 ml) baking soda
¼ teaspoon (1 ml) cinnamon
¼ cup (60 ml) honey
¼ cup (60 ml) corn oil
1 teaspoon (5 ml) *Vanilla
    Extract*
¾ cup (175 ml) buttermilk
2 large very ripe bananas
2 eggs, beaten

In a large mixing bowl, combine the dry ingredients. Place the honey, oil, vanilla, buttermilk and bananas in a blender and process on medium speed until smooth. (Do not blend eggs.) Add, along with the beaten eggs, to the dry ingredients. Stir lightly until combined.

Place batter in a lightly oiled 8½ × 4½-inch (22 × 11-cm) baking pan, and bake in a preheated 350° F. (175° C.) oven about one hour, until a cake tester comes out clean.

Try serving with a topping of fresh fruit.

Chapter 2

Let Your Blood Pressure Go Down

Looking at all the evidence together, one interesting fact about blood pressure emerges: Almost every dietary habit that is bad for any major system in our body is *also* bad for blood pressure. For instance:

•Having more than three drinks a day, which is harmful to the liver, *also* tends to elevate blood pressure.

•Being overweight, which predisposes toward diabetes and heart disease, *also* tends to elevate blood pressure.

•Eating excessive cholesterol, which can cause clogged arteries, *also* tends to elevate blood pressure.

•Eating too much fat, which hampers the circulation of the blood, *also* tends to elevate blood pressure.

In addition to the above, all of which are fairly well established, there is good evidence to suggest that:

•Eating meat and other animal products, which is believed to predispose toward heart disease and possibly cancer, *also* tends to elevate blood pressure.

•In laboratory animals, it's been shown that eating sugar, which stresses our blood sugar control mechanisms, *also* tends to make the blood pressure-raising tendency of fat even more pronounced.

•High residues of insecticides, which pollute our entire bodies, are *also* associated with higher blood pressures.

In a sense, then, we can say that high blood pressure can arise from the very same pattern of unwise eating (and habits like smoking) that is also associated with heart disease, diabetes, and other chronic illnesses.

There is one very important exception to that observation. *Salt.* Eating the amount of salt typically consumed in Western nations is not believed to be particularly harmful to most people except to the extent that it encourages high blood pressure (and resultant heart disease or stroke). And while the other dietary factors we mentioned may be very important, most scientists who have investigated the matter agree that excessive salt consumption is the number one dietary culprit when it comes to hypertension. If that is true, it means the salt that is so much a part of our dietary fabric is in fact a major cause of stroke, kidney disease and cardiac complications. Salt may well be to stroke what cholesterol is to heart attack. In fact, the two often do their evil work hand in hand. The hardening of the arteries involved in atherosclerosis can *create* the potential for high blood pressure, which salt then makes worse. It's also quite likely that high blood pressure can *aggravate* the effect of high cholesterol, encouraging the development of atherosclerosis and hardening of the arteries.

Yet, we all know people who eat a lot of salt, a lot of fat, and have other poor dietary habits and yet still have normal blood pressure. Others may have relatively good diets, or at least not as bad as the usual, and be diagnosed as hypertensive. So where does diet come in? What's more, if you did a study of 100 of your neighbors and found out how much salt they ate, and then took their blood pressure, you might not find any meaningful relationship between one and the other. Further, how can we explain the fact that while black people do not apparently consume any more salt than white Americans, they suffer from high blood pressure to a much greater extent?

For years, many doctors assumed that such facts meant the "salt theory" of hypertension had to be taken with a large grain of you-know-what. But now, we know better.

A QUESTION OF INDIVIDUAL VULNERABILITY

Yes, heredity is important, but only rarely does heredity *itself* produce high blood pressure. What it does is pass along either an inborn resistance to high blood pressure or an inbred vulnerability. When a person is resistant to high blood pressure, he can get away with a lot of bad eating, at least for most of his life. Often, however, the resistance seems to break down with advancing age, and blood pressure begins to climb. People who are *vulnerable* to salt-induced high blood pressure because of their heredity need only commit a few nutritional sins to find themselves in trouble. The more sins, the more trouble. However—and this is the really important point—*it's believed that if the vast majority of people who have an inherited vulnerability to high blood pressure ate more wisely, they would suffer no ill consequences from their vulnerability.* A pile of dry leaves may be extremely flammable, but only in the very rare instance of spontaneous combustion would it burst into flames unless someone put a match to the pile. With blood pressure, it's the same story. Salt is the match.

Here's why scientists believe that:

People who live on the islands of the South Pacific are closely related to each other genetically, but as you go from island to island and culture to culture, average blood pressures vary considerably. Extensive studies have shown that after all other possible factors are considered, the only difference between groups having different blood pressures is their salt consumption. High salt means high blood pressure. These observations have been repeated all over the world by various researchers who have pinpointed tribes living in close physical proximity, who are similar in all respects except that one tribe eats salt and the other doesn't. In tribes eating no salt, there is usually no high blood pressure whatsoever. In tribes that do eat salt, there *is* hypertension, and it usually becomes worse with advancing age, just as it does in the United States. A number of small societies have been found which do not use salt in cooking, but occasionally eat canned meat or fish that has been salted. Typically these people show a *moderate* tendency toward high blood pressure (*Ecology of Food and Nutrition,* vol. 2, 1973).

But why won't that kind of comparison work if you try it on your neighbors? The answer is simple: Once you consume more than a minimal amount of salt—probably in the vicinity of about half a teaspoon a day—blood pressure will begin to rise if the vulnerability is there. The average salt intake in the United States is estimated at about two teaspoons a day, and very few people eat less than one teaspoon a day. That probably sounds like a lot, but in fact, most of the salt in our diet, as you shall soon see, is hidden—put into almost every commercially sold food by processors. A person who never uses his saltshaker but who eats the usual supermarket variety of foods is likely to be well over the minimum amount of salt intake necessary to bring on hypertension. Once that minimum amount is reached, as we said, it doesn't matter that much if your salt intake from all sources is two teaspoons, three teaspoons or even four teaspoons. Not until the very high level of five teaspoons is reached—which it is in some areas of Japan—does more salt seem to make matters worse. At that level, the incidence of high blood pressure may reach 30 to 40 percent, which is extremely high, and stroke becomes the leading cause of death.

What about the question of why black people suffer more from hypertension than whites? If it isn't the amount of salt they eat, then what? That, too, could be a case of vulnerability—extreme vulnerability. Some scientists now believe that the systems of black people retain more salt than white people because of "selection" over a period of thousands of years. According to that theory, the early people of Africa had access to very little dietary salt, but needed some because of the extremely hot climate which encouraged perspiration. Those individuals whose bodies were better able to *conserve* salt had a definite survival advantage. So as the years passed, this trait of salt conservation became more and more common. That process may have been emphasized in women, who have a special need for salt during pregnancy and lactation. As a result, black women may have more of a tendency to retain sodium than black men. The development of these traits represents a very creative adaptation to a salt-poor environment. However, when that trait is transplanted to a country where the taste for salt may be freely satisfied, it turns against the people it had helped survive through the ages, and begins killing them. If this theory is correct, it would also explain why black women are even more susceptible to hypertension than black men.

Whether or not any particular theory is correct, the fact is that some people are salt-sensitive, showing elevation of blood pressure when their salt consumption reaches a mere fraction of what is ordinarily consumed in most modern societies. It is also a fact that "going a little easier on salt" accomplishes little in reducing blood pressure because the threshold of sensitivity is so low. On the positive side, if total salt consumption stays below about 800 to 1,000 milligrams a day, studies show that a significant drop of blood pressure in many hypertensives will occur quite rapidly. That is also the level of sodium consumption that seems to be the border line between populations who have zero or very little hypertension and those others who are well on their way to major problems.

WHAT INDIVIDUALS CAN DO FOR PROTECTION

At this point, you are probably asking yourself two questions. First, how do I know if *I* am a salt-sensitive person? In the most technical sense, you would have to undergo a recently devised test to study your metabolism, which at present is being used by only a very small number of physicians. But in a practical sense, most authorities agree that if your family has a history of high blood pressure, or if you have high blood pressure yourself, even if it is only moderately elevated, you would be very wise indeed to put yourself on a low-sodium diet. There are few, if any, single dietary changes that are likely to have as beneficial effect on your future well-being.

The second question is, just how *little* salt must I eat to pay the premium on my high blood pressure insurance policy?

Before we answer that directly, let's define our terms. You may have noticed that at first we were referring to salt, and then sodium. Let's clear up that matter right now. Table salt is composed almost entirely of sodium chloride. The chloride in that compound is no problem. What your body is sensitive to is the sodium. Some 39 percent of sodium chloride consists of sodium, a figure that is frequently rounded off to 40 percent. So 1,000 milligrams (1 gram) of sodium chloride, or table salt, contains about 400 milligrams of sodium. One level teaspoon of sodium chloride weighs about 5,500 milligrams, which means that 40 percent of that amount, or 2,200 milligrams, would be pure sodium. Actually, the true amount is a little bit less than that, 2,132 milligrams, because of the impurities in the table salt and because we have rounded off the percent of the sodium.

But sodium doesn't only occur in sodium chloride. Modest amounts are found naturally in many foods, although most vegetables and grains have very small amounts. If you were to eat a caveman-type diet, and your water supply wasn't contaminated with sodium (as are many water supplies including those that are "softened"), you would probably be taking in somewhere in the vicinity of 200 to 500 milligrams of sodium a day—and you would probably be much closer to the first amount than the second. If you are trying to stay below about 800 milligrams a day, that means, for all practical purposes, that you must avoid not only the saltshaker, but about 95 percent of all processed foods that contain added sodium. And those few sodium-added foods you *do* eat, you must eat in very limited quantities.

That is exactly our plan in this book. We use no salt as such, and the majority of recipes have no added sodium in any form whatsoever. A few recipes call for small amounts of cheese, Swiss or Jarlsburg, usually no more than one ounce, which contains only about 100 milligrams of sodium. The high-salt cheeses like feta and blue are strictly avoided. Sometimes we add a sprinkle or two of grated Parmesan, which is a very condensed cheese, high in salt, but the amounts used are so small that the sodium addition isn't more than 40 milligrams. Some of our recipes also call for tamari sauce, which is similar to soy sauce, and has the same salt content—which is very high. However, we never use more than half a teaspoon of tamari sauce per person so the maximum amount of sodium from this source is only 133 milligrams. And ordinarily, you would only be making a recipe with tamari a few times a week.

The result is that by following the recipes and food plans of this book, your daily sodium intake should remain below about 1,000 to 1,200 milligrams a day. On some days, it could be a few hundred milligrams higher, but more often, it will be in the vicinity of about 800 milligrams a day. It would be easy for us to bring the sodium content even lower, but that could do more harm than good. Any diet that is too severe or impractical is likely to be given up altogether in frustration. Based on available evidence, we believe that an average daily sodium intake of about 1,000 milligrams is sufficiently low to prevent the appearance of hypertension in the great majority of salt-sensitive people. There are a number of relatively primitive societies in the world who eat slightly more than this amount and have an extremely low rate of hypertension. We also feel that when the other dietary principles of this book are followed—very little fat and plentiful potassium, for example—it may not be necessary to be *quite* as strict about sodium as would otherwise be the case.

HOW LOW MUST YOU GO?

If you have already been diagnosed as having high blood pressure, or slightly elevated blood pressure, or if there is a history of high blood pressure or stroke in your family, you might well want to focus largely on recipes coded with the symbol indicating suitability for high blood pressure. Those recipes are very low in sodium indeed, and may offer other benefits as well, such as fiber and potassium. Stricter control of sodium intake is probably more necessary for those who already have high blood pressure than for those who want to prevent it. Exactly *how* strict you have to be is a subject of great debate, some of which is actually quite irrational. It seems that some doctors who believe that diuretic drugs are the one and only answer to high blood pressure wish to make it appear that only by restricting your diet to an incredibly small amount of sodium can you achieve any real benefits. But in fact, the evidence shows that significant benefits can be obtained in many if not all cases by limiting sodium intake to about 1,000 milligrams a day.

A study published by doctors from the Institute of Internal Medicine at the University of Bologna in Italy in 1976 showed that a diet containing about 1,175 milligrams of sodium a day reduced both systolic and diastolic blood pressure by about 10 to 12 points. That was sufficient to return the blood pressure value to normal in the majority of patients who had "mild" hypertension. Another group of patients with the same degree of hypertension (averaging about 162/100) were given diuretic drugs and their blood pressure did not fall any lower than the diet group. We might add that while diuretic drugs sometimes have unpleasant side effects (sometimes even raising cholesterol levels to a significant degree), restricting salt has no known side effect except that it often produces a slight weight loss because of less water retention.

However, note that this study was done on people with "mild" high blood pressure, not people with severe hypertension. If you are currently under treatment for hypertension, or if your doctor has given you dietary instructions, by all means discuss any proposed modifications with him or her. In some severe cases, your doctor may want you not only to strictly avoid all added sodium, but to use special low-sodium milk and limit your consumption of certain vegetables that are relatively high in natural sodium (artichokes, beet greens, beets, carrots, celery, dandelion greens, kale, mustard greens, spinach, Swiss chard and turnips). If that is the case, you'll certainly also want to avoid those recipes that call for tamari or cheese, even though they are used in very small amounts.

Perhaps this is an appropriate moment to reassure you that a diet using no table salt and scarcely any high-sodium foods does not have to be tasteless or dull. Right now, your taste buds are probably addicted to salt. They expect it in nearly everything. Foods simply taste funny without it. *That sensation of strange blandness is perfectly normal —and strictly temporary.* When you walk out of a movie theater into the bright sunlight, your eyes hurt, but you don't let that keep you in the dark for the rest of your life. You adapt to the light. And you will adapt to living without added salt. Or more accurately, you will adapt to the taste of real honest-to-goodness food because that's what you begin to taste about a week or two after you give up salt. We've seen that happen over and over again with people who begin following our way of eating. The sensations of eating fresh, natural, unsalted foods are so varied and intense that you would have no reason to go back to using salt even if it weren't dangerous to your health. But of course, it is. There is very little question but that many of the people who are killed or incapacitated by strokes and other complications of high blood pressure might never have gotten into trouble if they had strictly limited their salt intake before things reached the crisis stage. That knowledge, we think, should make it much easier for you to wean yourself away from salt.

The following portfolio of illustrations and tables is designed to give you new insight into why our customary diet is so loaded with salt, and where it's found.

Sodium in Natural vs. Processed Vegetables
(All values for ½ cup)

Fresh peas	Frozen peas	Canned peas	Pea soup
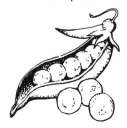	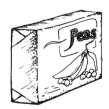	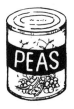	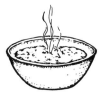
2 milligrams	92 milligrams	200 milligrams	450 milligrams

Fresh mushrooms	Cream of mushroom soup	Boiled potato	Hashed brown potatoes
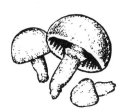	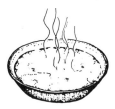	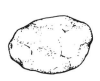	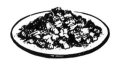
6 milligrams	477 milligrams	3 milligrams	223 milligrams

NOTE: 2,132 milligrams sodium = 1 teaspoon table salt.

Sodium in Natural vs. Processed Grains
(Values for ½ cup unless otherwise noted)

Brown rice (cooked without salt)	White rice (prepared per package instructions)	Spanish rice	Crisp rice breakfast cereal

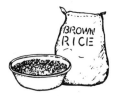 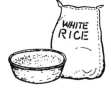 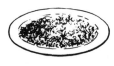 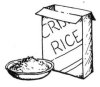

3 milligrams	383 milligrams	387 milligrams	192 milligrams

Fresh corn	Canned corn	Corn bread (1 serving)	Corn flakes

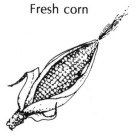 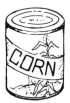 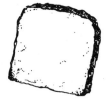 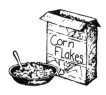

Barely a trace	302 milligrams	490 milligrams	126 milligrams

Rolled wheat (cooked without salt)	Bread (store-bought) (1 slice)	Saltines (4)	Waffles (1)

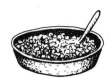 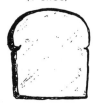 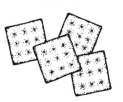 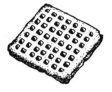

1 milligram	142 milligrams	123 milligrams	356 milligrams

NOTE: *2,132 milligrams sodium = 1 teaspoon table salt.*

Sodium in Natural vs. Processed Meats
(All values for ¼ pound as cooked)

Ground beef

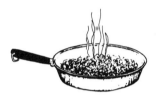

76 milligrams

Hamburger patty
(commercial type)

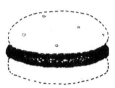

950 milligrams

Corned beef

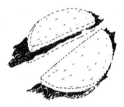

1,069 milligrams

Pork loin

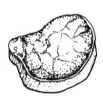

68 milligrams

Hot dogs (2)

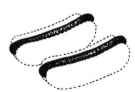

1,254 milligrams

Spiced ham

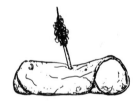

1,399 milligrams

NOTE: *2,132 milligrams sodium = 1 teaspoon table salt.*

Sodium Hidden by Shroud of Sugar and Fat

Apple	Apple pie (⅛ of pie)	Cherry pie (McDonald's)

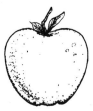
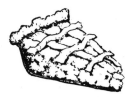
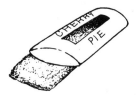

1 milligram	355 milligrams	456 milligrams

Chocolate cake	Gingerbread	Baked custard

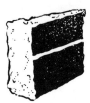
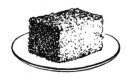
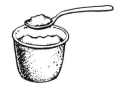

233 milligrams	277 milligrams	209 milligrams

Doughnut (large)	Danish pastry (1)	Chocolate shake (McDonald's)

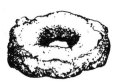
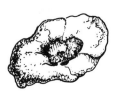
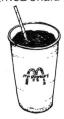

291 milligrams	238 milligrams	329 milligrams

The idea is not that these amounts of sodium are especially large (half a pizza has about 1,900 milligrams) but that these foods are collectively putting substantial sodium into your system without tasting salty.

NOTE: 360 milligrams sodium = ⅙ teaspoon table salt.

Sodium Content of Plant-Source Foods

Food	Portion Size	Milligrams	Food	Portion Size	Milligrams
Almonds	10	trace	Cherries		
Apple	1 medium	1	sweet	½ cup	1.5
Apricots	3	1	Coconut	1 piece	
Artichoke				(2 × 2 × ½ inch)	10
cooked	1 medium	36	Corn	½ cup	trace
Asparagus			Cranberries		
cooked	4 medium spears	1	raw, chopped	½ cup	1
Avocado	1 medium	9	Cucumbers		
Banana	1 medium	1	sliced	½ cup	3
Beans			Dates		
Green snap	½ cup	2.5	pitted	5	0.5
Kidney	½ cup	3	Eggplant		
Lima	½ cup	1	cooked	½ cup	1
Mung sprouts	¼ cup	1.25	Figs	3 medium	3
Beet greens			Filberts	10	trace
cooked	½ cup	55	Grapefruit	½ cup	1
Beets	½ cup	43	Grapes	10	2
Blueberries	½ cup	0.5	Lettuce		
Brazil nuts	3 large	trace	shredded	1 cup	5
Broccoli			Mushrooms		
cooked	1 medium stalk	18	raw	½ cup	5.5
Brussels sprouts	½ cup	8	Oatmeal		
Cabbage			salted	½ cup	262
cooked	½ cup	20	Oatmeal		
Cantaloupe	½	33	unsalted	½ cup	1
Carrot			Oil, vegetable	—	0
raw	1 medium	34	Onions		
Carrots			raw	1 tablespoon	1
cooked	½ cup	24	Orange	1 medium	1
Cashews			Orange juice		
unsalted	½ cup	10	frozen		
Cauliflower			concentrate	¾ cup	2
cooked	½ cup	5.5	Peach	1 medium	1
Celery			Peanuts	10 jumbo	1
raw, chopped	½ cup	75	Pear, Bartlett	1 medium	3

(continued on next page)

Sodium Content of Plant-Source Foods (continued)

Food	Portion Size	Milli-grams	Food	Portion Size	Milli-grams
Peas cooked	½ cup	1	Spinach raw	½ cup	19
Pepper sweet red	1 medium	10	Squash, summer cooked	½ cup	1
Pineapple diced	½ cup	1	Strawberries	½ cup	0.5
Plums	5	1	Sunflower seeds	¼ cup	11
Popcorn unsalted	1 cup	trace	Sweet potato cooked	1 medium	14
Potato baked	1	6	Tomato	1 medium	4
Prunes cooked	½ cup	5.5	Turnips cooked	½ cup	27
Raisins	1 tablespoon	2	Walnuts	1 tablespoon	trace
Rice, brown raw	½ cup	9	Watermelon	1 piece (10-inch diameter × 1 inch thick)	4
Spinach cooked	½ cup	45	Whole wheat flour	½ cup	4

NOTE: Food values, in general, are given throughout the book for the form in which the foods are commonly eaten. Unless otherwise noted, most food values have been adapted from Nutritive Value of American Foods in Common Units, *Agriculture Handbook No. 456, U.S. Department of Agriculture, 1975.*

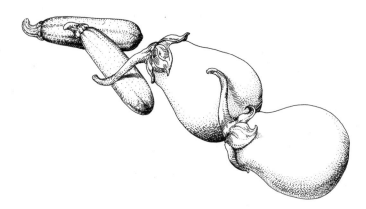

Sodium Content of Dairy Products

Food	Portion Size	Milli-grams	Food	Portion Size	Milli-grams
Butter			Cheese (continued)		
salted	1 pat	49	Provolone	1 ounce	248
Butter			Roquefort	1 ounce	513
unsalted	1 pat	0.5	Swiss	1 ounce	74
Buttermilk	1 cup	319	Swiss		
Cheese			pasteurized	1 ounce	388
American,			Cream		
process			Half-and-half	1 tablespoon	7
pasteurized	1 ounce	406	Heavy	1 tablespoon	6
Blue	1 ounce	396	Light	1 tablespoon	5
Cheddar	1 ounce	176	Ice cream		
Cottage			Hard	1 cup	84
Creamed	4 ounces	457	Soft	1 cup	109
Dry-curd	4 ounces	14	Ice milk	1 cup	89
2% low-fat	4 ounces	459	Milk		
Edam	1 ounce	274	Dry nonfat	¼ cup	161
Gouda	1 ounce	232	Low-fat	1 cup	150
Monterey	1 ounce	152	Skim	1 cup	127
Mozzarella	1 ounce	106	Whole	1 cup	122
Muenster	1 ounce	178	Yogurt		
Parmesan	1 tablespoon	93	Skim-milk	1 cup	115
	1 ounce	528	Whole-milk	1 cup	106

Sodium Content of Animal-Source Foods

Food	Portion Size	Milli-grams	Food	Portion Size	Milli-grams
Bacon	2 medium pc.	153	Lobster	4 ounces	238
Bacon, Canadian	1 thick slice	537	Oysters	4 ounces	83
Bluefish	4 ounces	118	Perch, ocean	4 ounces	174
Chicken	4 ounces	70	Pollock	4 ounces	126
Clams, cherrystone	1 dozen	432	Pork loin chop	4 ounces	68
Eggs	2 medium	108	Rabbit	4 ounces	47
Flounder	4 ounces	269	Round steak	4 ounces	80
Ground beef	4 ounces	76	Salmon	4 ounces	116
Haddock	4 ounces	201	Scallops	4 ounces	300
Halibut	4 ounces	152	Shrimp	4 ounces	211
Ham	4 ounces	64	Sirloin steak	4 ounces	64
Kidney	4 ounces	287	Stew meat	4 ounces	52
Lamb leg	4 ounces	70	Turkey	4 ounces	148
Liver	4 ounces	209	Veal loin	4 ounces	74

Sodium Content of Processed Foods

Food	Portion Size	Milli-grams	Food	Portion Size	Milli-grams
Asparagus, whole spears			Baby food (continued) Vegetables and		
canned	½ cup	285	ham	3½ ounces	360
			Beans		
Baby food			Beans and franks, canned	½ cup	687
Chicken	3½ ounces	263	Lima		
Oatmeal	3½ ounces	437	canned	½ cup	200

Sodium Content of Processed Foods (continued)

Food	Portion Size	Milli-grams	Food	Portion Size	Milli-grams
Beans (continued)			Macaroni and cheese		
White			canned	½ cup	365
canned	½ cup	431	Olives, green		
Beef			canned	5 large	463
Corned	4 ounces	1,069	Pancakes		
Potpie	⅓ of 9-inch pie	596	from mix	3 medium	456
Vegetable stew			Pickle, dill	1 medium	928
canned	½ cup	504	Pork sausage patty	1	259
Bologna	2 slices	338	Potato salad		
Boston cream pie	1 piece	192	with mayonnaise		
Bouillon cube	1 cube	960	and eggs	½ cup	600
Bread			Salad dressing,		
Italian	2 slices	352	commercial		
Rye	2 slices	278	French	1 tablespoon	219
White, soft	2 slices	284	Sardines		
Caviar, sturgeon	1 teaspoon	352	canned	2 ounces	282
Coffee cake	1 piece	465	Sauerkraut		
Corned beef hash,			canned	½ cup	877
with potato			Soup, commercial		
canned	½ cup	594	Asparagus, cream	1 cup	2,009
Crab			Bean with pork	1 cup	2,136
deviled	½ cup	1,040	Chicken gumbo	1 cup	1,940
Devil's food cake			Minestrone	1 cup	2,033
with chocolate			Tomato	1 cup	1,980
icing			Spaghetti with sauce		
frozen	1 4-inch piece	357	and cheese		
Ham, cured			canned	1 cup	955
chopped for			Tuna, canned in oil	4 ounces	907
lunchmeat	2 slices	1,480	Turkey potpie	1 piece	633
Ham, cured			Vegetable juice	6 ounces	366
picnic	4 ounces	909			
Hot dog	1	627			

Sodium in the Pantry

Food	Portion Size	Milli-grams	Food	Portion Size	Milli-grams
Baking powder	1 teaspoon	350	Pickle, dill	1 medium	928
Baking soda	1 teaspoon	1,123	Salad dressing, commercial		
Bouillon	1 cube	960	French	1 tablespoon	219
Ketchup	1 tablespoon	156	Salt	1 teaspoon	2,132
Mustard	1 teaspoon	65	Soy sauce	1 teaspoon	440
Olives, green, pickled	5 large	463	Steak sauce	1 tablespoon	273
			Tamari	1 teaspoon	267

Sodium Content of Beverages

Beverage	Portion Size	Milli-grams	Beverage	Portion Size	Milli-grams
Alcoholic Drinks			Carbonated Drinks		
Beer			Cola	12 ounces	3.5–7.0
Dark	12 ounces	15	Diet drinks	12 ounces	45–60
Light	12 ounces	56	Ginger ale	12 ounces	7–28
Regular	12 ounces	28	Grape	12 ounces	42
			Orange	12 ounces	81
Brandy	2 ounces	1.8	Pepsi	12 ounces	35–49
Gin	2 ounces	0.48	Root Beer	12 ounces	3.5–28
Port	4 ounces	11.2	Seven-Up	12 ounces	3.5
Rum	2 ounces	1.2	Juices		
Sherry	4 ounces	11.2	Apple	8 ounces	2
Whiskey	2 ounces	0.18	Apricot nectar	8 ounces	trace
			Cranberry	8 ounces	3
Wine			Grapefruit	8 ounces	2
Red	4 ounces	11.8	Orange	8 ounces	2
Rosé	4 ounces	8.9	Pineapple	8 ounces	3
White	4 ounces	8.3	Tomato, canned	8 ounces	486

NOTE: *Adapted from* Sources of Sodium in the Diet, *Water Quality Association, Illinois, 1978.*

Sodium Content of Typical Brand-Name Foods

Food	Portion Size		Milli-grams	Food	Portion Size		Milli-grams
Arthur Treacher's				*General Foods* (continued)			
Chips	4	ounces	396	Stove Top Stuffing			
Fish	4	ounces	348	Mix, Chicken	1	serving	550
Banquet Brand Dinners				*Gino's*			
Mexican Style	1	serving	3,114	Cheese Hero	1		739
Veal Parmigiana	1	serving	2,527	Cheeseburger	1		445
General Foods				*Jack In The Box*			
Bird's Eye Frozen				Jumbo Jack			
Vegetables				Hamburger			
Baby lima beans	1	serving	115	with cheese	1		1,665
Broccoli spears	1	serving	10	Super Taco	1	serving	968
Broccoli with				*Kentucky Fried Chicken*			
cheese sauce	1	serving	440	Potato Salad	4	ounces	600
Carrots with brown				Thighs	2		1,284
sugar glaze	1	serving	500	Vanilla Shake	1		283
Italian green beans	1	serving	4	*La Choy*			
Mixed vegetables	1	serving	45	Chicken Chow Mein	1	serving	924
Cafe Vienna	6	-ounce		Meat and Shrimp			
		serving	95	Egg Roll	1		322
Irish Mocha Mint	6	-ounce		Pork Chow Mein	1	serving	1,675
		serving	140	Won Ton Soup	1	serving	2,027
Jello's Instant				*Morton's Frozen*			
Pudding,				*Dinners*			
butterscotch	½	cup	385	Fried Chicken	1	serving	1,865
Log Cabin Pancake				Veal Parmigiana	1	serving	1,450
and Waffle Mix				Western Style	1	serving	1,650
Buttermilk	3	4-inch		*Myer's*			
		pancakes	645	Chicken and Noodles	4	ounces	455
Regular	3	4-inch		Creamed chipped			
		pancakes	475	beef	4	ounces	984
Post 40%				*Pillsbury Company*			
Bran Flakes	1	ounce	315	Blueberry Pancake			
Post Grape-Nut				Mix	3	4-inch	
Flakes	1	ounce	265			pancakes	875
				Devil's Food			
				Cake Mix	1	serving	370

SOURCE: *Information supplied by companies.*

Sodium Content of Bottled Waters

Spring and Mineral Waters	Milligrams (per 8 ounces)	Spring and Mineral Waters	Milligrams (per 8 ounces)
Apollinaris	91	San Pellegrino	1.8
Canada Dry Club Soda	37.8	Saratoga Vichy	123
Deer Park	0.5	Vichy Mineral Water	179
Glen Summit	0.25		
Mountain Valley	0.9		
Perrier	3.0		

NOTE: Adapted from "Elemental Composition of Household Water," Soil and Health Foundation Report, Rodale Press, March, 1979.

POTASSIUM, A POSSIBLE PROTECTOR

Even though added salt in the diet is probably the chief promoter of high blood pressure in people who are genetically vulnerable to it, it isn't the only factor. For many years, there has been a body of knowledge growing in sporadic bursts which suggests that even though sodium certainly predisposes to high blood pressure, the critical factor may be the *ratio,* or relationship, of sodium to another dietary mineral, potassium. In other words, although a high amount of sodium in the diet may be bad, it's even worse when potassium is low. Looking at it another way: it may be good to reduce the amount of sodium in your diet, but it's even better if you *also* increase the amount of potassium.

One common means of studying how much sodium or potassium a person habitually eats is to measure the amount of these minerals excreted in urine. When that was done in two recent studies, it was found that no strong relationship existed between the amount of sodium excreted and blood pressure, but there was a solid relationship between blood pressure and the ratio of excreted sodium to excreted potassium. In both instances, the higher the sodium in *relation to potassium,* the higher the blood pressure tended to be.

Why potassium apparently has this protective effect is not known for certain, although one researcher suggests that potassium may act as a natural diuretic to assist the kidneys in flushing excess salt from the body.

Some very interesting experiments with laboratory animals have been carried out for many years by George R. Meneely, M.D., professor of medicine at the Louisiana State University School of Medicine. One of his most important findings is that while giving extra potassium to laboratory rats on a high-salt diet does have "some protective effect on blood pressure," it isn't nearly as dramatic as the effect on their *longevity.* Consistently, Dr. Meneely found, rats fed a high-salt diet but with extra potassium added

Selected Good Sources of Potassium

Food	Portion Size	Potassium (milligrams)	Calories
Cantaloupe	½	682	82
Blackstrap molasses	1 tablespoon	585	43
Prunes	½ cup	559	206
Orange juice	1 cup	496	112
Soybeans	½ cup	486	117
Broccoli raw	1 medium stalk	481	47
Squash, winter baked	½ cup	473	65
Mango	1	437	152
Watermelon	1 piece (10-inch diameter × 1 inch thick)	426	111
Sweet potato	1	394	185
Potato	½ large	391	73
Beans, lima	½ cup	359	99
Pepper, green raw	1 large	349	36
Sunflower seeds	¼ cup	334	203
Chestnuts	10	331	141
Beans, kidney	½ cup	315	109
Peach	1 large	308	58
Apricots	3	301	55
Tomato	1 medium	300	27

outlived those who received only salt. In one experiment, the animals receiving the extra potassium lived an average of 7 months longer. When you consider that the oldest animal in the two groups only lived to be 34 months old, you can see the true extent of the benefit afforded by potassium. Curiously, *very* curiously, those potassium-supplemented animals even lived several months longer than another group of rats that was given a supposed "ideal" diet which did not contain *any* excess salt.

Few if any researchers in this area claim that the answer to the hypertension problem is simply to eat lots of potassium. Rather, what they say is that sodium should be cut way back while potassium is increased. It's likely, even though it hasn't been proved yet, that this strategy may be more effective than simply cutting back on sodium.

We've already talked about cutting way back on sodium, but how do you go about increasing the amount of potassium in your diet? Luckily, that's easy. There is no need to take potassium supplements or to go out of your way to eat special foods. Nearly all fresh fruits, vegetables and nuts contain generous amounts of potassium, as do potatoes and beans. These foods are used plentifully in hundreds of our recipes. So you'll automatically get large amounts of this beneficial mineral.

A little earlier, we presented a number of tables and illustrations showing the enormous extent to which our sodium intake is increased by food processing. And that, we suggested, could well be the reason why 20 percent of all Americans have high blood pressure, with the percentage rising to 40 percent in the higher age groups. But now take a look at this next table, and see what happens not just to the sodium, but to the *ratio* of potassium to sodium. You'll soon see that the severe distortion of the natural ratios existing between these minerals is one of the hallmarks of food processing.

One of the curious things about potassium is that the thiazide diuretics frequently given to people with high blood pressure cause the body to *lose* potassium. Some doctors advise their patients to make sure to eat an extra banana or orange every day to make up for this loss, but others don't, claiming that the amount of potassium lost is not important. Still others prescribe so-called potassium-sparing diuretics which do not create that problem—if it is a problem. In any event, the kinds of foods and recipes we use in this chapter—and indeed, throughout the book—tend to be quite high in potassium, so if you are trying to get more potassium into your diet because you're taking diuretics, you will do so easily. Potassium values of selected foods are given in the table "Selected Good Sources of Potassium." While many natural foods are high in potassium, these are among the very best sources. Besides being high in potassium, they are low in sodium. Fish, poultry and greens such as spinach and beet tops are excellent sources of potassium but have been omitted because they are naturally on the high side in sodium content. Those foods should not be eaten in great amounts by people with diagnosed high blood pressure, although they will create no problems for someone with normal pressure. Because potassium is easily lost in cooking water, you can get the most from foods by eating them raw, when possible, or drinking the liquid or broth from the food that's cooked. If you boil potatoes, cooking them in their skins saves much of the potassium that would otherwise be lost.

Besides sodium and the potassium/sodium ratio, there are a few other observations about diet and high blood pressure which we feel are worth sharing. Your doctor or dietitian is not very likely to mention these findings, but you can decide for yourself if they seem worthwhile.

Sodium-Potassium Ratio of Selected Foods

The lower the ratio, the smaller the chances that the food will raise blood pressure, according to some leading researchers.

Food	Portion Size	Sodium (milligrams)	Potassium (milligrams)	Ratio (sodium divided by potassium)
Apple	1 medium	1	152	**0.007**
Apple pie	⅛ pie	355	94	**3.78**
Bread flour	⅙ cup	0.5	22	**0.02**
Bread, white	1 slice	134	33	**4.06**
Chicken	8 ounces	150	622	**0.24**
Chicken a la king	1 cup	760	404	**1.88**
Corn	½ cup	1	152	**0.006**
Corn flakes	½ cup	126	15	**8.4**
Ham				
fresh (uncured)	3 ounces	48	220	**0.22**
Hot dog	1 large	627	125	**5.02**
Milk, whole	1 cup	122	351	**0.35**
Cream cheese	1 tablespoon	35	10	**3.5**
Cheddar cheese	1 ounce	198	23	**8.61**
Peach	1 large	2	308	**0.006**
Peaches				
canned	½ cup	2.5	167	**0.015**
Peach pie	⅛ pie	316	176	**1.80**
Peanuts	¼ cup	1.75	252	**0.007**
Peanuts				
salted	¼ cup	150	243	**0.62**

VEGETARIAN DIETS SEEM PROTECTIVE

The first observation is that vegetarians tend to have lower blood pressures than people who aren't. What's more, the *strictest* vegetarians have the lowest pressures of all.

Like so many other findings about diet and health, the original observation about vegetarianism and blood pressure was made many years ago but pointedly ignored for half a century. In 1926, a California researcher by the name of A. N. Donaldson published in a medical journal his finding that while nonvegetarian male college students he tested had an average blood pressure of 126/75, lacto-ovo vegetarian students had blood pressures of only 113/65. A lacto-ovo vegetarian is one who eats dairy products and eggs, abstaining from meat products. Donaldson also reported that when meat was added to the diets of the vegetarians, their blood pressures went up after 11 days.

Apparently, there wasn't much follow-up on this discovery in the United States, but in Europe several doctors published studies showing that Donaldson's findings had real significance. A Yugoslavian study showed that not only hypertensive patients, but elderly people with blood pressures within the normal range, both experienced a drop of pressure after two or more months on a diet that restricted meat, fish and eggs to only five percent of calories. That's roughly equivalent to eating meat or fish about once or twice a week.

In our own era, Frank M. Sacks, M.D., and colleagues published a study in 1974 in the *American Journal of Epidemiology* showing that vegetarians do indeed have lower blood pressure. The Sacks group studied a total of 210 men and women living in communal households in the Greater Boston area, following the macrobiotic diet, which has an extremely low content of animal products. Most of the people studied, in fact, were strict vegans, meaning they ate no animal products at all—not even milk, butter or eggs. The macrobiotic diet emphasizes whole grains and beans above all else, rounding out the diet largely with vegetables, various edible seaweeds, and a small amount of fruit. Sugar, caffeine and other highly refined foods are shunned. Interestingly, though, sodium in the form of sea salt (which to our way of thinking is scarcely different from regular salt) is used in moderate amounts in cooking, and salty condiments such as miso and tamari are used in soups and as seasonings.

Keeping in mind that by American standards, a perfectly normal blood pressure is generally expressed as 120/80, here are the blood pressures found in these vegetarians: in the age group from 16 to 29, 106/65; from age 30 to 39, 110/70; and over 40 years of age, 114/72.

Those blood pressures are typical of "primitive" people who usually have zero incidence of high blood pressure (and very little heart disease as well). Perhaps of most interest, the blood pressure average of 114/72 found in the oldest group studied seems more typical of teenagers than people in their 40s.

We mentioned before that macrobiotic dietary principles allow for the use of a certain amount of salt-rich condiments. They are used both in cooking and as seasonings. In addition, macrobiotic adherents eat rather substantial amounts of seaweed, which is also high in sodium. (A macrobiotic leader told one of the present authors that just enough miso or tamari should be added to give food the right flavor, but "it should not taste salty.") Nevertheless, this addition of sodium to the diet does not prevent them from enjoying low blood pressure. In fact, Dr. Sacks found that while some of the people he studied added more salty seasoning at the table, and others didn't, those who did add the salt did *not* tend to have higher blood pressure. In fact—and this may be the most important part of all—the *only* dietary variable correlating with blood pressure at all was the percentage of animal food products that were eaten. Those who said they ate less than five percent of their diet in the form of animal foods had lower blood pressures than those who ate that much or more.

Now of course, it's possible that people living in communes and following a very special way of life and diet aren't very good subjects for a study about blood pressure in *all* people. Aside from any psychological considerations, it is against the principles of those who follow the macrobiotic way of life to smoke, use drugs or drink coffee. Their average weight was also quite modest, averaging about 140 pounds for men and 112 pounds for women. Still, the fact those who were the strictest vegetarians had the lowest blood pressure at least *suggests* there is something more at work here than general life-style.

Lending strength to the idea that vegetarians have lower blood pressure than other people is a study from Australia, which found that vegetarian Seventh-day Adventists have lower blood pressure than nonvegetarians living in the same general area of Australia. While Seventh-day Adventists had average blood pressures of approximately 129/76, the meat eaters had average blood pressures of 139/85. Echoing similar findings in Boston, the vegetarians who tended to have higher blood pressure were those who ate eggs. Coffee and tea drinking also seemed to be associated with slightly higher blood pressure. The Australian physicians who conducted the study suggest that one explanation for this trend could be the amount of saturated fat in the diet, or perhaps simply animal products, whether meat or eggs (*American Journal of Epidemiology,* vol. 105, no. 5, 1977).

GOOD OILS AND BAD CHEMICALS

There are several other important clues about blood pressure and diet that relate to eating more foods from vegetable sources. We mentioned in the previous chapter that polyunsaturated oil seems to have beneficial effects on cholesterol and platelet aggregation. The same study we cited then, which involved 50 hypertensive men and women, found that after one month of eating an increased amount of polyunsaturated oil, their average blood pressure fell from 147/91 to 139/86. That's not a phenomenal decrease, but it's certainly helpful. The people in that study got the additional polyunsaturates from eating sunflower seed oil and other products made from sunflower seeds, one of the richest natural sources of polyunsaturated oil (*Preventive Medicine,* March, 1979).

Within months of the publication of that report came another one, from Germany, confirming that polyunsaturates do indeed play an important role in regulating blood pressure. Scientists at the University of Heidelberg biopsied one ounce of fat from each of 650 men and analyzed its content of polyunsaturates. When they compared the relative amount of this oil in the men to their blood pressure, they found a very striking relationship: those with the highest amount of polyunsaturates in their fat tended to have the lowest blood pressures and vice versa (*Research in Experimental Medicine,* vol. 175, no. 3, 1979).

These findings do not necessarily mean it is wise to consume an especially large amount of polyunsaturate-rich sunflower or corn oil. We feel, as a number of scientists do, that the best course of action is to use the polyunsaturated oils *in place of* other oils and animal fats, rather than as simple additions to the diet. These oils are high in calories, after all, and most of us would be better off limiting our total consumption of fats and oils anyway. But certainly, moderate amounts of sunflower oil, as well as nuts and seeds, can be added without fear to salads or other appropriate dishes. Whole grains and legumes such as corn and soybeans are also rich in polyunsaturates and since such foods are staples in our dietary approach, you will be getting a substantial amount in your regular menu. Tuna and salmon also contain valuable polyunsaturates.

In 1977, it was reported at a major meeting of experimental biologists that people who had higher levels of pesticide residues in their blood also tended to have higher blood pressure. The most obvious implication of that finding is that growing your own organic food might be a good way to help keep your blood pressure down. But it may be worth knowing that another study has found that vegetarians, on the average, have lower levels of pesticide residues in their systems than nonvegetarians. Animal products, being at the top of the food chain, tend to accumulate the many chemical toxins used in modern agriculture. Vegetable products, even though they may have been treated chemically themselves, don't *accumulate* pesticides over a period of months or years. It's conceivable, at least, that the consumption of lower amounts of chemicals could be one of the factors playing a role in the lower blood pressures of vegetarians such as those studied.

One specific pollutant that has been linked to high blood pressure is cadmium, a heavy metal found in automobile exhaust, cigarette smoke, and runoff water from mines and industry which eventually enters our own water and food supply. Medical specialists not long ago found that besides having higher amounts of cadmium in their blood, people with high blood pressure tended to have a higher ratio of cadmium to zinc. Zinc, unlike cadmium, is a mineral essential to health, which is involved in many metabolic processes. It's possible that zinc fights the ill effects of cadmium somehow, and that when cadmium gets the upper hand, blood pressure goes up.

Here we may have yet another example of how food processing can lead to high blood pressure, because zinc is often lost in the process of "refining"—which more correctly ought to be called "degrading." Yet, that same process may not remove any of the cadmium. Changing whole wheat into white flour is a good example. While whole wheat has a zinc to cadmium ratio of over 100 to 1, white flour has a ratio of only about 17 to 1. The same is true for rice and probably other grains. The thing to do here, of course, is to stick with natural, undegraded foods. (The macrobiotic diet referred to previously calls for the use of whole grains exclusively, and in very abundant quantities.) We should also note that many animal experiments have shown vitamin C to be highly protective against the toxic effects of cadmium.

FOOD FIBER MAY HELP, TOO

If, in fact, vegetarians tend to have lower blood pressure, and those who eat very little cheese, eggs or dairy products have the lowest blood pressure of all, the explanation conceivably could have less to do with meat or even animal fat than with dietary *fiber.* If you are on a vegetarian diet and exclude milk, cheese and eggs, you have no choice but to be on a high-fiber diet, getting your protein from grains, beans, potatoes and vegetables. But does fiber really have an effect on blood pressure? Actually, not much attention had been given to that question until 1978, when a group of scientists with the U. S. Department of Agriculture and the University of Maryland discovered, almost by accident, that when dietary fiber goes up, blood pressure tends to go down.

The study, by June L. Kelsay, Ph.D., and colleagues tried primarily to find out what effect the addition to the diet of moderate amounts of fiber from fruits and vegetables has on the absorption of nutrients. In doing that, they had the same group of volunteers on a low-fiber diet for about a month and then on a high-fiber diet. Neither diet was remarkably different from what many people eat, which makes their discovery about blood pressure all the more interesting. What they found was that the average blood pressure of all 12 men in the study went down slightly on the high-fiber diet, but not enough to be statistically significant. However, there *was* an important change in 6 of those 12 men whose diastolic pressure (the second value, which is more important than the first, called systolic blood pressure) was higher than 80. In that group, the average blood pressure fell from 123/88 on the low-fiber diet to 118/78 on the high-fiber diet.

Although it's true that only six men were involved, which makes this more of an observation than a real study, a drop of 10 points in diastolic blood pressure may have very real health benefits (*American Journal of Clinical Nutrition,* July, 1978). Each degree rise of blood pressure above normal increases the chances of death. Even a pressure of 140/95, considered only a very mild elevation, means the statistical risk of death has increased two-and-a-half times. A person with a diastolic pressure over 105 is four times more likely to suffer a first major heart attack than a person whose diastolic pressure is 85 or below. Looking at it the other way, every time you can bring your diastolic pressure down a notch, you're putting the odds in your favor.

At least one doctor has suggested that his own clinical experience shows that a large percentage of *raw* foods in the diet may also be beneficial to blood pressure. John M. Douglass, M.D., avoids red meat and fish so his diet winds up being a high-fiber vegetarian one consisting largely of vegetables, seeds, nuts, various fruits and some milk products.

Although there are many theories and conflicting observations about diet and blood pressure, what they all pretty much boil down to is that processed food tends to create high blood pressure, while natural food prevents and alleviates it. It isn't necessary for a moment to pick and choose between the various approaches to lower high blood pressure we've discussed—low-salt, low-meat, high-potassium, high-fiber and so forth. If you set out to avoid added salt, for instance, you will be forced to avoid processed food at the same time. If you set out to eat foods high in potassium, you will automatically wind up eating lots of fresh, unprocessed fruits and vegetables (*also* high in vitamin C). If you set out to eat a lot of raw foods, you will automatically wind up eating a lot of vitamin C from fruits and vegetables, which are also high in fiber.

And if you follow the recipes in this book, especially those with the blood pressure symbol, you will get the whole show.

Just as important, you may have realized that if you set out to eat a diet which evidence suggests is good for your blood pressure, you will to a very large extent *also* be eating a diet good for your heart. As we mentioned briefly at the beginning of this chapter, the same fat that is bad for your arteries is no friend to your blood pressure, either. And the low-fat, vitamin-rich vegetables that are good for your heart are just as good for your blood pressure. So the two dietary approaches are natural companions from both the medical and culinary points of view.

BREAKFASTS

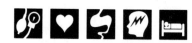

Choo-Choo Granola (Muesli)

Makes 10 servings
2 cups (500 ml) rolled oats
⅔ cup (150 ml) wheat germ
½ cup (125 ml) sunflower seeds
½ cup (125 ml) walnuts,
    chopped
½ cup (125 ml) pumpkin seeds
½ cup (125 ml) figs, chopped
½ cup (125 ml) dried apricots,
    chopped

This tasty breakfast—actually a muesli—gets its name from two characteristics: one, it makes you use your jaws, and two, it goes through you like a freight train.

Combine dry ingredients and keep in a sealed bottle in refrigerator. When ready to serve, add milk as required and top with several slices of fresh apple.

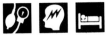

Nutty Oatmeal

Makes two servings
1½ cups (375 ml) water
1 tablespoon (15 ml) peanut
butter
⅔ cup (150 ml) rolled oats
1 banana, cubed
1 teaspoon (5 ml) honey

Bring water to a boil in a medium saucepan and stir in peanut butter and rolled oats. Stir over medium heat about three to six minutes until mixture is thickened and creamy.

Remove from heat, cover and set aside. Stir banana pieces and honey into cooked oatmeal. Serve plain or with skim milk.

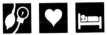

Date-Nut Porridge

Makes one serving
¾ cup (175 ml) water
3 pitted dates, chopped
2 teaspoons (10 ml) walnuts,
chopped
dash cinnamon
⅓ cup (80 ml) rolled oats

Place water, dates, nuts and cinnamon in a small pan, and bring to a boil. Stir in oats and simmer until thickened, stirring occasionally. Remove from heat, cover, and let stand a minute or two.

Serve hot with skim milk or orange juice.

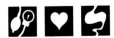

Pear Porridge

Makes one serving
¾ cup (175 ml) pear juice
⅓ cup (80 ml) rolled oats
1 tablespoon (15 ml) raisins
dash cinnamon

Bring pear juice to a boil in a saucepan. Stir in rolled oats and raisins, and cook until thickened. Add cinnamon to taste.

Note: The sweetness of the juice will eliminate the need for honey.

Variation: Try other unsweetened, natural fruit juices, such as apple cider, pineapple, etc., in place of the pear juice.

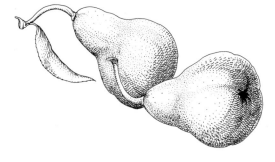

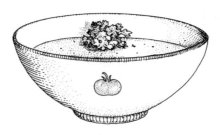

SOUPS

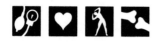

Cream of Tomato Soup

Makes two servings
3 large, ripe tomatoes
⅛ teaspoon (0.5 ml) basil
⅛ teaspoon (0.5 ml) oregano
1 clove garlic
½ cup (125 ml) dry-curd unsalted cottage cheese
chopped scallions, *Whole Wheat Croutons* or minced fresh parsley (garnish)

Seed tomatoes and place them in a blender with the herbs and garlic. Process on low speed until smooth. Place ingredients in a saucepan and bring to a boil over medium heat. Simmer for 10 to 15 minutes. Stir in cottage cheese and heat through. Return soup to the blender and process until creamy. Serve hot with chopped scallions, croutons or parsley for garnish.

Pureed Garden Soup

Makes six servings
2 teaspoons (10 ml) corn oil
6 carrots, thinly sliced
1 medium onion, thinly sliced
1½ cups (375 ml) thinly sliced potatoes
1 cup (250 ml) *Vegetable Stock*
1 cup (250 ml) skim milk
1 tablespoon (15 ml) sesame tahini

In large skillet or Dutch oven, place oil and carrots, onion and potatoes. Saute until tender, adding small amounts of water, if necessary, to prevent vegetables from sticking to the pan. Set aside one cup (250 ml) of the vegetables. Place the remaining vegetable mixture in a blender, adding stock and milk. Puree on low speed until smooth. Stir in reserved cup of vegetables and tahini. If not all of the soup is to be served immediately, freeze or refrigerate some when cooled. To serve remainder, return to skillet or Dutch oven and heat through before serving. Makes about four cups (1 l).

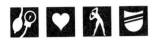

Peachy Plum Soup

Makes two servings

2 large, ripe peaches
3 ripe plums
  yogurt
  dash freshly grated nutmeg

Place the pitted fresh fruits, washed but with their skins, in a blender and process on medium speed until smooth. Place in mugs and chill. Serve with a dollop of yogurt on each, and dust with freshly grated nutmeg.

SALADS

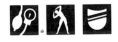

Orange-Date Salad

Makes two servings

2 oranges, cubed
1 unpeeled apple, cubed
2 pitted dates, finely chopped
2 tablespoons (30 ml) yogurt
1 tablespoon (15 ml) wheat germ
  dash cinnamon

Toss fruit together in a medium bowl with yogurt. Place in two serving bowls, and sprinkle with wheat germ and a dash of cinnamon.

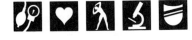

Molded Fruit Salad

Makes eight servings

1 cup (250 ml) orange juice
1 cup (250 ml) water
2 tablespoons (30 ml) gelatin
½ teaspoon (2 ml) *Vanilla Extract*
2 cups (500 ml) chopped melon
1 large banana, chopped
1 orange, chopped
½ cup (125 ml) pitted dates, chopped
¼ cup (60 ml) walnuts, chopped
  mint leaves (garnish)

Combine the orange juice and ½ cup (125 ml) of the water in a medium saucepan. Bring to a boil. Remove from heat. Soften the gelatin in the remaining ½ cup (125 ml) of cold water, then dissolve the mixture in the hot liquid. Add the vanilla. Allow to cool, then chill just until the mixture begins to thicken.

In a large bowl, fold the fruit and nuts into the gelatin. Pour into a large, lightly oiled mold and chill until firm. Turn out onto a serving plate, garnish with mint leaves, and serve.

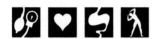

Millet, Fruit and Vegetable Salad

Makes four servings
½ cup (125 ml) corn
1 cup (250 ml) cooked millet
½ sweet red pepper, chopped
1 large banana, cubed
2 teaspoons (10 ml) lemon
    juice
2 tablespoons (30 ml) walnuts,
    chopped
2 tablespoons (30 ml) sunflower
    seeds, toasted
Lemon Vinaigrette Dressing
spinach leaves

Briefly simmer corn in water to cover until tender. Combine with millet and pepper.

Toss banana with lemon juice. Mix banana with corn mixture and add nuts and sunflower seeds. Toss salad with enough dressing to moisten. Serve on a bed of spinach leaves.

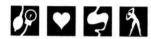

New Potato and Onion Salad

Makes two servings
2 cups (500 ml) baked new
    potatoes, halved
½ cup (125 ml) yogurt
¼ cup (60 ml) diced onions
1 teaspoon (5 ml) dillweed
¼ teaspoon (1 ml) garlic powder
⅛ teaspoon (0.5 ml) coriander

Many people find this potato salad tastes far better than the usual kind, and it saves you about 100 calories per serving in the bargain.

Depending on the size of your new potatoes, it will probably take about 6 to 10 to yield two cups (500 ml) after they are cut in half. If you wind up with a little more or less, don't worry about it. Just adjust the amount of the other ingredients.

Bake the potatoes at 350° F. (175° C.) for about 35 minutes or until done. (If more convenient, boil them.) Cut the potatoes in half and allow them to cool for about 5 minutes. Place in a medium bowl and add the yogurt, onions, dillweed, garlic and coriander. Mix well.

New potatoes are very flavorful and this dish probably tastes better if eaten while they are still warm. Garlic powder is used rather than whole garlic because it's a lot easier to mix into a dish like this, which isn't cooked after the garlic is added. You might want to add some chopped celery or sprinkle on some paprika.

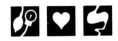

Chick-pea and Corn Salad

Makes four servings
1 cup (250 ml) cooked
    chick-peas
1 cup (250 ml) cooked corn
1 scallion, chopped
2 tablespoons (30 ml)
    Vinaigrette Dressing
lettuce or spinach leaves

Combine chick-peas, corn and chopped scallion. Toss with dressing. Serve on a bed of lettuce or spinach.

Vinaigrette Dressing

Makes ¾ cup (175 ml)
¼ cup (60 ml) cider vinegar
1 teaspoon (5 ml) Dijon-style
    mustard
½ cup (125 ml) corn oil or
    mixture of corn oil and
    olive oil

In a blender, process the vinegar and mustard until combined. Add the oil in a slow stream while the blender is running on low speed. Refrigerate the unused portion.

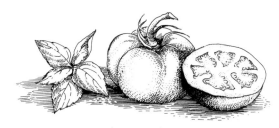

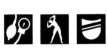

Basil Tomatoes

Makes four servings
2 large, ripe tomatoes
2 tablespoons (30 ml) fresh basil,
    minced

A colorful and flavorful summer harvest treat.

Slice tomatoes and arrange on a large serving plate. Sprinkle with minced basil. Chill, covered, before serving.

Note: These can be eaten as is, or with *Tofu Mayonnaise* on the side.

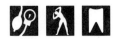

Makes two servings
1 cup (250 ml) shredded
    cabbage
⅓ cup (80 ml) white or red
    grapes, halved
2 tablespoons (30 ml) walnuts,
    chopped
Sesame-Fruit Dressing

Cabbage-Grape Salad

Combine ingredients in a medium bowl and toss with *Sesame-Fruit Dressing* to taste. Makes two servings.

Variation: Pineapple cubes can be substituted for the grapes.

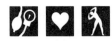

Makes four servings
1 medium cucumber, peeled
    and cubed
½ cup (125 ml) seedless grapes,
    halved
1 teaspoon (5 ml) *Tarragon
    Vinegar*
½ cup (125 ml) yogurt
2 teaspoons (10 ml) fresh mint,
    minced
1 clove garlic, minced
    spinach leaves
    mint sprigs (garnish)

Grape-Cucumber Salad

Our taste-testers were intrigued with the interesting flavor combination.

Combine cucumber with grapes in a medium bowl. Toss with remaining ingredients. Serve on a bed of spinach with a sprig of mint as garnish.

Makes ½ cup (125 ml)
3 tablespoons (45 ml) red wine
    vinegar
3 tablespoons (45 ml) orange
    juice
2 teaspoons (10 ml) paprika
2 cloves garlic
1 tablespoon (15 ml) sunflower
    oil

Sunshine Salad Dressing

Combine ingredients in blender on high speed, or crush garlic and shake in covered jar until blended. Delicious served over spinach salad with orange segments, or as a marinade for sliced oranges and thinly sliced red onions.

BREADS

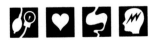

Barley Bread

Makes two loaves
½ cup (125 ml) barley
2 cups (500 ml) water
1⅔ cups (400 ml) skim milk
1 tablespoon (15 ml) active
 dry yeast
¼ cup (60 ml) lukewarm water
¼ cup (60 ml) medium
 unsulfured molasses
2 tablespoons (30 ml)
 sunflower oil
6–7 cups (1.5–1.75 l) whole
 wheat flour

An exceptionally fine bread with a taste and texture you'll love.

In a medium saucepan, bring barley and water to a boil; reduce heat and simmer until barley is tender. Drain well and set aside. Scald the milk and allow to cool to room temperature. Dissolve the yeast in the lukewarm water in a large mixing bowl, and add the milk, molasses and oil. Stir to combine. Add two cups (500 ml) of the flour and beat with the liquid ingredients. Add two more cups (500 ml) of flour by the half cup (125 ml), beating after each addition, until the batter is elastic and smooth. Then, knead in barley and enough remaining flour by hand to make a smooth, but not stiff, dough. Sprinkle some flour on your working surface and continue kneading bread dough until it becomes elastic. Place dough in a lightly greased bowl in a warm place until it is double in bulk, about an hour or more. Divide the dough into two oiled 8½ × 4½-inch (22 × 11-cm) bread pans. Cover with a damp towel and let dough rise until not quite double in size. Bake in a pre-heated 375° F. (190° C.) oven for 45 minutes. The bread will continue to expand in the oven, producing a high loaf.

Remove from pans and place on a cooling rack. Allow to cool before slicing.

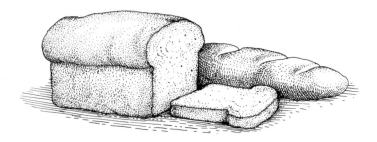

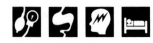

Quick Yeasted Date Bread

Makes one loaf

1 cup (250 ml) lukewarm
   water
1 tablespoon (15 ml) active
   dry yeast
1 tablespoon (15 ml) honey
2 cups (500 ml) whole wheat
   flour
¼ cup (60 ml) soy flour
¼ cup (60 ml) brewer's yeast
¾ cup (175 ml) sunflower
   seeds
1 egg, beaten
¼ cup (60 ml) honey
¾ cup (175 ml) pitted dates,
   chopped
1½ teaspoons (7 ml) cinnamon
½ teaspoon (2 ml) cardamom

This makes a hearty bread with a fine taste.

Thoroughly mix the water, yeast, honey and one cup (250 ml) of the whole wheat flour in a large bowl. Set aside in a warm place.

Meanwhile, in another bowl, combine remaining cup (250 ml) of whole wheat flour with the soy flour and brewer's yeast. Place the sunflower seeds in a blender and process in short bursts at high speed until they are ground into meal. Stir the sunflower seeds into the flour mixture.

When the yeast mixture is light and frothy, add the flour mixture, the egg, honey, dates and spices. Stir until thoroughly combined. Place the batter in a lightly oiled 8½ × 4½-inch (22 × 11-cm) bread pan and allow to rise until nearly double in bulk. Bake in a preheated 350° F. (175° C.) oven for 50 to 60 minutes, until done.

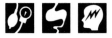

No-Knead Dill Bread

Makes one loaf

½ cup (125 ml) skim milk
1 tablespoon (15 ml) honey
1 tablespoon (15 ml) corn oil
1 tablespoon (15 ml) active
   dry yeast
½ cup (125 ml) lukewarm
   water
2½ cups (550 ml) whole wheat
   flour
½ small onion, minced
2 tablespoons (30 ml) fresh
   dillweed
½ teaspoon (2 ml) dill seed

A very quick and delicious herb bread.

Scald the milk and stir in the honey and oil. Set aside to cool to lukewarm. Place yeast and warm water in a large bowl. When yeast is dissolved, add warm milk mixture, one cup (250 ml) flour, onion and herbs. Beat well with a wooden spoon. Add remaining flour by the half cup (125 ml), beating after each addition until batter is smooth.

When all the flour has been incorporated into the batter, place bowl in a warm place and allow the dough to rise until it triples in size, about 45 minutes. Beat again with a wooden spoon until batter is smooth and compact. Turn dough into lightly oiled 8½ × 4½-inch (22 × 11-cm) bread pan and allow to rise in a warm place for 10 minutes before placing in a preheated 350° F. (175° C.) oven. Bake one hour. Remove bread from pan and cool on rack before slicing.

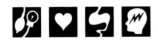

Quick Whole Wheat Bread

Makes one loaf
1 cup (250 ml) skim milk
2 tablespoons (30 ml) active
   dry yeast
½ cup (125 ml) lukewarm water
1 tablespoon (15 ml) honey
4 cups (1 l) whole wheat flour
⅛ teaspoon (0.5 ml) mace

Scald the milk and set aside to cool. In a large bowl, dissolve the yeast in the warm water and add the honey. When the yeast is dissolved and has begun to foam, add the lukewarm milk and two cups (500 ml) of the flour. Stir with a wooden spoon to combine, then beat the batter until smooth. Continue to add flour by the half cup (125 ml), beating after each addition. Add the mace. When the dough becomes stiff, the remaining flour can be added as you knead by hand. When all the flour is incorporated into the dough, cover the bowl with a towel and set in a warm place. When the dough has tripled in bulk, about 45 minutes, punch down and beat again. Place the batter in an oiled 8½ × 4½-inch (22 × 11-cm) bread pan, and allow to rise in a warm place about 8 to 10 minutes. Place bread in a preheated 350° F. (175° C.) oven and bake about one hour. Remove from oven, take bread from pan and cool on a rack before slicing.

MAIN DISHES

Crunchy Chicken Tropicana

Makes two servings
8 ounces (225 g) chicken
   breast, skinned and
   boned
¼ cup (60 ml) *Chicken Stock*
2 tablespoons (30 ml) lemon
   juice
2 tablespoons (30 ml) pineapple
   juice
1 teaspoon (5 ml) blackstrap
   molasses
2 cloves garlic, crushed
1 cup (250 ml) diced pineapple
½ cup (125 ml) peanuts
2 cups (500 ml) cooked brown
   rice

Loaded with potassium, B vitamins and protein.

Cut chicken in thin strips. Put stock, juices, molasses and garlic in a hot wok. When steaming, put in the chicken and stir vigorously for several minutes, until nearly done. Add pineapple and peanuts and continue stirring for another minute. Then add brown rice and mix well. Turn down heat and let steam until dish is hot. Serve immediately.

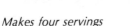

Poached Fish Fillets Italian-Style

Makes four servings

2 cups (500 ml) water
1 small onion, chopped
1 tablespoon (15 ml) minced
    fresh parsley
2 whole cloves
1 bay leaf
1 tablespoon (15 ml) cider
    vinegar
1 tablespoon (15 ml) olive oil
1½ pounds (675 g) fish fillets
    lemon wedges (garnish)

In a large covered skillet, bring the water, onion, parsley, cloves, bay leaf, vinegar and oil to a boil. Reduce heat and simmer for 15 minutes. Remove the bay leaf and cloves.

Cut the fish into four serving pieces. (Haddock, halibut, cod, hake, red snapper, grouper, pollock and flounder are all good here.) Place the fish in the liquid, cover, and simmer for about 10 minutes, just until the fish is opaque.

Serve hot with the broth and lemon wedges.

Broiled Tuna Melt

Makes one serving

2 ounces (55 g) unsalted
    water-packed tuna,
    drained
1½ tablespoons (25 ml) dry-curd
    unsalted cottage cheese
1 slice whole wheat bread

Mash tuna with fork, combine with cottage cheese, and spread evenly over bread slice. The bread can be toasted beforehand, if desired. Broil until tuna mixture is hot. Serve as a luncheon dish.

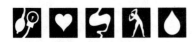

Lentil Stew

Makes six servings

1 cup (250 ml) dried lentils
5 cloves garlic, crushed
2 onions, chopped
1 green pepper, chopped
4 cups (1 l) tomato juice
1 tablespoon (15 ml) chili
    powder
1 teaspoon (5 ml) cumin
    powder
½ teaspoon (2 ml) basil
¼ teaspoon (1 ml) oregano
¼ teaspoon (1 ml) thyme

A zesty basic lentil stew can be used in many ways. Try it with Corn Pone *or* Tortillas Buenas. *Good, too, served over brown rice.*

Wash lentils, drain and set aside. In a heavy skillet, place the garlic, onions and pepper with a few spoonfuls of water and steam-stir about 5 minutes, until slightly tender. Add the tomato juice, chili powder, cumin and herbs. Stir in the lentils. Bring to a boil, reduce heat and simmer 45 to 50 minutes until lentils are tender. Makes four cups (1 l).

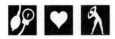

Lentil-Tomato Sauce

This thick sauce is nice over stuffed peppers.

Makes three cups (750 ml)
2½ cups (625 ml) tomato juice
½ cup (125 ml) small dried
  red lentils
1 medium onion, finely
  minced
3 cloves garlic, minced
1 teaspoon (5 ml) basil or
  mixed herbs
1 tablespoon (15 ml) fresh
  parsley
  dash cayenne pepper

Place ingredients in a saucepan or skillet and simmer until lentils are quite tender, about 20 minutes. Place ingredients in a blender and process on medium speed until smooth. Return to saucepan and heat before serving.

Variation: For spaghetti, you may want to add ½ green pepper, seeded and chopped, to the saucepan. Also, after the mixture has been pureed, cooked mushroom slices can be added.

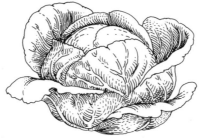

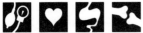

Scalloped Cabbage

A new look at cabbage!

Makes six servings
12 cups (3 l) sliced cabbage,
  (about 2 pounds
  [1 kg])
3 tablespoons (45 ml) corn oil
4 tablespoons (60 ml) whole
  wheat flour
2 teaspoons (10 ml) brewer's
  yeast
2 cups (500 ml) skim milk
1½ cups (375 ml) dry-curd
  unsalted cottage cheese
2 cups (500 ml) soft whole
  grain bread crumbs

Place cabbage in a large saucepan and steam in a small amount of water until slightly tender, but still firm. The cabbage should retain some crispness. Prepare a white sauce by placing oil in a heated skillet. Add flour and brewer's yeast, stirring to combine. Slowly add milk, stirring to make a paste with each addition. When all of the milk is incorporated, stir over medium heat three or four minutes until mixture thickens.

In a large, lightly oiled casserole dish, place a layer of cabbage, some each of the cottage cheese, bread crumbs, and white sauce. Repeat in layers, ending with the white sauce and a topping of bread crumbs. Bake in a preheated 350° F. (175° C.) oven 30 to 40 minutes, until cabbage is tender.

SIDE DISHES

Ratatouille

Makes six to eight servings
1 tablespoon (15 ml) sesame
   oil
4 cups (1 l) cubed eggplant
   (1 small)
2 cups (500 ml) cubed
   zucchini (1 medium)
1½ cups (375 ml) coarsely
   chopped onions
2 green peppers, seeded and
   cubed
3 cloves garlic, minced
2–3 medium tomatoes, coarsely
   chopped
3 tablespoons (45 ml) minced
   fresh parsley

A wonderful party dish, as it can be prepared the day before, and seems to gain in flavor on being reheated. It is also a delightful Mediterranean way to serve fresh vegetables of the summer season.

Place half the sesame oil in a heavy skillet and heat. Saute the eggplant in small enough quantities that there is just one layer in the pan, and remove when soft. Add remaining oil to saute rest of eggplant. Set aside.

Saute the zucchini in the same way, but add a few spoonfuls of water rather than oil if it sticks to the pan. Combine the zucchini with the eggplant.

In the skillet, steam-stir the onions and the peppers in a few spoonfuls of water until they are tender, but not browned. Stir in the garlic.

Place the tomatoes over the onions, peppers and garlic in the skillet and cover. Cook over low heat for five minutes, or until the tomatoes begin to release their juices. Uncover and stir the vegetables over medium-high heat until the juices have nearly evaporated. Stir in the parsley and remove the vegetables from the flame.

In a casserole dish, layer the tomato mixture with the eggplant and zucchini mixture, beginning and ending with tomatoes.

Cover the casserole and bake in a 350° F. (175° C.) oven for 15 to 20 minutes. The casserole can also be prepared in advance and chilled before baking. In this case, be sure casserole is heated through before serving, increasing the baking time.

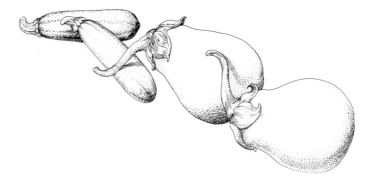

Zucchini Fiesta

Makes four servings
3 small zucchini
6 cherry tomatoes, halved
1 clove garlic, crushed
1 teaspoon (5 ml) basil or
    marjoram

A lively, low-calorie vegetable dish.

Slice zucchini in thin rounds and place in a skillet with remaining ingredients. Begin cooking over slow heat, and stir until juices are released. Continue cooking over medium heat until zucchini is tender and the liquid is absorbed.

Note: If you have fresh basil, substitute one to two tablespoons (15 to 30 ml) for the dried herb.

"Grownup" Green Beans

Makes six servings
3 cups (750 ml) green beans
½ cup (125 ml) water
1 clove garlic, minced
    dash cayenne pepper

Snap beans in half and place in a saucepan with the water. Sprinkle with the garlic and just a little cayenne pepper. Bring to a boil and allow to steam, covered, just until tender. Serves about six, though for green bean lovers at the peak of the season, it might serve only two.

Reserve the broth for later use in soups or sauces.

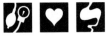

Mashed Potatoes with Green Beans

Makes two servings
2 cups (500 ml) mashed
    potatoes
1 cup (250 ml) sliced green
    beans, cooked

This dish was a regular on the dinner table when Sharon's husband grew up in southern Holland.

Combine hot mashed potatoes with hot cooked green beans. Serve immediately.

Variation: This combination can also be enhanced by boiling some finely chopped onions with the green beans.

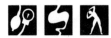

Steamed New Potatoes

Makes two servings
4 small new potatoes
 chopped fresh parsley
 yogurt

Steam potatoes in a small amount of water until tender. They will have a flakiness and a taste superior to boiled potatoes.
Cube and toss with a little parsley and yogurt.

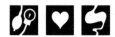

Potato Cakes

Makes four servings
2 cups (500 ml) mashed
     potatoes
1 egg, beaten
1 small onion, grated
1 tablespoon (15 ml) chopped
     fresh parsley
½ teaspoon (2 ml) basil,
     crumbled
 dash freshly grated nutmeg
 wheat germ

Combine all ingredients except wheat germ in a medium mixing bowl, and form into eight cakes. Dredge cakes in wheat germ to coat and place on a lightly oiled baking sheet. Bake 20 to 25 minutes in a preheated 350° F. (175° C.) oven. Serve hot.

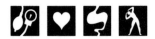

Corn on the Cob

Makes four servings
4 ears corn

This simple preparation produces juicy ears of corn steamed in their husks.

Preheat oven to 350° F. (175° C.). Place corn, unhusked, directly on baking rack. Bake 30 minutes. Remove husk and corn silk and serve immediately.

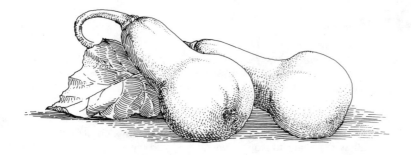

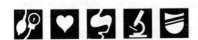

Baked Butternut Squash

Makes four servings
1 butternut squash
½ teaspoon (2 ml) corn or
     sunflower oil
1 unpeeled apple, chopped
1 teaspoon (5 ml) honey
4 tablespoons (60 ml) apple
     juice
     cinnamon

Cut butternut squash in half and remove seeds and stringy pulp. Rub the cut surface of each half with ¼ teaspoon (1 ml) oil. Place half of the apple in each of the squash cavities. Drizzle with honey and apple juice. Sprinkle with cinnamon.

Cover the squash halves with aluminum foil and place in a baking dish with ½ inch (1 cm) of water. To keep the squash level, you may have to place a folded piece of aluminum foil at the neck end.

Bake in a preheated 350° F. (175° C.) oven for 1½ hours. Remove foil, scoop out apple filling and cut the squash halves in two, lengthwise. Spoon the filling into each cavity and serve.

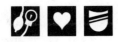

Fruited Baked Squash

Makes six servings
4 cups (1 l) peeled, cubed
     butternut squash
1 unpeeled apple, chopped
1 orange, chopped
     dash freshly grated nutmeg
¼ cup (60 ml) apple juice or
     cider

Combine squash with apple and orange. Toss with nutmeg and fruit juice. Place in a medium, covered casserole dish.

Bake in a preheated 350° F. (175° C.) oven about one hour, until squash is tender. If browning is desired, remove lid during last 15 minutes or so of baking.

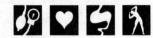

Polenta

Makes six servings
6 cups (1.5 l)
1½ cups (375 ml) whole grain
   cornmeal

Here's a traditional Italian dish which can be easily combined with any number of vegetables you might happen to have. Cheap, too!

Bring water to a boil in a heavy saucepan over high heat. Pour the cornmeal slowly into the boiling water, stirring constantly. Do not allow the water to stop boiling as you add meal.

Reduce the heat, and simmer the polenta 20 to 30 minutes. Stir frequently. When it is thick (it should support a wooden spoon upright in the center), remove it from the heat. Serve hot with *Good Gravy* or with a good tomato sauce.

Some or all of the polenta can also be spooned, while hot, into a lightly oiled baking dish and smoothed with a wooden spoon. Cool and refrigerate. To serve, cut in oblong cakes and bake or broil until heated through.

MISCELLANEOUS

Vegetable Stock

Makes 3½ cups (875 ml)
2 cups (500 ml) vegetable
   trimmings
1 bay leaf
4 cups (1 l) water

When preparing vegetables for cooking, set aside onion skins and trimmings, carrot trimmings or peelings, potato skins (if you prefer to remove them before cooking), scallion tops, celery leaves or trimmings, mushroom pieces or other vegetable parts. These can be frozen until you have sufficient quantity for a stock.

Avoid cabbage, broccoli, cauliflower or brussels sprouts, as these vegetables will impart their distinctive taste to the entire stock.

Bring the trimmings, bay leaf and water to a boil in a large saucepan, reduce heat and simmer gently about 45 minutes. Strain through cheesecloth, discarding the vegetable trimmings. If the stock is not to be used immediately, cool, then refrigerate. Stocks made without salt will not keep for long in a refrigerator, so freeze the stock if you will not use it within a day or two.

Variation: Save the water from cooked vegetables, and place in a container in the refrigerator or freezer. By combining vegetable broths, you will have a nutritious liquid for cooking rice, adding to soups, etc.

Chicken Stock

Makes one quart (1 l)
bones of 4 whole chicken
    breasts
6 cups (1.5 l) water
1 onion, sliced
1 carrot, sliced
2 stalks celery, sliced
1 bay leaf
2 tablespoons (30 ml) fresh
    parsley
2 teaspoons (10 ml) lemon
    juice
½ tomato, seeded and chopped
    (optional)
1 mushroom, sliced (optional)

Avoid highly salted stocks by making your own.

In a large kettle, place the bones; add water and the remaining ingredients. Bring to a boil, reduce heat, and simmer, covered, about 1½ to 2 hours. Strain through cheesecloth. Store, covered, in the refrigerator. To use, skim off any fat and add to recipes.

Note: If the stock will not be used within about two days, place in the freezer. Stock made without salt will spoil more rapidly than salted stocks.

Variation: Purchase necks or backs to add to the stockpot. Also, keep a bag in the freezer to store chicken bones (raw or cooked) and vegetable trimmings. For a richer stock, use about two pounds (1 kg) of bones or chicken pieces and two cups (500 ml) of vegetable trimmings for 6 cups (1.5 l) of water.

Barbeque Sauce

Makes ⅔ cup (150 ml)
⅔ cup (150 ml) tomato paste
2 cloves garlic, crushed
2 teaspoons (10 ml) blackstrap
    molasses
2 tablespoons (30 ml) lemon
    juice
2 tablespoons (30 ml) finely
    chopped onions
1 teaspoon (5 ml) basil
½ teaspoon (2 ml) chili powder
¼ teaspoon (1 ml) cumin
    powder
¼ teaspoon (1 ml) thyme
⅛ teaspoon (0.5 ml) ginger

Can be used for glazing chicken breasts prior to baking, or as a sauce for grilled vegetables, broiled fish or meat 'n' vegetable loaves.

Combine ingredients. Refrigerate in a glass jar.

Baba Ghannouj

Makes two cups (500 ml)
1 large eggplant
2 cloves garlic
¼ cup (60 ml) sesame tahini
4–5 tablespoons (60–75 ml)
        lemon juice
    dash cayenne pepper
    parsley sprigs (garnish)

Try this Arabian dip with some flat, whole wheat Pita Bread *broken into bite-size pieces. If you are like so many others who develop a fondness for the dish, you will understand its Arabic name: "Father of Greediness."*

Char the eggplant under the broiler or with a fork over the flame of a gas stove. When the skin is blackened and the eggplant begins to soften, run cold water over the eggplant and peel. Place the eggplant in cheesecloth or a kitchen towel and squeeze out moisture. Place pulp with the remaining ingredients in a blender and process on low speed until smooth. Serve in a bowl sprinkled with a little cayenne and garnished with parsley. This will keep in the refrigerator at least a week.

Hot Pepper Sauce

Makes one cup (250 ml)
3 sweet red peppers
4–5 cloves garlic
2 tablespoons (30 ml) olive or
        safflower oil
¼ teaspoon (1 ml) cayenne
        pepper

Based on the Mediterranean "rouille," our sauce gives a lift to soups (especially fish), stews and vegetables.

Place washed, whole peppers over an open flame on the gas stove or under a broiler, and turn as the skin chars. The skin of the pepper must be blackened on all sides. When this is done, wrap the charred peppers in a wet kitchen towel for 10 minutes.

Unwrap the peppers and, one at a time, hold them under a slow stream of water from the faucet and remove the skins. Cut the peppers open and remove the seeds and stems.

Place the pepper pulps in a blender with the garlic, oil and cayenne. Process on medium speed until smooth.

To serve, place a few spoonfuls in soup or on vegetables.

Herbal Seasoning Mix

Makes ½ cup (125 ml)
2 tablespoons (30 ml) basil
2 tablespoons (30 ml) paprika
2 tablespoons (30 ml) thyme
2 tablespoons (30 ml) marjoram
1 tablespoon (15 ml) ginger
2 teaspoons (10 ml) finely
    grated lemon rind
1 teaspoon (5 ml) dry mustard
1 teaspoon (5 ml) sage
¼ teaspoon (1 ml) cayenne
    pepper

Put all ingredients in a blender and process on low speed until combined. Spoon into a shaker-top container. Put a piece of waxed paper inside the lid to keep it airtight. Remove to shake. Store in the refrigerator.

Season with Reason

Makes ¼ cup (60 ml)
2 tablespoons (30 ml) sunflower
    seeds
2 tablespoons (30 ml) sesame
    seeds
1 teaspoon (5 ml) brewer's
    yeast
1 teaspoon (5 ml) marjoram
1 teaspoon (5 ml) basil
½ teaspoon (2 ml) thyme
½ teaspoon (2 ml) oregano
½ teaspoon (2 ml) paprika
    dash cayenne pepper

No need for salt when you give your food a lift with a tasty mixture of seeds and herbs.

In a blender, grind the sunflower and sesame seeds with short bursts at high speed. Combine with the remaining ingredients, place in a tightly covered jar, and store in the refrigerator.

Makes 1½ cups (375 ml)
½ cup (125 ml) finely chopped
   onions
2 teaspoons (10 ml) sesame oil
2 cups (500 ml) chopped ripe
   tomatoes or Italian plum
   tomatoes
4 tablespoons (60 ml) tomato
   paste
1 teaspoon (5 ml) basil, crushed
1 teaspoon (5 ml) blackstrap
   molasses

*Makes 2 ½ tablespoons
(35 ml)*
3 teaspoons (15 ml) coriander
1 teaspoon (5 ml) cumin
   powder
1 teaspoon (5 ml) turmeric
1 teaspoon (5 ml) paprika
½ teaspoon (2 ml) mustard
   powder
½ teaspoon (2 ml) cardamom
½ teaspoon (2 ml) cinnamon
¼ teaspoon (1 ml) mace
⅛ teaspoon (0.5 ml) allspice

Mediterranean Tomato Sauce

This can be simmering on a back burner while you prepare the rest of your meal. It makes a small quantity, suitable for two, to be served over pasta. Or try it over cooked vegetables, polenta, cooked beans or cooked brown rice.

Saute onions in the oil until translucent. Add remaining ingredients and simmer, covered, about 40 minutes, stirring occasionally. If a smooth sauce is desired, press through a sieve or puree in a blender.

Curry Powder

Combine spices in a cup measure and funnel into a small spice jar. You can design your own curry to suit your tastes. Other spices you may think of including are: ginger, celery seed, cayenne pepper, garlic powder or chili powder.

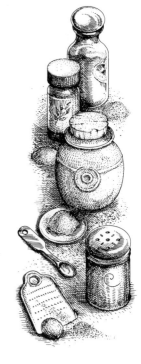

Light Chicken Broth

Makes one quart (1 l)

2 small onions, chopped
  skins from 2 whole chicken
  breasts
1 stalk celery with leaves
2 bay leaves
2 carrots, chopped
4 cloves garlic, crushed
½ teaspoon (2 ml) rosemary
  pinch thyme
5 cups (1.25 l) water

In a heavy skillet, steam-stir onions in a small amount of water until they are translucent. Add the chicken breast skins and saute until they begin to brown.

Add the remaining ingredients, transferring to a larger pot, if necessary, and bring to a boil. Reduce heat, and simmer gently 1½ to 2 hours. Strain broth and refrigerate. Skim fat from surface and use in soups, stews and sauces.

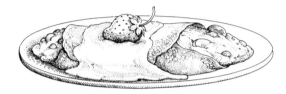

DESSERTS

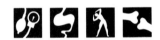

Buckwheat Crepes with Cheese-Fruit Filling

Makes four servings

Crepes:

1 cup (250 ml) buckwheat flour
⅓ cup (80 ml) pear juice
1 cup (250 ml) yogurt
2 eggs

Desserts can't get much more nutritious than this and still taste like dessert. Try it too for breakfast or brunch.

Combine ingredients in a mixing bowl, beating until smooth. To make crepes, place about three tablespoons (45 ml) of batter on a hot, lightly oiled crepe or omelet pan. Swirl uncooked batter around quickly to coat the bottom of the pan in a thin layer. Cook over medium heat until bubbles appear on the surface, and surface appears dry. This should take only about two minutes. Turn and cook other side about 30 seconds. Remove and place to cool on a kitchen towel atop a cooling rack. Repeat procedure to produce eight crepes.

Filling:

½ cups (375 ml) low-fat cottage
  cheese
¾ cup (175 ml) strawberries,
  chopped
¾ cup (175 ml) seedless grapes,
  chopped
2 large bananas, chopped
  dash freshly grated nutmeg

Combine cottage cheese with chopped fruit in a medium bowl and add a dash of nutmeg. To fill, place equal amounts of the cheese mixture on the edge of each crepe, placed first-cooked side down, and roll. Place seam-side down on serving plates.

To serve, top rolled crepes with a few dollops of *Maple Applesauce* in the center of each.

Maple Applesauce

Makes one cup (250 ml)
2 large unpeeled apples,
    chopped
¼ cup (60 ml) apple juice
2 tablespoons (30 ml) maple
    syrup

Place apples in a blender with the remaining ingredients. Process on medium speed until smooth.

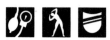

Fresh Strawberry Pie

Makes eight servings
4 cups (1 l) strawberries
    9-inch (23-cm) prebaked
    No-Roll Pie Crust
1 cup (250 ml) apple juice
2 teaspoons (10 ml) lemon
    juice
1 tablespoon (15 ml) agar-agar
    flakes
2 teaspoons (10 ml) maple
    syrup or honey
¼ teaspoon (1 ml) *Vanilla
    Extract*
    Whipped Tofu Topping

Arrange whole, hulled berries in pie shell and chill. Place apple and lemon juice, agar-agar and sweetening in saucepan and bring to a boil. Simmer five minutes. Remove from heat, stir in vanilla, and allow to cool slightly. (If mixture cools too thoroughly, it will solidify in the pan, in which case it should be reheated.) Spoon mixture over chilled berries in pie shell. Return to refrigerator and chill until firm. Before serving, top with dollops of *Whipped Tofu Topping*.

Strawberry-Rhubarb Pie

Makes eight servings
2½ cups (625 ml) chopped
    rhubarb
1 cup (250 ml) apple juice
2 tablespoons (30 ml)
    agar-agar flakes
1 tablespoon (15 ml) honey
2 cups (500 ml) whole
    strawberries
    9-inch (23-cm) prebaked
    No-Roll Pie Crust

Place rhubarb and apple juice in a medium saucepan and bring to a boil. Simmer until rhubarb begins to soften, about five minutes. Sprinkle agar-agar on rhubarb sauce, add honey, and simmer five minutes more. Remove from heat and allow to cool slightly. Stir in strawberries. When mixture is cool, but before it begins to gel, pour strawberry-rhubarb mix into a prebaked pie shell. Chill before serving.

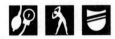

Jeweled Raspberry Pie

Makes eight servings
3 cups (750 ml) red or black
    raspberries
9-inch (23-cm) prebaked
    No-Roll Pie Crust
2 cups (500 ml) apple juice
2 heaping tablespoons (40 ml)
    agar-agar flakes

A sparkling beauty of a pie, with no whipped cream or heavy sweeteners to offset the nutrient bonus of this fine summer fruit. Serve it for company or to cap a special family dinner. Combine red and black raspberries to enhance the jeweled effect.

Pick over and wash raspberries and drain; place berries in pie shell and chill while preparing filling. In a saucepan, bring apple juice to a boil and sprinkle with agar-agar. Simmer five minutes. Remove from heat and cool slightly. Spoon apple juice mixture over raspberries in chilled pie shell. Return to refrigerator until firm.

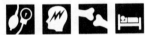

Lemon Chiffon Pie

Makes eight servings
 1 teaspoon (5 ml) finely grated
    lemon rind
½ cup (125 ml) lemon juice
½ cup (125 ml) apple juice
 2 tablespoons (30 ml)
    agar-agar flakes
18 ounces (500 g) tofu
1½ teaspoons (7 ml) *Vanilla
    Extract*
¼ cup (60 ml) honey
 2 very ripe bananas
    9-inch (23-cm) prebaked
    No-Roll Pie Crust
    lemon slices (garnish)

Place lemon rind and juices in a small saucepan and sprinkle with the agar-agar. Bring to a boil, reduce heat, stir, and simmer for five minutes. Remove from heat and cool slightly.

Place half of the lemon juice mixture with half of the tofu, vanilla, two tablespoons (30 ml) honey, and one banana in a blender and process on low speed until smooth. Repeat with the remaining lemon mixture, tofu, honey and banana. Place the blended mixtures in the cooled pie shell, and when it is room temperature, chill until firm.

To serve, garnish with very thin lemon slices.

Frozen Banana Pop

Makes one serving
1 small, very ripe banana
  Carob Syrup
  wheat germ or chopped nuts

Peel banana and place on a stick. Wrap in plastic wrap or foil and place in a freezer until solid.

To serve, dip in *Carob Syrup* and dust with wheat germ or nuts. Frozen bananas can also be dipped and coated, then rewrapped and popped back into the freezer for enjoying later.

Baked Currant-Pears

Makes four servings
4 firm pears
3 tablespoons (45 ml) currants
2 tablespoons (30 ml) sunflower
    seeds
1 tablespoon (15 ml) lemon
    juice
1 teaspoon (5 ml) honey
¼ cup (60 ml) apple juice
    dash freshly grated nutmeg

Halve, core, but do not peel pears. Combine currants and sun-flower seeds and stuff pear halves. Combine lemon juice, honey and apple juice in a small bowl. Place stuffed pear halves in a shallow casserole dish, drizzle honey-juice mixture over each half, and dust with nutmeg. Cover, and bake in a preheated 350° F. (175° C.) oven 30 minutes.

These stuffed pears make an attractive dessert dish.

Variation: Top with *Sesame-Fruit Dressing* instead of honey-juice mix-ture. Also, raisins and sesame seeds can be substituted for currants and sunflower seeds.

Frozen Banana Yogurt

Makes four servings
1 banana
½ unpeeled apple
1½ tablespoons (25 ml) medium
    unsulfured molasses
1 teaspoon (5 ml) lemon juice
1 teaspoon (5 ml) *Vanilla
    Extract*
1 cup (250 ml) yogurt

Cut banana and apple in pieces and place in blender with re-maining ingredients. Process at medium speed until smooth. Pour into freezer tray and cover with aluminum foil. Place in freezer and chill until firm, about three hours. To serve, place frozen mixture in blender and process on low speed until slightly softened.

Creamy Dessert Sauce

Makes 1½ cups (375 ml)
1 banana
½ cup (125 ml) strawberries or
    unpeeled chopped
    apples
1 tablespoon (15 ml) tahini
2 tablespoons (30 ml) apple
    juice
½ cup (125 ml) yogurt
    mint sprigs (garnish)

Combine ingredients in a blender on medium speed and process until smooth.

Try this over a slice of *Banana Pound Cake* or tossed with a fresh fruit salad. Just combine melon cubes, strawberries, blueberries, peach slices, cubed apples, grapes, orange sections or other fruit; add some dessert sauce and serve in individual bowls. Garnish with mint.

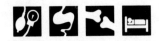

Tofu-Rice Pudding

Makes four servings

3 cups (750 ml) cooked brown rice
6 ounces (170 g) tofu
3 tablespoons (45 ml) maple syrup
½ teaspoon (2 ml) finely grated lemon rind
½ teaspoon (2 ml) *Vanilla Extract*
⅛ teaspoon (0.5 ml) cardamom
½ cup (125 ml) raisins

Place rice in a mixing bowl. In a blender, combine tofu, maple syrup, lemon rind, vanilla and spice. Blend on low speed until smooth. Pour over brown rice, add raisins and stir to combine. Chill before serving. Makes 3½ cups (875 ml).

Chapter 3

Better Digestion, Top to Bottom

There are probably millions of people today—yes, *millions*—who could escape the discomfort, pain and danger of chronic digestive disorders by a relatively simple change of diet. Unfortunately, they don't know this—possibly because they haven't been to a physician in years, or perhaps because the medical advice they're getting is old-fashioned.

We are, in fact, just now coming out of what might be called the Dark Ages of Digestion. It's not just that we didn't know anything about the relationship between nutrition and digestion, but rather that many of the things we believed were the *exact opposite* of the truth! And since we often turned those beliefs into advice, it is easy to imagine that more harm than good was done in many cases.

Consider two conditions that are very common: chronic constipation, and diverticular disease of the colon (which hospitalizes hundreds of thousands of people in America each year and causes many others to suffer from episodes of cramping pains and sometimes worse). To give you an idea of what was being said about constipation just about 25 years ago, let's take a look at the July, 1954, issue of *Consumer Reports.* In its best sanctimonious voice, the magazine declared that "so often [the causes of constipation] originate in infancy and childhood, with intensive psychotherapy offering the only possibility of a permanent cure."

Psychotherapy for constipation? Yes, and *intensive* psychotherapy, too! The article in question goes on to advise that a good way to help a child overcome constipation is to give him or her more sugar and less protein. (In fact, giving a child more sugar and thereby pushing fibrous foods out of the diet is one of the best ways to *encourage* constipation.) In the case of the "spastic type of constipation," the article says that "doctors prefer a diet which is low in residue or bulk-producing foods, especially whole grain cereals, bread, bran and fibrous vegetables." This is really an astonishing piece of work, because the authors have managed to recommend precisely the kind of diet that is now believed to *cause* an irritable, spastic colon, while warning people away from precisely those foods known to improve the condition.

Well, that's some of the advice a popular magazine was passing along for constipation in those days. What about the medical press? Skimming through some old issues of the *Journal of the American Medical Association*, it didn't take us long to find a real doozy. In the issue of March 15, 1958, there was a brief report recommending the use of broad-spectrum antibiotics along with other drugs for the treatment of constipation. If psychotherapy for constipation is stupid, antibiotics are insane. But since psychotherapy and antibiotics were the two hottest medical fads of the 50s, maybe it shouldn't be that surprising to find them both recommended for a condition no one seemed to understand in those days.

But the question is, do we understand it any better today? Some of us do, thank goodness. But we may still be in the minority, according to a study published in the December, 1978, issue of the *Journal of the American Geriatrics Society* by researchers at the University of Maryland School of Pharmacy. Their work revealed that laxatives are *the* most frequently prescribed drugs in nursing homes, and that almost no constipated patients are advised to increase their intake of fiber. Of some 73 elderly patients included in this study, no less than 50 used laxatives (16 were actually using more than one). Not a single patient was being managed with dietary advice. How many of those 50 should have been taking laxatives? Quite possibly, none, scientists say, pointing out that "valid indications for the use of laxatives are limited." The best treatment for constipation, they say, "involves the use of naturally laxative foods such as the fruits and vegetables, oatmeal, cracked wheat bread or bran."

Laxatives, we might add, were also recommended in that *Consumer Reports* article we mentioned. So were enemas. Which is worth talking about, because—as we have just seen—there is still a lot of bad practice going on these days in relation to managing constipation. As for laxatives, the most popular kind contain an element that chemically stimulates or irritates the bowel (such as the herb senna). Take a laxative of that kind long enough and the bowels actually begin to lose their inborn reflex to contract at appropriate times. In fact, that reflex can be *completely* eradicated in some incidences, doctors believe. At that point, of course, the person is literally addicted to laxatives, even more profoundly than a drug addict is dependent on drugs. As for enemas, they aren't much better because once again, an outside force is being used to replace a normal reflex, which when not used becomes weaker and weaker, just like unused muscles.

All of which brings us down to the recommendation given by the Maryland pharmacists that *food* be used as the treatment of choice in constipation. At last, it seems, we have arrived at some common sense. *At last?* Listen to this: the true cause of constipation is "food which leaves little residue; very completely digested food . . . fecal matter too small to duly excite peristalsis." There it is in a nutshell: low-fiber food is the cause of constipation. If the quote sounds just a little old-fashioned, it's because it was written in 1886 by a Dr. W. B. Cheadle in the *Lancet* (2, 1063). After psychotherapy, antibiotics, laxatives and all the rest, we are finally beginning to catch up with good old Dr. Cheadle.

The key phrase in Dr. Cheadle's remarks is "food which leaves little residue." Today, we know it's not just the residue of the food that is important in providing sufficient bulk to provoke peristalsis or normal bowel movements, but the ability of that food residue to hold water. To the extent that it holds water, it actually gains in bulk and exerts gentle pressure on the lining of the bowel, inducing it to make gentle, rhythmic contractions. The problem, of course, is in knowing which foods have relatively high residues, with water-holding capacity.

WHY SO MANY PEOPLE ARE CONSTIPATED

So much for theory. What about practice?

One woman at a workshop told us she thought the reason for her constipation must have been purely psychological, as she had a good appetite and ate what she considered to be a perfectly normal, well-balanced diet. Just exactly what *do* you eat? we asked her.

"Well, for breakfast, I have a large glass of orange juice, two eggs, bacon, buttered toast and coffee. Isn't that a good breakfast? Doesn't it have all the food groups?"

"The food groups are old-fashioned and an inadequate way of judging a diet," we pointed out. "Particularly when it comes to inducing regular, easy bowel movements, what we are looking for is fiber. Now that orange juice you drank had lots of vitamin C, but it had no fiber at all. There was no fiber in the eggs. No fiber in the bacon, no fiber. . . ."

"No fiber in bacon? It seems to have fiber in it."

"No meat has fiber in it, not even a five-pound roast. No fiber in the coffee, either—naturally. Or in the milk, if you use milk with it. The only fiber at all you had in your breakfast was in the toast, and if it was white toast, barely a trace."

"I think the bread I use is enriched. Does that mean anything?"

"It means very little as far as vitamins go and absolutely nothing when it comes to fiber. When whole wheat is refined into white flour, so much fiber is removed in the process that you'd have to eat eight pieces of white bread to get the amount of crude fiber that naturally occurs in one piece of whole wheat bread."

Shortening the rest of this discussion, it turned out that our friend skipped lunch altogether, and for dinner had a piece of fish or meat, a vegetable or two, a green salad and occasionally some dessert. One or two cocktails rounded out her daily nutritional intake. That meant the only fiber she was getting during the course of an entire day was the trace of fiber in her white toast and the fiber in the vegetables and greens she ate for dinner.

"But don't plenty of people eat like that?" she wanted to know.

"Certainly. But you happen to be a little more vulnerable to constipation than the average person. There is so little fiber in your diet, that you don't have to be extremely vulnerable, just slightly. However, another person could eat the same as you and just happen to be naturally resistant to constipation. The point is, if you eat a reasonable amount of fiber, it doesn't matter whether you are vulnerable or not. Unless you have a serious illness or some kind of emotional crisis, you will have good bowel movements."

"But I've been taking a laxative for years. I *need* it."

"You can't say that until you give fiber a chance. The easiest way to do that for a person like yourself who follows a rigid dietary routine would be simply eating about two teaspoons of unprocessed bran every day. Mix it in with some yogurt or cooked cereal. However you take it, just make sure that you also drink *at least* one extra glass of water a day to make sure that the bran has enough moisture to absorb."

"And the next morning, I'll be back on schedule?"

"No! Bran doesn't work like that. Only laxatives do. It will take at least two or three days before the bran begins to work. It may take even longer. Every couple of days, increase the amount of bran you are eating a little bit until you feel that everything is working fine. Be patient, because in the beginning you may find that the bran gives you a little gas. But that will go away after a couple of weeks as your body adjusts."

"How much bran am I going to need?"

"Probably no more than about two tablespoons a day. Maybe three at the most. Actually, you'd be better off getting your fiber from a variety of sources, using maybe one tablespoon of bran and making sure that you are eating plenty of whole grains like brown rice, oats, whole wheat bread and plenty of fruits and vegetables, like carrots, peas, broccoli and beans."

"How about prune juice?"

"Forget about prune juice. Prune juice contains a natural chemical which stimulates the bowel just as the herb senna does. The idea is to get enough fiber and water in you so that your bowels work by themselves."

Before we bid a final farewell to the land of constipation and sail on to some of the more troublesome horizons of digestive difficulties, let us pause for a moment and consider why we have even bothered writing about something as seemingly unimportant as constipation. First of all, constipation isn't just a meaningless deviation from the national norm of bowel movements. Part of our definition of constipation is a definite feeling of discomfort and the need to strain. And that, friends, is no joke. No one talks about it much, but ask any cardiologist and he will tell you that a significant number of heart attacks occur in the john. Why? Because when people strain to move their bowels, they may significantly reduce the amount of blood reaching their heart and trigger abnormal heart rhythms.

But there is another, larger dimension to constipation. Even if it doesn't cause any particular problem or discomfort, constipation is often emblematic of a diet unhealthful for *many* reasons: deficient in whole grains, beans, vegetables and fruits, and top-heavy with fiberless sugars and fats and possibly alcohol. That's why we say that while the simplest approach may be to just add some bran to your diet, you're better off cleaning up your whole act.

EASING PAINFUL BOWEL PROBLEMS

Constipation is only a kind of junior varsity version of a problem afflicting millions of people today. That problem, which goes by various names, generally involves painful cramps, irregularity (constipation, chronic diarrhea or alternating bouts of *both*), painful elimination, bloating, gas, and sometimes heartburn to boot. When many of these problems are present but x-rays can reveal nothing structurally wrong with the digestive tract, the term "irritable bowel syndrome" is often used. If x-rays reveal the presence of tiny pouches in the wall of the large intestine, the term *diverticulosis* is used. That term comes from the Latin word *diverticulum,* which as one British text put it, "means a way-side house of ill-fame and these way-side houses certainly live up to their evil reputation." When the diverticula (the plural for the other word) become inflamed and extremely painful, the condition is at that point called *diverticulitis.* At its worst, diverticulitis can be so painful as to be totally disabling and may also cause systemic infection. After a few recurring bouts of diverticulitis, you usually become a candidate for surgery.

An editorial in the British medical journal *Lancet* (June 2, 1979) points out that until recently diverticular disease "was thought to be due to stagnation of feces in the colon and treatment was aimed at keeping the colon as empty as possible by means of a low-residue diet and a regular purgation [treatment with laxatives]." However, the journal goes on to point out, Dr. Neil Painter and colleagues showed that the less that was in the colon, the *greater* the pressure, the greater the pain, and the greater all the other problems of diverticular disease. It goes on to explain, in short, that the old-fashioned idea of avoiding roughage *causes* rather than improves diverticular disease.

A few years ago, we visited Dr. Painter at the Manor House Hospital in London and as he put it, "it's perfectly plain that in the digestive tract there is nothing rough about 'roughage' or dietary fiber. When it is moist, bran becomes 'softage.' "

And what does bran, one of the most concentrated forms of fiber, do for diverticular disease and its nasty cousins? At the Manor House Hospital, a study was made of the bowel habits of 62 diverticular patients who were put on Dr. Painter's high-fiber dietary regime—bran, whole wheat bread, minimum intake of sugar and sugar-loaded foods, some increase in raw fruits and vegetables, and an extra pint of fluid daily. Before going on this regime, 28 of the diverticular patients customarily moved their bowels infrequently (every other day, every third day, or more irregularly), while three had frequent small stools and attacks of diarrhea. After a period on the high-fiber, bran diet, *all* patients customarily had normal bowel movements once, twice or three times a day. The bran also made the stools softer and easier to pass. At the start of the diet, only 8 of the 62 patients were able to move their bowels without straining. Once on the fiber regimen, 51 said straining had become "a thing of the past." A further benefit: while the majority of these patients had been accustomed to taking laxatives, on a bran diet 55 found that they could do without medication, and the remaining 7 resorted to laxatives only occasionally.

Most important: although at least 10 of these patients had pain severe enough to indicate surgery, "all recovered without surgery and remain well since on bran."

Several years after our interview with Dr. Painter, the surgeon published an article in a European surgery journal reviewing his experience and mentioned that the fiber regimen, when employed in a number of British hospitals, resulted in a dramatic reduction in surgery for diverticular disease. At the Royal Berkshire Hospital in Reading, for instance, one operation for diverticular disease—which in the past had been performed once every three weeks—is now being done only about once a year because patients are being put on the bran-fiber diet. Emergency operations for diverticulitis have fallen almost 50 percent at that hospital (*Acta Chirurgica Belgica,* November, 1979). Further evidence comes from the department of surgery at the Royal Liverpool Hospital in England where two surgeons tracked the progress over a period of five years of 100 patients admitted with acute diverticular disease. Seventy-five of the patients were treated with nothing but a high-fiber diet (two tablespoons of bran plus whole wheat bread, oats, vegetables, etc.) while 25 had surgery and were subsequently put on the high-fiber diet. In the entire group of 100 patients, 91 became and remained symptom-free, even after five years. Just as important, only 1 patient in the entire group developed a serious complication related to diverticular disease (*British Journal of Surgery,* February, 1980).

A number of British surgeons who have been at the forefront of fiber research have pointed out that if the colon was designed to function best on a high-fiber diet, then it only stands to reason that the rest of the digestive tract functions best on that same diet. To take one very obvious example, Dr. Painter has found that his bran-rich diet normally gives complete relief to patients with mild "first-degree" hemorrhoids, and is also successful with some more serious cases. Even when surgery may be necessary, he puts the patient on a bran diet before and after the operation.

The same low-fiber diet that can produce constipation, diverticular disease and hemorrhoids may also be involved in the genesis of appendicitis, gallbladder problems and hiatal hernia, other doctors believe. There even seems to be a definite connection between a low-fiber diet and varicose veins. A survey in one English hospital showed that patients with diverticular disease are more than twice as likely to have varicose veins as other people who are the same age and sex. As we explain in more detail in our special entry, "Varicose Veins," it seems that straining at stool forces blood down the leg veins, rendering certain crucial valves unable to function.

Selected Dietary Sources of Fiber

Food	Portion Size	Total Fiber (grams)	Food	Portion Size	Total Fiber (grams)
Spinach			Peanuts	¼ cup	3.0
cooked	1 cup	11.4	Orange	1 medium	2.9
Corn	1 cup	7.8	Rolled oats	1 cup	2.8
Peas,			Kale		
raw	1 cup	7.6	cooked	1 cup	2.8
Blackberries	1 cup	7.4	Coconut		
Sweet potato	1 medium	7.2	shredded	¼ cup	2.7
Apple	1 medium	6.8	Brown rice	1 cup	2.6
Whole wheat bread	2 slices	5.4	Apricots	4 medium	2.6
Potato	1 medium	5.3	Celery	2 stalks	2.4
Broccoli			Asparagus		
cooked	1 cup	5.2	chopped	1 cup	2.4
Almonds	¼ cup	5.1	Cabbage		
Raisins	½ cup	5.0	raw, shredded	1 cup	2.2
Zucchini	1 cup	5.0	Barley	½ cup	2.2
Plums	4 medium	4.6	Cucumbers		
Kidney beans	½ cup	4.5	sliced	1 cup	2.2
Carrots			Peaches	2 medium	2.0
cooked	1 cup	4.4	Cauliflower		
Squash, summer	1 cup	4.4	cooked	1 cup	1.8
White beans	½ cup	4.2	Tangerine	1 medium	1.8
Lentils	½ cup	3.7	Cherries	1 cup	1.7
Brussels sprouts	1 cup	3.6	Pineapple	1 cup	1.6
Pear	1 medium	3.5	Onions		
String beans	1 cup	3.4	cooked	½ cup	1.6
Banana	1 medium	3.2	Walnuts	¼ cup	1.6
Strawberries	1 cup	3.1	Tomato	1 medium	1.4
Pinto beans	½ cup	3.1	Lima beans		
Beets	1 cup	3.0	dried	½ cup	1.4

SOURCES:

1. "Composition of Foods Commonly Used in Diets for Persons with Diabetes," Diabetes Care, September/October, 1978.

2. McCance and Widdowson's The Composition of Foods, Elsevier/North-Holland Biomedical Press, 1978.

It's worth pointing out here that food fiber is not all the same. Some fiber seems especially valuable in prompting brisk functioning of the colon: whole wheat, with its bran, is probably the best example. Other forms of fiber, such as the pectin in apple, are valuable in helping to reduce cholesterol. Very recent research indicates that oat bran (which at this writing is not yet available commercially) can reduce virtually all blood fats, including triglycerides. Whole corn and rice seem to be unusually effective in slowing down the absorption of glucose, which makes them particularly valuable for people with blood sugar metabolism problems. Actually, we are still at the very beginning of the process of understanding which food fibers do what and we cannot produce a comprehensive list of foods whose fibers are valuable for particular purposes. That seems to be at least several years off. In the meantime, though, as far as better digestion is concerned, the evidence suggests that whole grains, carrots and peas are particularly valuable. Don't forget to drink extra water as well. Salad greens, by the way, are not at all effective for achieving easier or more regular movements. If this is a problem for you, by all means use one of our breakfast mixes containing bran, or eat our bran muffins or other bran foods.

EATING FOR TWO: YOU AND YOUR ULCER

Ulcers. Now there's a disease that even the medical establishment admits should be treated with diet. Bland, soft foods; frequent feedings; milk or cream when trouble seems to be brewing. Oh, there is drug therapy, too—and surgery if that fails—but we all know that doctors frequently advise ulcer patients to watch their diets.

What we don't all know, unfortunately, is that the dietary advice most commonly dispensed to ulcer patients is as scientifically mushy as the food they are supposed to thrive on.

It's probably tradition more than anything else that is responsible for the popularity of the "Sippy" or bland diet for ulcers, which features such foods as soft cereals, puddings, poached eggs and lots of milk. Despite its popularity, this diet has long been suspected of uselessness. In 1975 the medical journal, *Digestion* (vol. 13), took a scientific look at the question. Three Brazilian researchers studied 15 patients with ulcers. During the study, the patients spent a day eating a normal diet and a day eating a bland diet. Several times during each day, the researchers measured the acidity of the patients' digestive juices. They found that the normal diet generated no more acidity than the bland diet. "Based on our findings, we assume that there is no actual reason why the ulcer patient should be deprived of the varied appetizing meal in favor of a restricted diet of which no therapeutic advantage could so far be demonstrated," the researchers asserted.

What about the idea of frequent feedings? According to Jon I. Isenberg, M.D., of the Veterans Administration Wadsworth Medical Center in Los Angeles, frequent feedings raise gastric acidity by making the stomach work more often, leading to further lining erosion (*Journal of the American Medical Association,* February 2, 1979). Dr. Isenberg adds that more than three out of four hospitals make the mistake of putting patients on a bland diet/frequent feeding regimen.

That leaves milk. Surely milk cannot be bad for ulcer patients, can it? What could possibly be more soothing than milk? Or so it would seem. But body chemistry is often full of surprises, and when scientists got around to measuring the effect milk really has, they discovered that while it does in fact neutralize acid at first, after a few minutes milk actually *increases* the amount of gastric acid (*Annals of Internal Medicine,* March, 1976). This "rebound" effect of milk is now widely recognized by medical researchers, although the information seems to be taking its time in reaching the average doctor.

What *is* reliably known about healing or at least soothing ulcers with diet? Not much, to tell you the truth. But certainly one of the more intriguing studies we have seen —dating back to the 1940s—involves, of all things, cabbage juice. Garnett Cheney, M.D., treated 13 ulcer patients with a mixture of four to five ounces of fresh cabbage juice and one to two ounces of celery juice five times daily. In 11 of 13 cases the ulcers disappeared in six to nine days (*California Medicine,* January, 1949). Seven years later, Dr. Cheney and his associates healed over 90 percent of 45 ulcer patients with a cabbage juice concentrate derived from fresh pressed raw cabbage. In 1963, a Hungarian study appeared in the *Journal of the American Medical Women's Association* (vol. 18, no. 6), in which the "great majority" of 162 ulcer patients enjoyed "complete relief from pain" after receiving a raw cabbage juice derivative.

Dr. Cheney used one quart of cabbage juice a day to heal his patients. To render the juice more palatable, he added celery juice made from both stalks and greens, pineapple juice, tomato juice or citrus juice. Chilling the juice, he said, helps to improve the flavor.

At this point, you may well be wondering how it could be possible that a bland diet and milk regimen, which seems so reasonable and is so popular, could be largely useless, while something as silly sounding and unknown as cabbage juice therapy might actually work. We got some insight into this paradox when we talked with Dr. Cheney several years ago. When he and his colleagues were carrying out their work, he told us, they found that other doctors regarded cabbage juice as "a joke." Particularly at that time —the early 50s—when miracle drugs were all the rage, cabbage juice seemed hopelessly primitive. Trying to overcome the prejudice against it, the doctors came up with the idea that there was a "factor" in cabbage juice that was specifically for healing ulcers, a factor that they dubbed "vitamin U," the "U" standing for ulcers. They hoped the new terminology might win new respect for their research, but it didn't.

To our knowledge, this early work has never been confirmed or disproved by other Western scientists. So make of it what you will. You could certainly do worse than to enjoy a salad of fresh raw cabbage leaves before your nonbland dinner. In fact, chewing those cabbage leaves could do you a world of good even if vitamin U turns out to stand for "useless." Dr. Isenberg, whom we mentioned before, has reported that animal research findings indicate that food not chewed thoroughly does not have the chance to mix properly with urogastrone, a substance secreted by the salivary glands. Urogastrone protects the intestinal lining from erosion in experimental animals, so chewing food thoroughly may be the best safeguard against peptic ulcer.

One of the problems with ulcer research—and why there are so many unanswered questions about the best treatment for ulcers—is that the condition often heals itself with time. It's also likely that a substantial number of cases involve emotional factors and the stresses of home or workplace.

But regardless of the underlying cause of stomach ulcers, their healing still requires the proper nutrition, for the obvious reason that the new tissue which must be synthesized by the body to heal the erosion has an absolute requirement for certain nutrients. As you will see in more detail later in this book, where we discuss recuperation, the chief nutrients involved in healing are vitamins A and C and the mineral zinc. In fact, there is some indication that zinc may be of special importance to ulcer patients. According to Donald J. Frommer, M.D., of the department of gastroenterology at the Prince of Wales Hospital in Sydney, Australia, zinc can speed the healing of gastric ulcers even in patients who show no signs of zinc deficiency (*Medical Journal of Australia,* November 22, 1975).

Recognizing that emotional factors play an undeniable role in the development and healing of ulcers, Dr. Frommer conducted a double-blind study. Rather than simply giving ulcer patients some zinc and observing how rapidly they improved, he simultaneously gave another group of patients capsules that appeared to be identical but were actually placebos, or inert pills containing nothing but milk sugar. And to be sure he did not distort the results by any preconceptions he had, he made certain that he and other doctors did not know the difference between the capsules either. Only the hospital pharmacist knew which patients were receiving zinc and which were receiving the placebo.

The patients—all of whom had been x-rayed—were told to take one capsule three times a day before meals. They were also advised to reduce—or if possible to stop —smoking and drinking alcohol. They were also advised not to take aspirin, since aspirin can aggravate ulcers. Three weeks later, at the end of the trial, a second series of x-rays were taken. It was determined that 4 of 10 patients who took zinc (150 milligrams a day) had *complete* healing of ulcers. Only 1 out of 8 patients given placebos had complete healing. In addition, all 10 of the zinc group showed *some* degree of healing, while 2 out of 8 in the placebo group showed no healing. These results are not exactly overwhelming, but they do suggest, at the very least, that anyone worried about healing up an ulcer should do a quick audit of his or her zinc status. Foods rich in zinc include, among others: meat, cheese, eggs, wheat germ and other whole grain products, sunflower seeds, pumpkin seeds and nuts. There is no way, however, that you can get 150 milligrams of zinc a day from food—unless you were to eat lots of Atlantic oysters, which are exceptionally high in zinc, but which we don't recommend because of the possibility of pollution. What you could do, though, is to put more zinc in your diet from nuts and seeds and perhaps some meat and cheese, although you don't want to go overboard on fats. You might also want to think of zinc supplements.

HEARTBURN, HIATAL HERNIA AND OTHER UPSETS

Chronic indigestion after eating may erupt from bad food, bad table manners, or bad vibes. Or none of the above. So make sure you see your doctor if you have chronic indigestion. Your physician may be able to get a handle on your problem faster than you think. If your answer is yes to an inquiry about smoking, you already have one good clue as to what might be causing your heartburn. And if your doctor sees that your waistline could be measured in yards as well as inches, you'll probably be told that you may lose your problem as you lose weight. In fact, you could lose it even sooner, because it may simply be the sheer size of the meals you're packing down that is causing your distress. And if gas is your problem, your doctor may point out that learning not to swallow air as you eat could turn off that darn bubble machine.

As we mentioned in our brief discussion of ulcers, trying to reduce stomach acidity by eating bland foods or drinking milk usually doesn't work. Frequently, neither do antacids. Doctors at the Veterans Administration Wadsworth Medical Center and the University of California at Los Angeles, found that antacids provide no more relief for ulcer pain than do worthless placebos (*Gastroenterology,* January, 1977). Besides that, a review in the *New England Journal of Medicine* (March 7, 1974) by two doctors at the University of Wisconsin Medical School points out that "no antacid is free of hazard. Severe side effects can be expected from all commonly used preparations if they are used to excess." Among those hazards are sodium overload (from sodium bicarb) and excessive loss of phosphorus as a result of binding by aluminum hydroxide, another common antacid ingredient (which can also cause constipation).

Actually, it's no wonder that so many Americans suffer from heartburn. According to researchers at the University of California at Los Angeles, the two major promoters of stomach acid are protein and dairy products. While fat by itself does not stimulate acid production, it can lead to a different kind of indigestion, because the digestive juices have to work harder to cut through fat. And while they are working, they may call out reinforcements in the form of hydrochloric acid, which besides attacking the food you just ate, may also attack your stomach wall or cause heartburn.

In practical terms, what all this means is that fat-rich meat, the kind most people eat, is an invitation to heartburn. Eat a particularly large piece of fatty meat—with all that protein and fat—and you're giving indigestion an engraved invitation. And if you follow the main course with a big portion of ice cream (which you hope will take care of all that acid) you could be in for even worse trouble when your stomach develops acid rebound from that big shot of calcium.

Or, looking at it in a more positive light, to the extent that you stay away from a high-protein meal (which basically means staying away from large servings of meat, poultry or fish) and stay away from fats (in meat, butter, mayonnaise, dressings and such), you'll be making it a lot harder for heartburn to light its fire. Luckily, there's no shortage of recipes in our book that are moderate in protein and very low in fat.

Oddly enough, our old friend bran may be helpful to some folks with heartburn and nausea, at least when those conditions are present along with diverticulosis. Dr. Painter and his colleagues reported in the *British Medical Journal* (April 15, 1972) that among 70 patients with diverticular disease of the colon, 11 often felt nauseated. But after several weeks of taking an average of two tablespoons of bran daily, 7 of those patients reported their nausea had simply disappeared. Two others said their symptoms were relieved. Many cases of heartburn were also relieved by the bran regimen. In another study, 19 out of 22 patients complaining of nausea were either completely or largely relieved after taking bran (*British Medical Journal,* February 21, 1976). As to why bran should have a beneficial effect on heartburn, Dr. Painter and his colleagues propose a commonsense theory: If fiber-rich foods such as bran are necessary for the normal function of the lower bowel, then they are probably also needed for the health of the whole digestive tract.

If you happen to live in an area where you can obtain fresh papaya, you may find that this delectable food can make your digestion a little sweeter. That's because papaya naturally contains a group of enzymes known as papain—one of which has a special function of breaking down protein while another is an especially potent enzyme that helps break down *all* food in the stomach. Papaya also has several supplementary enzymes—including amylase, lipase and pectase. The presence of these accompanying enzymes is very desirable, because they increase the digestive activity of papain. Lipase, for instance, specializes in breaking down fatty tissue, which in some cases prevents the protein-attacking enzymes from doing their work.

You may also want to put papaya enzymes to work for you by sprinkling some powdered papain on lean, tough cuts of meat before cooking. The enzymes go to work as the food cooks and make it considerably more tender and more digestible. However, make sure that the papain you buy is not mixed with salt or monosodium glutamate.

BREAKFASTS

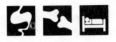

Powerhouse Pancakes

Makes three servings
1 cup (250 ml) whole
   wheat flour
1½ teaspoons (7 ml) *Baking
   Powder*
⅓ cup (80 ml) bran
½ cup (125 ml) soy flakes
2 tablespoons (30 ml)
   honey
1 tablespoon (15 ml)
   safflower oil
1¾–2 cups (425–500 ml)
   buttermilk
2 eggs, beaten

Mix dry ingredients together. Add remaining ingredients to beaten eggs. Combine the two mixtures in a medium bowl. Adjust buttermilk to thickness of batter desired.

Spoon pancakes on griddle over moderate heat until bubbles appear over the top. Turn once to finish cooking. Makes 8 to 10 pancakes.

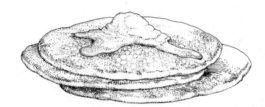

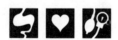

Fruit-full Cereal Bowl

Makes one serving
1 unpeeled apple
½ banana
¼ cup (60 ml) white or red
   grapes, halved
½ cup (125 ml) rolled oats
1 tablespoon (15 ml) bran
1 tablespoon (15 ml) wheat
   germ
1 teaspoon (5 ml) sunflower
   seeds

Cube the fruit into a cereal bowl, then sprinkle with the oats, bran, wheat germ and sunflower seeds. Serve plain, just tossing the cereal with the fruit to moisten, or with milk or orange juice.

Variation: Try any seasonal fruits that suit your fancy: oranges, pineapples, pears, strawberries, melons and plums are a few suggestions.

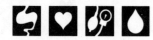

Orange-Cinnamon Cracked Wheat Cereal

Makes four to six servings
1 cup (250 ml) cracked wheat
4 cups (1 l) water
½ teaspoon (2 ml) cinnamon
½ cup (125 ml) raisins
  freshly squeezed orange juice

Because of its nutty flavor and the addition of orange juice, this cereal can be served quite nicely without milk or honey.

To shorten cooking time, the cracked wheat can be soaked in the water overnight. In the morning, combine the cracked wheat, water, cinnamon and raisins in a heavy saucepan and bring to a boil. Lower heat and simmer until the wheat is tender, from 10 to 30 minutes. Add juice to taste. Serve hot.

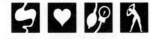

Sunshine Oatmeal

Makes two servings
1½ cups (375 ml) water
⅔ cup (150 ml) rolled oats
5–6 pitted prunes, chopped
  dash cinnamon
1 tablespoon (15 ml)
    sunflower seeds,
    toasted
1 teaspoon (5 ml) honey
  freshly squeezed orange
    juice

Bring water to a boil. Stir in oats, prunes and cinnamon. Simmer four to five minutes until oatmeal is thick. Stir in sunflower seeds and honey.
Serve hot with freshly squeezed orange juice instead of milk.

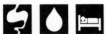

Creamy Apple Porridge

Makes two servings
½ unpeeled apple, coarsely
    chopped
⅓ cup (80 ml) rolled oats
¾ cup (175 ml) water
¼ teaspoon (1 ml) cinnamon

Place apple in a blender and process on low speed until smooth. Place applesauce with the oats in a medium saucepan with the water, add cinnamon, and cook about 5 to 10 minutes, until the oatmeal is creamy.

SOUPS

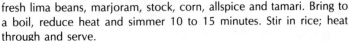

Fresh Lima Chowder

This is a nice soup to make in quantity. Freeze a portion for later use, if desired.

Saute onions and peppers in oil until slightly tender. Add the fresh lima beans, marjoram, stock, corn, allspice and tamari. Bring to a boil, reduce heat and simmer 10 to 15 minutes. Stir in rice; heat through and serve.

Variation: Add one cup (250 ml) sliced okra when adding the lima beans.

Makes 10 servings
1 cup (250 ml) chopped red onions
1 cup (250 ml) chopped sweet red peppers
1 tablespoon (15 ml) corn oil
2 cups (500 ml) lima beans
1½ teaspoons (7 ml) marjoram
4 cups (1 l) *Chicken Stock* or *Vegetable Stock*
1 cup (250 ml) fresh or frozen corn
¼ teaspoon (1 ml) allspice
2 teaspoons (10 ml) tamari
1 cup (250 ml) cooked brown rice

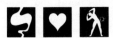

Browned Potato and Cabbage Soup

This soup became an instant favorite, a demonstration of how simple ingredients can be transformed into sought-after fare.

In a kettle or stockpot, cook the potatoes and cabbage in the water until tender. While these vegetables are simmering, place onions in a large skillet with the oil and saute until golden. Add flour and toss until onions are coated. Continue to cook and stir over medium heat for a minute or two, then add milk slowly, stirring after each addition until milk is incorporated. Add tamari. Stir onion sauce into undrained potatoes and cabbage. A dash of cayenne pepper can be added for flavoring. Simmer soup an additional 10 to 15 minutes over low heat. For a thicker soup, remove one cup (250 ml) of vegetables and process in a blender on low speed until smooth, and stir into the soup. Serve hot. Reheated, the soup is even more delicious.

Makes six servings
3 cups (750 ml) cubed potatoes
6–7 cups (1.5–1.75 l) chopped cabbage (about 1 pound [450 g])
1 cup (250 ml) water
3 cups (750 ml) chopped yellow onions
2 teaspoons (10 ml) corn oil
2 tablespoons (30 ml) whole wheat flour
2½ cups (625 ml) skim milk
1 tablespoon (15 ml) tamari
dash cayenne pepper

Potato-Buttermilk Soup

Makes four servings

1½ cups (375 ml) cubed
    potatoes
1 small carrot, sliced
1 small onion, finely chopped
1 clove garlic, minced
1 teaspoon (5 ml) tamari
1 tablespoon (15 ml) fresh
    parsley
¼ cup (60 ml) bran
1 cup (250 ml) buttermilk
freshly grated nutmeg

Place potatoes, carrot, onion, garlic, tamari and parsley in a saucepan with water to cover. Bring to a boil; reduce heat and simmer ingredients until they are tender, adding bran to the simmering vegetables in the last three to five minutes of cooking. Place buttermilk in a blender and add half of the vegetable mixture. Process on low speed until smooth. Return blended mixture to saucepan and heat, but do not boil. Serve the soup hot, topped with a dash of nutmeg. Makes about 3½ cups (875 ml) of soup.

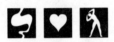

Tomato-Lentil Soup

Makes six to eight servings

⅔ cup (150 ml) dried lentils
4–5 cups (1–1.25 l) water
½ head garlic (8–10 cloves)
2 stalks celery, sliced
3 carrots, sliced
1 teaspoon (5 ml) tamari
⅔ cup (150 ml) tomato paste
1 tablespoon (15 ml) fresh
    parsley, chopped
1 teaspoon (5 ml) basil
½ teaspoon (2 ml) marjoram

Place lentils and four cups (1 l) of water in a saucepan or large skillet. Bring to a boil, reduce heat and simmer. Peel and mince garlic; add with celery and carrots to lentils. Simmer until vegetables and lentils are tender. Stir in tamari, tomato paste, herbs and enough additional water to make desired consistency. Leftovers can be frozen for later use.

Variation: For *Chili-Lentil Soup,* add one tablespoon (15 ml) of chili powder and ½ teaspoon (2 ml) of cumin powder.

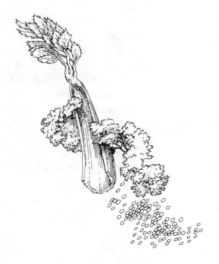

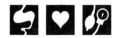

Lentil Soup with Dill

Makes four servings

1 tablespoon (15 ml) sunflower
 oil
2 onions, chopped
3 cloves garlic, minced
2 carrots, thinly sliced
1 cup (250 ml) dried lentils
1 quart (1 l) *Chicken Stock* or
 Vegetable Stock
½ cup (125 ml) fresh dillweed
¼ teaspoon (1 ml) thyme
¼ teaspoon (1 ml) celery seeds
 pinch cloves
 pinch allspice

Warm the oil in a large skillet or heavy-bottom saucepan. Saute onions and garlic until onions are translucent.

Add carrots, lentils and stock. Bring to a boil. Add seasonings, reduce heat, cover and simmer for about 40 minutes, until the lentils and vegetables are tender. Serve hot.

Note: Two tablespoons (30 ml) of dried dillweed can be substituted if no fresh dill is available.

SALADS

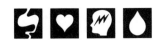

Three Bean Salad

Makes six servings

1½ cups (375 ml) cooked black
 beans
1½ cups (375 ml) cooked
 kidney beans
1 cup (250 ml) cooked green
 beans
2 scallions, chopped
1 tablespoon (15 ml) chopped
 fresh parsley
⅓ cup (80 ml) cider vinegar
1 teaspoon (5 ml) tamari
1 teaspoon (5 ml) honey
1 tablespoon (15 ml) sesame
 tahini
 lettuce or spinach leaves
 parsley sprigs (garnish)

Combine beans, preferably while still hot from cooking, in a large mixing bowl with scallions and parsley. Place vinegar in a small saucepan and heat, adding tamari, honey and tahini when vinegar comes to a boil. Simmer one minute while stirring to combine, and then pour over the bean combination. Refrigerate until well chilled before serving. Makes four cups (1 l). Serve on a bed of lettuce or spinach, and garnish with parsley.

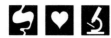

Green Pea Salad

Makes four servings
2 cups (500 ml) green peas
¼ cup (60 ml) finely chopped
   scallions
1 unpeeled tart apple, finely
   chopped
1 tablespoon (15 ml) minced
   mint leaves or fresh
   parsley
Creamy Garlic Dressing

This recipe takes advantage of complementary flavors. Toss with Creamy Garlic Dressing *for a colorful, tasty dish.*

Cook the green peas in a small amount of water, three to seven minutes, just until tender. Drain, reserving liquid for later use.

Add the scallions, the apple and the mint. Toss with enough dressing to moisten. Chill before serving.

Chick-pea Salad

Makes four servings
1 cup (250 ml) shredded
   cabbage
1 cup (250 ml) cooked
   chick-peas
½ cup (125 ml) mung bean
   sprouts
2 tablespoons (30 ml) olive oil
2 tablespoons (30 ml) mild
   vinegar
1 teaspoon (5 ml) basil
   lettuce
   parsley (garnish)

Combine cabbage, chick-peas and sprouts in a serving bowl. Mix olive oil, vinegar and basil together and pour over salad. Toss and serve on a bed of lettuce. Garnish with parsley.

Variation: For a main dish, add one cup (250 ml) of cooked brown rice to the cabbage, and stir one tablespoon (15 ml) of yogurt into the dressing. Serve chilled.

Cabbage and Pineapple Salad

Makes four servings
2 cups (500 ml) shredded
   cabbage
½ cup (125 ml) chopped
   pineapple
2 tablespoons (30 ml) yogurt
⅛ teaspoon (0.5 ml) thyme
   dash freshly grated nutmeg

Toss cabbage and pineapple with the yogurt, thyme and nutmeg. Serve chilled.

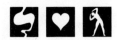

Garlic Bean Salad

Makes four servings

1 cup (250 ml) dried baby lima
   beans
1 stalk celery, finely chopped
2 tablespoons (30 ml) minced
   scallions
1 glove garlic, crushed
1 tablespoon (15 ml) minced
   fresh parsley
¼ cup (60 ml) *Vinaigrette*
   Dressing

Soak dried beans overnight. Drain, rinse and cover with water. (Or, wash beans and place with water in a saucepan. Bring to a boil, cook for one or two minutes, remove from heat and cover. Allow to stand for one hour.) Then cook beans until tender. Drain, and set aside to cool.

Combine celery, scallions, garlic and parsley in a small bowl. Toss with beans and pour on *Vinaigrette Dressing.* Place in the refrigerator and marinate three to four hours or overnight. Serve chilled.

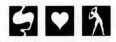

Cumin Cabbage Salad

Makes six servings

4 cups (1 l) finely shredded
   cabbage
¼ cup (60 ml) minced green
   peppers
1 tablespoon (15 ml) minced
   fresh parsley
2 tablespoons (30 ml) safflower
   oil
1 tablespoon (15 ml) lemon
   juice
2 teaspoons (10 ml) yogurt
½ teaspoon (2 ml) cumin
   powder

Combine cabbage with green peppers and parsley in a large bowl. Thoroughly mix oil, lemon juice, yogurt and cumin and pour over salad. Toss to combine.

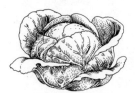

BREADS

Poppy Seed Rolls and Cinnamon-Raisin Bread

*Makes one dozen rolls and
one loaf*
2 tablespoons (30 ml) active
dry yeast
½ cup (125 ml) lukewarm
water
6 tablespoons (90 ml)
honey
2½ cups (625 ml) lukewarm
buttermilk
1 tablespoon (15 ml) tamari
1½ cups (375 ml) wheat
germ
6–6½ cups (1.5–1.6 l) whole
wheat flour
6 tablespoons (90 ml) soy
or corn oil
poppy seeds
2 teaspoons (10 ml)
cinnamon
¾–1 cup (175–250 ml) raisins

Something a little different: here we're making two specialty breads at the same time from one basic recipe. Both are beautiful to look at, delicious to eat.

Dissolve the yeast in the water in a large bowl, and stir in the honey. When the yeast is bubbly, add the buttermilk, tamari, wheat germ and 2 cups (500 ml) of the flour. With a hand mixer on high speed, mix the wheat germ, flour and yeast mixture for five minutes. Add ¼ cup (60 ml) of the oil and the remaining wheat flour, 1 cup (250 ml) at a time, stirring after each addition. When the dough holds together, turn it out onto a floured surface and knead until smooth, adding only enough flour to keep the dough from sticking. Oil a large bowl or kettle, and turn the ball of dough around in the oil until it is coated. Cover the container and allow dough to rest in a warm place until doubled in bulk. Punch the dough down until it collapses, form again into a ball, and cover, returning to a warm place. When the dough has doubled a second time, punch the air out again, and turn the dough onto a floured surface.

For *Poppy Seed Rolls,* make small balls of dough, about two inches (5 cm) in diameter, and coat them with a little of the remaining two tablespoons (30 ml) of oil. Place the balls (about 12 will do) in the bottom of a lightly oiled 8-inch (20-cm) round cake pan. Sprinkle generously with poppy seeds and set aside to rise.

For *Cinnamon-Raisin Bread,* sprinkle cinnamon over the remaining dough a little at a time as you knead the raisins into the dough. Try to incorporate as many raisins as possible, or they may look sparse once the dough has risen. Place dough in a lightly oiled 8½ × 4½-inch (22 × 11-cm) bread pan.

When the rolls have risen almost double in bulk, place them in a preheated 400° F. (200° C.) oven. After 15 minutes, turn the oven down to 350° F. (175° C.) and bake the rolls about 20 minutes longer, until they are browned and baked through. When *Cinnamon-Raisin Bread* has risen to almost double in bulk, place the bread in the oven for about 45 minutes, just until browned and baked through.

When each of the breads is done baking, remove from the oven and turn out on cooling racks. The *Poppy Seed Rolls* will break apart easily for serving.

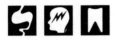

Pumpernickel Bread

Makes two loaves

1 tablespoon (15 ml) active dry yeast
¼ cup (60 ml) lukewarm potato stock (water in which potatoes have been cooked)
2 tablespoons (30 ml) corn oil
2 tablespoons (30 ml) blackstrap molasses
2 teaspoons (10 ml) finely grated lemon rind
1 tablespoon (15 ml) caraway seeds
1 teaspoon (5 ml) kelp powder
1 teaspoon (5 ml) tamari
1 tablespoon (15 ml) carob powder
2 cups (500 ml) skim milk or buttermilk
½ cup (125 ml) gluten flour
2 cups (500 ml) whole wheat flour
2 cups (500 ml) rye flour
1 cup (250 ml) bran
½ cup (125 ml) wheat germ

Dissolve yeast in the potato stock. Place oil, molasses, lemon rind, caraway seeds, kelp, tamari and carob powder in a large mixing bowl. Scald milk and add to mixture, stirring to combine. When the milk mixture is lukewarm, add the yeast, gluten flour and 1 cup (250 ml) whole wheat flour. Beat with an electric mixer for 5 minutes. Add ½ cup (125 ml) whole wheat flour, then the rye flour, 1 cup (250 ml) at a time, beating after each addition. Add bran and wheat germ, stirring until dough is smooth. Place remaining whole wheat flour on kneading surface and turn the dough out to knead. Incorporate flour until dough is no longer sticky. When dough has been kneaded until smooth and elastic, place in a large, oiled bowl, cover and leave to rise until double in size, 1½ to 2 hours. Punch down dough. Divide between two 8½ × 4½-inch (22 × 11-cm) bread pans and let rise until double, about 1 hour. Bake 50 minutes in a preheated 375° F. (190° C.) oven. Remove from pans and cool on a rack before slicing.

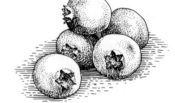

Blueberry Corn Bread

Makes 10 servings

2 cups (500 ml) whole grain cornmeal
½ cup (125 ml) bran
1 teaspoon (5 ml) baking soda
1 teaspoon (5 ml) *Baking Powder*
1 cup (250 ml) blueberries
2 eggs
¼ cup (60 ml) maple syrup
1½ cups (375 ml) yogurt

Combine dry ingredients in a large mixing bowl; add blueberries and toss to coat. In a medium mixing bowl, beat eggs, adding maple syrup and yogurt. Add to dry ingredients, stirring just enough to combine. Some lumps can remain. Place in a lightly greased 8 × 8-inch (20 × 20-cm) baking pan. Bake in a preheated 425° F. (220° C.) oven for about 25 minutes, until golden brown.

Sunflower-Buckwheat Bread

Makes one loaf

½ cup (125 ml) sunflower
   seeds
2 cups (500 ml) buckwheat
   flour
1½ teaspoons (7 ml) baking
   soda
½ teaspoon (2 ml) *Baking
   Powder*
⅛ teaspoon (0.5 ml) mace
1¾ cups (425 ml) buttermilk
¼ cup (60 ml) honey
1 teaspoon (5 ml) tamari

Place sunflower seeds in a blender and grind with short bursts on high speed.

Mix the dry ingredients together in a medium mixing bowl. Stir together the buttermilk, honey and tamari, and add to the dry ingredients, stirring until combined. Place the batter in a lightly oiled 8½ × 4½-inch (22 × 11-cm) bread pan and bake in a preheated 350° F. (175° C.) oven for about 50 minutes.

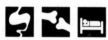

Potato-Corn Muffins

Makes one dozen

1 cup (250 ml) whole grain
   cornmeal
4 teaspoons (20 ml) *Baking
   Powder*
2 teaspoons (10 ml) brewer's
   yeast
¼ teaspoon (1 ml) freshly grated
   nutmeg
1 egg, beaten
1 cup (250 ml) soft mashed
   potatoes
2 tablespoons (30 ml) corn oil
1 cup (250 ml) yogurt
1 tablespoon (15 ml) honey
1 teaspoon (5 ml) medium
   unsulfured molasses

Here's a good way to use leftover mashed potatoes. If the potatoes are stiff, add some yogurt and beat until fluffy.

Stir together the cornmeal, *Baking Powder,* brewer's yeast and nutmeg in a medium mixing bowl. Add egg and remaining ingredients. Beat until smooth.

Lightly oil a muffin pan and divide batter between the 12 muffin cups. Bake in a preheated 350° F. (175° C.) oven about 30 to 35 minutes.

Currant-Buckwheat Muffins

Makes one dozen
1 cup (250 ml) buckwheat flour
¼ cup (60 ml) whole grain
    cornmeal
2 teaspoons (10 ml) *Baking
    Powder*
½ cup (125 ml) currants
1 cup (250 ml) skim milk
2 tablespoons (30 ml) corn oil
2 tablespoons (30 ml) medium
    unsulfured molasses
2 eggs, beaten

Combine dry ingredients in a medium mixing bowl and add currants. In a separate bowl, add milk, corn oil and molasses to the eggs and stir into the flour mixture until smooth. Place batter in 12 lightly oiled muffin cups and bake at 375° F. (190° C.) for 20 minutes.

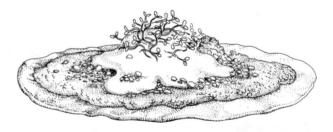

MAIN DISHES

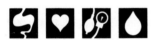

Zucchini Tortilla

Makes one serving
1 corn tortilla
½ cup (125 ml) *Mexican Lentils*
½ medium zucchini, shredded
3 tablespoons (45 ml) yogurt
2 tablespoons (30 ml) alfalfa
    sprouts

You don't have to be Mexican to love this dish. Our taste-testers were unanimous in their verdict: Olé!

Heat corn tortilla briefly in a hot skillet or under the broiler. Place on serving plate and cover with *Mexican Lentils,* or any moist bean recipe. Top with zucchini, spoon yogurt over zucchini and crown with alfalfa sprouts.

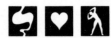

Bean Enchiladas

Makes four servings

1 cup (250 ml) cooked kidney, pinto or black beans
1 cup (250 ml) cooked soybeans
1 small onion, chopped
2 cloves garlic, minced
1 tablespoon (15 ml) chili powder
1 teaspoon (5 ml) cumin powder
1 teaspoon (5 ml) tamari
1 tablespoon (15 ml) lemon juice
8 corn tortillas
3 cups (750 ml) *Hot Taco Sauce*
½ cup (125 ml) shredded sharp cheese

Mash or process beans in a blender on low speed until smooth. Steam-stir onion and garlic in a small amount of water until they begin to brown. Add spices, tamari, lemon juice and beans. Soften corn tortillas by dipping each one briefly into boiling water in a small skillet. Place about ⅓ cup (80 ml) of bean mixture on each tortilla, and roll up. Place seam-side down in a casserole dish and cover with *Hot Taco Sauce*. Sprinkle with cheese. Bake in a preheated 350° F. (175° C.) oven for 15 to 20 minutes, or until sauce bubbles and cheese melts. The remaining bean mixture can be used to thicken soups or to spread on sandwiches.

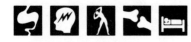

Spaghetti with Herbed Cheese

Makes four servings

1 cup (250 ml) ricotta cheese
4 cloves garlic, crushed
½ cup (125 ml) walnuts, ground
¼ cup (60 ml) minced fresh basil
2 tablespoons (30 ml) minced fresh parsley
1 tablespoon (15 ml) grated Parmesan cheese
1 teaspoon (5 ml) kelp powder
¾ pound (340 g) whole wheat spaghetti
1 cup (250 ml) peas

"Great! Nice change from a sauce," said those encountering this pasta dish.

In a medium bowl, blend together the ricotta cheese and garlic, using a wooden spoon. Grind the walnuts in a blender with short bursts at high speed. Add walnuts, herbs, cheese and kelp powder to ricotta and stir to combine.

Bring a large kettle of water to a boil and cook the pasta until firm-tender. At the same time, cook the peas in a small amount of water, or steam them just until tender. Drain the pasta and peas, and toss in a serving bowl with enough herbed cheese to thoroughly coat. Serve hot.

Note: If fresh basil is unavailable, substitute ¼ cup (60 ml) minced fresh parsley for the basil, and add one tablespoon (15 ml) of dried basil to the mixture. (Eliminate the two tablespoons (30 ml) of fresh parsley called for in the original recipe.)

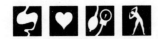

Lentil Risotto

Makes six servings
2 yellow onions, chopped
1 cup (250 ml) brown rice
½ cup (125 ml) lentils
3 cups (750 ml) *Chicken Stock*
     or *Vegetable Stock*
dash cloves

Serve as is, or use as a basis for spaghetti sauce or a Mexican dinner by adding tomato sauce and herbs, or garlic and spices. High in protein.

Place the onions in a heavy-bottom saucepan, and steam-stir in a little water until translucent. Add the brown rice, and continue stirring another minute. Add the lentils and broth, and flavor with a small pinch of ground cloves.

Bring to a boil, reduce heat and simmer uncovered about 35 minutes, until most of the water is absorbed. Do not stir. Cover pan and place over very low heat until remaining water is absorbed. This should take about 5 minutes.

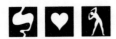

Pasta Sauce with *Lentil Risotto*

Makes three servings
1 small onion, chopped
¼ cup (60 ml) finely chopped
     carrots
2 cups (500 ml) *Lentil Risotto*
⅔ cup (150 ml) tomato paste
1 cup (250 ml) *Chicken Stock*
     or *Vegetable Stock*
1 tablespoon (15 ml) grated
     Parmesan cheese
2 teaspoons (10 ml) oregano
2 teaspoons (10 ml) basil
1 teaspoon (5 ml) tamari
½ pound (225 g) whole wheat
     pasta

Steam-stir the onion and carrots in a few spoonfuls of water until tender. Stir in *Lentil Risotto* and tomato paste until combined. Add stock, cheese, herbs and tamari. Simmer over low heat until flavors are combined, about 20 minutes.

To cook pasta, bring a large kettle half-filled with water to a boil, stir in pasta and cook until pasta is tender, but still firm. Drain and serve with sauce.

Note: To cut calories, try this idea: for each serving, briefly simmer one cup (250 ml) of mung bean sprouts. Drain and use in place of pasta.

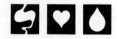

Makes six servings

Loaf:

2 cups (500 ml) cooked lentils
1 cup (250 ml) cooked brown
      rice
½ cup (125 ml) chopped green
      peppers
½ cup (125 ml) chopped onions
½ cup (125 ml) chopped
      tomatoes
¼ cup (60 ml) chopped celery
2 tablespoons (30 ml) yogurt
4 tablespoons (60 ml) tomato
      paste
3 tablespoons (45 ml) minced
      fresh parsley
½ cup (125 ml) soft whole grain
      bread crumbs
2 teaspoons (10 ml) basil
1 teaspoon (5 ml) oregano
½ teaspoon (2 ml) marjoram
¼ teaspoon (1 ml) dried hot red
      pepper flakes
2 eggs
1 egg white

Topping:

1 scallion, chopped
1 teaspoon (5 ml) blackstrap
      molasses
1 clove garlic
¾ cup (175 ml) *Vegetable Stock*
4 tablespoons (60 ml) tomato
      paste
¼ cup (60 ml) yogurt

Lentil Loaf with Tomato Topping

Combine all ingredients, except eggs, in large mixing bowl. Place eggs and egg white in a blender and add one cup (250 ml) of the lentil mixture. Process on low speed until smooth. Stir into lentil mixture and turn into a lightly oiled casserole dish.

Combine topping ingredients, and process in blender on medium speed until smooth.

Coat loaf with topping, reserving extra for use as a sauce, and bake in a preheated 350° F. (175° C.) oven for 45 minutes.

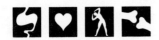

Autumn Cabbage Pie

Makes six servings

1 small onion, chopped
1 tablespoon (15 ml) sesame oil
4 cups (1 l) finely chopped
    cabbage
1 teaspoon (5 ml) oregano
1 teaspoon (5 ml) basil
    dash cayenne pepper
1 pound (450 g) tofu
3 eggs, separated
2 teaspoons (10 ml) tamari
    9-inch (23-cm) unbaked
      No-Roll Pie Crust

Saute the onion in the oil in a large skillet until it is translucent. Add the cabbage, oregano and basil; sprinkle with a few grains of cayenne, and stir occasionally over medium heat until the cabbage begins to soften, about 15 to 20 minutes. Remove from heat.

Combine the tofu, egg yolks and tamari in a blender and process on low speed until smooth. Beat the egg whites until stiff. Fold the tofu mixture into the slightly cooled cabbage. Stir to combine thoroughly. Fold in the beaten egg whites, then pour the entire mixture into the unbaked pie crust.

Bake in a preheated 350° F. (175° C.) oven for 45 minutes. Allow to cool slightly before serving. This pie is also tasty the following day. Let the pie return to room temperature if it has been refrigerated. It will serve well for packed lunches or picnics.

Zucchini Pie

Makes six to eight servings

1½ cups (375 ml) mashed
    potatoes
1 tablespoon (15 ml) sesame
    tahini
3 cups (750 ml) shredded
    zucchini
½ cup (125 ml) yogurt
¼ cup (60 ml) grated onions
2 eggs, beaten
½ teaspoon (2 ml) marjoram
½ teaspoon (2 ml) basil
½ teaspoon (2 ml) oregano
2 tablespoons (30 ml) grated
    Parmesan cheese

Combine mashed potatoes (they should be on the dry side) and sesame tahini. Press into a lightly oiled 9-inch (23-cm) pie plate as for a crust. Combine zucchini with remaining ingredients, except the cheese. Pour mixture into the potato crust and place pie in a preheated 350° F. (175° C.) oven for about 55 minutes. Sprinkle with the cheese about 45 minutes after the pie has been baking, and return to oven for remaining 10 minutes.

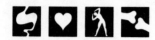

Potato Pizza

Makes six servings

3 cups (750 ml) cubed potatoes
1 cup (250 ml) whole wheat
    flour
1 large, ripe tomato
1 small onion
½ cup (125 ml) tomato paste
1 tablespoon (15 ml) olive oil
2 teaspoons (10 ml) oregano
1 clove garlic
1 cup (250 ml) ricotta cheese
2 tablespoons (30 ml) grated
    Parmesan cheese

Scrub potatoes, but do not peel before cutting into cubes. Boil until soft, then mash, and add flour until quite stiff. Spread mashed potato mixture in the bottoms of two lightly oiled 8 × 8-inch (20 × 20-cm) baking pans, or on the bottom of a lightly oiled cookie sheet with sides. Place in a preheated 400° F. (200° C.) oven for 15 minutes while preparing sauce.

In a blender, combine the tomato, onion, tomato paste, oil, oregano and garlic. Process on low speed until smooth.

After 15 minutes, remove crust from oven. Break up ricotta, and sprinkle evenly over the crust. Top with the sauce and sprinkle with Parmesan. Return to the oven for 15 or 20 minutes, until done. Serve hot.

SIDE DISHES

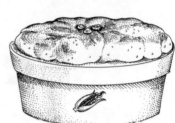

Corn Souffle

Makes six servings

1 tablespoon (15 ml) corn oil
2 tablespoons (30 ml) whole
    wheat flour
1 tablespoon (15 ml) brewer's
    yeast
1 cup (250 ml) skim milk
2 cups (500 ml) fresh or frozen
    corn
2 egg yolks, beaten
    dash cayenne pepper
2 egg whites, beaten stiff

Corn and brewer's yeast are both helpful in hypoglycemia. This souffle can be served with poached fish and a crisp, colorful salad.

Heat oil in a skillet, and stir in flour and brewer's yeast. Stir over medium heat for 2 or 3 minutes, then add milk gradually, stirring all the while, to avoid lumping. Bring to the boiling point and stir in corn and egg yolks. Cook about 10 minutes, stirring frequently to avoid sticking. Flavor with a few grains of cayenne pepper.

Remove from heat. Gradually fold in egg whites. Pour into an ungreased souffle dish and bake in a preheated 350° F. (175° C.) oven for 30 minutes. Serve immediately.

Minted Peas and Carrots

Makes two servings
1 cup (250 ml) sliced carrots
½ cup (125 ml) water
½ cup (125 ml) fresh or frozen
   peas
1 teaspoon (5 ml) chopped
   fresh mint
2 tablespoons (30 ml) yogurt

Bring carrots to a boil in the water. Cook until nearly tender, about 10 minutes. Add peas and cook just a couple of minutes longer, until the peas are slightly cooked, but still firm. Most of the water should have been absorbed during cooking. Drain, if necessary, saving liquid for stock, and stir in fresh mint and yogurt. Serve hot.

Oven-Baked French Fries

Makes four servings
4 medium potatoes
1 tablespoon (15 ml) sesame
   tahini

People can't believe these delicious "fries" haven't been deep fried. A terrific introduction to more natural foods.

Slice the potatoes in thin strips with a sharp knife. Place in a bowl and toss with the tahini until the potato strips are well coated. Place the potatoes on a lightly oiled baking sheet and place in a pre-heated 450° F. (230° C.) oven. Bake about 30 to 40 minutes, turning them several times as they bake. When they are well browned and tender, place them in a serving dish.

Sesame Baked Potatoes

Makes two servings
2 Idaho or other baking potatoes
2 teaspoons (10 ml) sesame
   tahini
   wheat germ

Wash, dry, but do not peel potatoes. Prick them with a fork or knife. Coat with sesame tahini and roll in wheat germ. Wrap each potato tightly in foil and bake in a 350° F. (175° C.) oven for one hour.

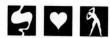

Basic Boiled Potatoes

Makes two servings
2 medium potatoes
1½ cups (375 ml) boiling water

Wash potatoes well, removing spots and sprouts, but do not peel. Cube potatoes and drop into boiling water. Cook covered 15 to 20 minutes, until tender. Drain well, reserving the potato water for use in soups or breads.

A folded towel can be placed over the pot for five minutes after draining the potatoes, to produce a mealy consistency.

Serve with a little yogurt, chopped parsley or chives.

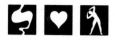

Potato-Sauerkraut Casserole

Makes six servings
1 medium onion, chopped
1 pound (450 g) sauerkraut
6 medium unpeeled potatoes, cubed
   yogurt, warmed

Place onion and sauerkraut in a large saucepan with enough water to generously cover. Place potatoes in another saucepan, covering with water.

Bring both pots to a boil, reduce heat, and simmer until potatoes are tender. Turn off heat. Drain potatoes and mash with enough yogurt to make a creamy, yet firm consistency. Drain sauerkraut well. (This will remove much of the sodium.)

In a large, lightly oiled casserole dish, place half of the mashed potatoes. Add the sauerkraut in a layer, then top with the remaining mashed potatoes.

Place casserole in a preheated 375° F. (190° C.) oven for 20 minutes, or until top is lightly browned. Serve hot.

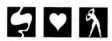

New Potatoes in Garlic Broth

new potatoes
Garlic Broth
dash tamari

If you have a garden, you will find tiny new potatoes just right for stovetop steaming in *Garlic Broth*. Wash them, but do not peel. Place potatoes in a saucepan or skillet, add enough *Garlic Broth* to keep the potatoes from sticking, and scoot the little fellas around the bottom of a pan with a wooden spoon until they are tender. Add only a drop or so of tamari per person to be served. The seasonings are delicate enough to allow the freshness to come through undisturbed. Serves as many as your supply of potatoes will allow.

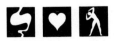

Mashed Potatoes with Yogurt

Makes two servings
2 medium potatoes
1½ cups (375 ml) boiling water
¼ cup (60 ml) yogurt, warmed

Wash potatoes well, removing spots and sprouts. Do not peel. Cube the potatoes and drop into boiling water. Cook covered 15 to 20 minutes, until tender. Drain well, reserving the water for use in soups or breads.

Mash potatoes with a fork or potato masher, adding just enough yogurt to make a moist, fluffy consistency. To make them even fluffier, the mashed potatoes can be left in the pan and placed over very low heat for four to five minutes.

Note: A little grated onion, chopped parsley, chives, watercress or a dash of freshly grated nutmeg can be added to the mashed potatoes.

Cabbage Topped with Cheese

Makes eight servings
10 cups (2.5 l) cabbage, thinly sliced (about 1½ pounds [675 g])
2 cloves garlic
1 teaspoon (5 ml) oregano
1 teaspoon (5 ml) basil
2 tablespoons (30 ml) grated Parmesan cheese

Place cabbage in a large saucepan along with garlic and spices in water to cover. Cook for 20 to 30 minutes, until tender. Stir occasionally, adding a little water if necessary to prevent scorching. Place cabbage, which should have cooked nearly dry, in a lightly oiled shallow baking pan. Sprinkle with the Parmesan cheese and place under a broiler until cheese begins to brown. Makes about six cups (1.5 l).

Steamed Cabbage Vinaigrette

Makes four servings
4 cups (1 l) finely shredded cabbage
2 tablespoons (30 ml) safflower oil
1 tablespoon (15 ml) cider vinegar
¼ teaspoon (1 ml) Dijon-style mustard

Steam the cabbage three to four minutes, just until crisp-tender. Combine oil, vinegar and mustard and pour over hot cabbage. Serve immediately or chill.

Stovetop Bulgur Stuffing

Makes four servings
1 small yellow onion, finely
    chopped
1 stalk celery with leaves,
    finely chopped
1 teaspoon (5 ml) basil
½ teaspoon (2 ml) oregano
½ teaspoon (2 ml) sage
½ teaspoon (2 ml) thyme
½ teaspoon (2 ml) marjoram
⅔ cup (150 ml) bulgur
1½ cups (375 ml) *Chicken
    Stock* or *Vegetable
    Stock*
1 cup (250 ml) soft whole
    grain bread cubes
1 tablespoon (15 ml) minced
    fresh parsley

Steam-stir onion and celery in a small amount of water in a medium skillet, until tender. Add a little water as necessary to prevent scorching.

Add herbs, bulgur and stock. Cook, covered, about 15 minutes until stock is absorbed and bulgur is soft. Stir in bread cubes and parsley, heat and serve.

MISCELLANEOUS

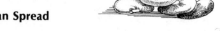

Pinto Bean Spread

Makes 1½ cups (375 ml)
1 cup (250 ml) cooked pinto
    beans
½ cup (125 ml) *Yogurt Cream
    Cheese*
½ teaspoon (2 ml) tamari
¼ teaspoon (1 ml) coriander
¼ teaspoon (1 ml) cumin
    powder
¼ teaspoon (1 ml) hot
    Hungarian paprika or
    dash cayenne pepper
½ clove garlic, crushed

We think this is one of the greatest spreads ever! Try it the next time a natural-foods friend visits.

Beans can be mashed with a fork and hand-blended with remaining ingredients. Chill. Use this spread on sandwiches or to fill celery stalks.

Potluck Sandwich Spread

Tofu Mayonnaise
Pinto Bean Spread
Hummus Tahini or *Soybean*
    Tahini Dip
Eggplant Dip
etc.

This is a grand way to make a clean sweep of the leftovers. When the end of the week rolls around, and little containers in your refrigerator are harboring remnants, gather them together to make a new creation. Unless things have been lying in wait too long, you may find the sum is tastier than its parts! Add only enough *Tofu Mayonnaise* to make the combination spreadable, unless you plan to serve a dip.

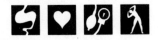

Makes 2½ cups (625 ml)
1 cup (250 ml) dried chick-peas

Oven-Baked Chick-peas

Soak chick-peas about 24 hours in enough water so that they remain covered as the peas expand. Place in a medium-size baking pan. Cover with water to one inch above chick-peas. Place aluminum foil over the baking dish to allow some steam to escape.

Bake in a preheated 350° F. (175° C.) oven for 2 to 2½ hours, until tender.

Note: Make best use of oven heat by adding chick-peas with other baking. If not quite tender when other baking is completed, leave for 30 minutes in the turned-off oven. Chick-peas can also be finished by simmering atop the stove.

High-Protein No-Roll Crust

Makes one 9-inch (23-cm) pie
crust
¾ cup (175 ml) whole wheat
    flour
2 tablespoons (30 ml) soy flour
2 tablespoons (30 ml) wheat
    germ
¼ cup (60 ml) soy oil
2 tablespoons (30 ml)
    buttermilk

Combine ingredients in a 9-inch (23-cm) pie plate. Toss with a fork until all the ingredients are combined, then press with fingers along bottom and sides of the plate. Fill and bake according to desired recipe.

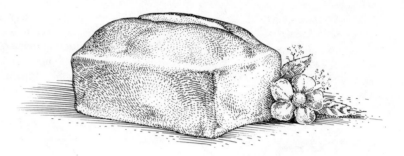

DESSERTS

Golden Light Pound Cake

Makes one loaf
2¼ cups (550 ml) whole wheat
     pastry flour
1½ teaspoons (7 ml) *Baking*
     Powder
½ teaspoon (2 ml) baking soda
¼ teaspoon (1 ml) cinnamon
¼ cup (60 ml) honey
¼ cup (60 ml) corn oil
1 teaspoon (5 ml) *Vanilla*
     Extract
2 eggs, beaten
1 cup (250 ml) buttermilk

A scrumptious pound cake with a nice density, just like the traditional loaf. But it's so much lighter than the traditional version (which calls for a pound of everything: butter, sugar, eggs!) that we're tempted to call it "Ounce Cake."

In a large mixing bowl, combine the dry ingredients. Beat liquid ingredients together in a medium bowl and stir into flour mixture until combined. Place batter in a lightly oiled 8½ × 4½-inch (22 × 11-cm) bread pan. Bake in a preheated 350° F. (175° C.) oven for 40 minutes. Makes 20 slices.

Serve plain or with a topping of fresh fruit and a dab of *Whipped Tofu Topping*. This also makes a fine breakfast cake.

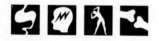

Whipped Tofu Topping

Makes one cup (250 ml)
½ cup (125 ml) tofu
½ cup (125 ml) *Yogurt Cream*
     Cheese
1 tablespoon (15 ml) maple
     syrup

Combine ingredients in a blender on low speed. Serve on fruit pies, fresh fruit or whole wheat pancakes.

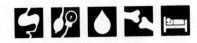

Whole Wheat Bread Pudding

Iron, calcium, protein, fiber—a great taste, too.

Makes eight servings

2½ cups (625 ml) whole grain
     bread cubes
1 unpeeled apple, diced
½ cup (125 ml) raisins
1 cup (250 ml) chopped
     pineapple
2½ cups (625 ml) yogurt
2 eggs, beaten
3 tablespoons (45 ml) medium
     unsulfured molasses
½ teaspoon (2 ml) cinnamon
1 teaspoon (5 ml) *Vanilla*
     Extract

Choose stale, whole wheat bread for cubes and place on a baking sheet in a 200° F. (95° C.) oven until dried. Combine ingredients in a large mixing bowl and place in a lightly oiled two-quart (2 l) casserole dish. Bake in a preheated 350° F. (175° C.) oven for 45 minutes.

Plum Kuchen

Makes eight servings

2 cups (500 ml) whole wheat
     flour
1 cup (250 ml) bran
1 cup (250 ml) wheat germ
2 teaspoons (10 ml) *Baking*
     Powder
½ teaspoon (2 ml) baking soda
1 egg
1½ cups (375 ml) yogurt
⅓ cup (80 ml) maple syrup
1 tablespoon (15 ml) sesame
     tahini
½ teaspoon (2 ml) *Vanilla*
     Extract
6–8 plums, sliced in thin
     sections

Combine dry ingredients in a large mixing bowl. In another bowl, beat egg into yogurt and add syrup, tahini and vanilla. Add wet ingredients to flour mixture and stir lightly, just until combined. Place half of the batter in a lightly oiled 8 × 8-inch (20 × 20-cm) baking pan. Place half of the plums in rows across surface of the batter. Add remaining batter and top with rows of remaining plums. Bake in a preheated 400° F. (200° C.) oven for 30 minutes. Cool before slicing.

Chapter 4

Take a Load Off Your Nerves

Psychologists have told us so much about how we drive ourselves crazy with our words and thoughts that the idea that emotional disturbances can result from food and drink probably strikes many intelligent people as ridiculous. Quackery. Seventeenth-century stuff. But that kind of thinking is itself old-fashioned today. At least it should be in this new age of holistic health. Unfortunately, even many physicians routinely ignore the possibility of a link between the patient's diet and his or her emotions.

Few doctors who have made the tranquilizers Librium and Valium best-selling drugs are aware, for instance, of such a simple, everyday fact as this one, stated in an editorial in the *British Medical Journal* (July 30, 1977):

Too much coffee produces symptoms indistinguishable from those of anxiety neuroses: recurrent headaches, mental irritability, cardiac arrhythmias and gastrointestinal disturbances.

Those are strong words to use about something as commonplace as coffee. But it is the very familiarity, the ho-humness of coffee, that makes it so dangerous. We take our coffee-drinking habit so much for granted that it has become practically invisible, even to many medical people.

Example: John F. Greden, M.D., reported the case of a 27-year-old Army nurse who visited a base clinic complaining of light-headedness, headache, restlessness, irregular heartbeat and a sense of anxiety that had developed over a three-week period (*American Journal of Psychiatry,* October, 1974). After a number of laboratory tests turned up nothing of any significance, the nurse was referred to the psychiatric clinic. Following the usual interviews and tests, the doctors there delivered their diagnosis: "anxiety reaction (probably secondary to a fear that her husband would be transferred to Vietnam)." The nurse thought this was nonsense, and decided to take a closer look at her diet, something the clinic doctors had ignored altogether. She realized that since the purchase of a drip coffeepot, which produced much better-tasting coffee, she had been drinking 10 to 12 cups a day. Her anxiety had begun just after she bought the pot. Putting two and two together, she quit drinking coffee, and her symptoms disappeared within 36 hours.

In another case reported by Dr. Greden, a 34-year-old Army personnel sergeant was driving the base medical staff crazy with frequent clinic visits. He complained of severe headaches and anxiety. Three complete medical exams in two years turned up nothing. The exams, of course, were not so thorough that they included questions about the sergeant's diet. So it was not until he was referred to the psychiatric clinic that someone thought to ask him about his caffeine intake. The sergeant was a heavy coffee drinker, and had been taking 8 to 10 caffeine-containing headache pills a day as well. When he cut back his use of caffeine, the headaches *and* anxiety disappeared.

All these cases and others led Dr. Greden to conclude that excessive coffee drinking can produce classic symptoms of anxiety. Yet, he found in a random survey of 100 outpatient psychiatric records at a major medical center that not *one* of them listed coffee- or tea-drinking habits, even though 42 records referred to anxiety symptoms.

Verner Stillner, M.D., M.P.H, a psychiatrist who also has had experience dealing with people whose minds are disturbed by high doses of caffeine, put it this way: "I think that, around the world, caffeine is the most utilized and most abused drug."

Certainly the average American is consuming caffeine at dangerous levels. In its discussion of caffeine, the American Pharmaceutical Association *Handbook of Nonprescription Drugs* (5th edition, 1979) says, "Doses larger than 250 milligrams often cause insomnia, restlessness, irritability, nervousness, tremor, headaches, and, in rare instances, a mild form of delirium manifested as perceived noises and flashes of light."

How much coffee must you drink to exceed the danger point of 250 milligrams? The average cup of coffee will deliver about 100 milligrams of caffeine, so it only takes two-and-a-half cups to make you a candidate for insomnia, nervousness, and all the rest. A survey sponsored by the International Coffee Organization found that Americans aged 10 and over drink coffee at the rate of 2.06 cups per day, so you can see that you don't really have to be a coffee hound to exceed the 250-milligram mark. If you want to get more specific about the caffeine in coffee, it's worth noting that since caffeine is soluble in hot water, the longer the coffee (or tea) is exposed to hot water, the more caffeine is extracted. A five-ounce cup of perked or boiled coffee will probably contain about 120 milligrams of caffeine. Drip or vacuum methods will yield a lower caffeine count, probably in the vicinity of about 90 milligrams per cup. Instant coffee is even weaker, averaging about 70 milligrams a cup. Decaffeinated coffee, of course, has very little caffeine, only about 3 milligrams per serving.

Coffee, however, is far from being the only source of caffeine in our diet. A strongly brewed good cup of tea, for instance, may have 107 milligrams of caffeine, while a medium-strong cup will have about half that much. A 12-ounce can of Coca Cola contains about 65 milligrams of caffeine, while Pepsi contains only 43 (related, possibly, to the greater commercial success of Coke?). An Excedrin tablet has as much caffeine as a Coke. (A No-Doze tablet has 100 milligrams of caffeine, a Vivarin 200.)

What few people realize is that chocolate also contains caffeine: not really large amounts, but enough to be meaningful—especially to the nervous system of a child. A single ounce of milk chocolate contains, according to our calculations, 8.4 milligrams of caffeine. That's just a little less than the amount found in a cup of prepared cocoa. Now, let's imagine that a child with a sweet tooth and fairly permissive parents consumes three ounces of milk chocolate a day. That's 25 milligrams of caffeine. Compared to the 250-milligram level we mentioned before, that doesn't sound like much, until we realize that the child we're talking about only weighs about one-third as much as an adult, so the *effect* of that caffeine on his or her nervous system is going to be equivalent to the effect of 75 milligrams or so of caffeine on an adult: the amount in one cup of instant coffee.

But caffeine isn't the only "hidden ingredient" in chocolate. A related chemical, called theobromine, is found in chocolate products in even larger amounts than caffeine. There's seven times more theobromine in milk chocolate, for instance, than caffeine. Theobromine is not as powerful a stimulant to the nervous system as caffeine, but it is still a stimulant.

So, there are 25 milligrams of caffeine plus 175 milligrams of another "upper" in those 3 ounces of milk chocolate. Now, let's assume that same child also consumes two 12-ounce bottles of Coca Cola a day (which many young children do). The soda means an additional 130 milligrams of caffeine. Together with the 25 milligrams from the chocolate, the child has a total caffeine intake of 155 milligrams a day. Multiply *that* by three to compensate for the child's small size, and you get an equivalent adult dose of 450 milligrams—almost twice the threshold dose which can create everything from restlessness to "a mild form of delirium." Is it any wonder so many mothers think their children are out of control?

While we were working on this chapter, someone asked us a good question: *how long does caffeine stay in your system?* Interesting, because many people—like our questioner—can tolerate one or two cups of coffee a day only if the effect has worn off by bedtime.

Our research found more agreement among scientists on how fast caffeine gets to work on you than on how fast your system can get rid of it. Caffeine is absorbed very rapidly into the system, and within minutes comes into contact with the central nervous system as well as other body tissues. Peak plasma levels are reached in about one hour, but that is an *average* value. In one study of nine people, peak caffeine saturation level was reached in five subjects after just 30 minutes, and at one hour in three subjects. But in one person, the maximal caffeine level wasn't reached for two hours. If you happen to be similar to that last individual, be warned: the cup of coffee you had at your friend's house at 10:30 P.M. on Sunday night is going to hit peak power in your nervous system at 12:30 A.M. Monday morning.

By the time caffeine is thoroughly distributed throughout your body, the metabolic machinery that cleans up toxins has already swung into action. Depending on which authority you choose to believe, about half of the caffeine in your system has been swept out in anywhere from 3 to 10 hours. Why all the confusion? Actually, scientists didn't know why they kept getting such varying results until two medical scientists at McGill University in Montreal discovered that the speed at which the body breaks down caffeine depends, among other things, on whether or not you are a smoker. The half-life of caffeine in a young *nonsmoker* is about 6 hours, Allen H. Neims, M.D., Ph.D., told us. Half-life diminishes the concentration of caffeine by one-half of *what's left* every 6 hours. Drink four cups in the morning, for instance, and half the caffeine is gone by suppertime. Half the remainder, for a total of 75 percent, by bedtime. However, Dr. Neims said, in smokers, the half-life of caffeine is only 3½ hours. It seems that the smoke in cigarettes causes an increase in a certain enzyme which enhances caffeine metabolism. It's quite possible, in fact, that the reason smokers seem to drink more coffee than others is that they metabolize it faster and must consume more in order to keep their caffeine stimulation at the desired level.

Showing just the opposite trend, caffeine in pregnant women during the last few months of pregnancy has a half-life of 18 hours. And in newborns, caffeine has a half-life of *four days.*

Let's assume that you are neither a newborn baby nor a pregnant woman and that you are a nonsmoker. And let's assume that during the course of the morning and the early afternoon, you put down four cups of coffee. What's a dose like that going to do to your sleep? Well, in approximate terms, by suppertime, you'll have the equivalent of two cups of coffee still in you, and by midnight, one cup. So if your system is sensitive to one cup, you *will* have trouble sleeping, even though you haven't had coffee since lunchtime. If you aren't sensitive to one cup of coffee, or if your rate of clearing caffeine is faster than average (there's a lot of individual difference), the caffeine won't keep you up.

Surprisingly, the "coffee nerves" story doesn't end with caffeine. Research has revealed that besides having a direct irritant effect on nerves, coffee also burns up our precious supply of thiamine, or vitamin B$_1$, the nutrient so necessary for tranquillity. Two Swiss researchers found that after drinking a quart of coffee in a three-hour period, much of the body's thiamine had been destroyed. Curiously, the suspected offender was not caffeine, but another constituent of coffee called chlorogenic acid (*International Journal for Vitamin and Nutrition Research,* vol. 46, 1976). A similar study at the University of Hawaii revealed that tea also causes a mild thiamine deficiency (*Federation Proceedings,* March 1, 1976). Scientists in Thailand discovered that the actual amount of thiamine destroyed by one quart of tea was about 2.1 milligrams—or almost *twice* the amount of thiamine recommended by the government as adequate for an adult woman (*Nutrition Reports International,* May, 1974).

In other words, if you are a heavy coffee or tea drinker, the chances are you are suffering from a deficiency of thiamine.

And what will that do to you? It could cause you to be nervous and irritable and to complain of such problems as nervous exhaustion, fatigue, loss of appetite, loss of memory, depression, constipation, inability to concentrate and feelings of inadequacy. What it will give you, in short, is a terrible case of "coffee nerves." It may even lead you to a doctor who—not believing that any person who eats a "normal" diet needs more vitamins—will give you any one of a variety of extremely popular stimulants, tranquilizers, or mood levelers.

If you feel that your coffee- or tea-drinking habits through the years may have created a thiamine deficiency, which is not at all unlikely, stay tuned for further information on how to get more of this important vitamin into your diet.

HOW TO EASE AWAY FROM CAFFEINE

Okay. You see yourself or another member of your family in the caffeine story, and you want out. And for good reason: how many things are more precious than tranquillity? But please, before you decide that you never want to drink another cup of coffee again, stop for a minute and make a plan. Coffee drinking, after all, is a habit, just like smoking. Now, in our experience, weaning yourself from coffee isn't nearly as difficult as freeing yourself from tobacco. Just the same, if you do it too abruptly, you may run into big problems.

Quite a few people who drink more than just two or three cups a day find that when they suddenly give up coffee altogether, they develop caffeine-withdrawal headaches. We discuss this in more detail under the section on "Headaches," but we can tell you that these headaches generally don't last more than a few days, if that long. In fact, you may not get a headache at all. You may only be bothered with a feeling that you're not quite awake, or a kind of fuzziness or a lack of sharpness. Eventually, all that will pass, but you can minimize the shock to your system when you give up coffee if you do it gradually, by degrees.

A very logical way to ease off the caffeine habit is one step at a time. If you've been drinking perked coffee, for instance, switch to drip. From drip, move down to instant. Meanwhile, cut back your daily number of cups by one or two each week. Substitute fruit juice, spring water or herb tea. When the going begins to get a little rough, you will find that there are more natural and healthful ways to stimulate your nervous system than injecting it with caffeine. Take a 20-minute walk in the fresh air. Listen to some music. Maybe just relax and take a snooze. If it's tea that's your main source of caffeine, apply the same tactics. The most caffeine is extracted from tea when the tea is loose and it's brewed for a long time. Made from a bag, or with the help of a tea infuser, less caffeine winds up in the drink. And the sooner you separate the tea leaves and the water, the less caffeine you're going to get. You can also move down from brands of tea containing large amounts of caffeine to those containing less. One recent study found that Twinings English Breakfast Tea had a very high content of caffeine—107 milligrams when brewed strong. At the other end of the scale were Lipton and Tetley, with only 70 milligrams when made strong. Here's another trick: since caffeine is soluble in hot water, you can try getting the *flavor* of tea without the caffeine by simply soaking two tea bags in a quart of water overnight. Add some fresh peppermint and lemon wedges to perk up the taste, and enjoy it hot or cold the next day.

Herb teas can do a lot to get you off your caffeine habit. At first, try substituting an herb tea for one cup of coffee or black tea a day, gradually eliminating caffeine. Start off with peppermint or spearmint tea, which have robust flavors. After that, experiment with one or more of the many blends on the market. Some contain a whole host of exotic ingredients such as camomile, lemon grass, orange blossoms and rose petals. Other blends may consist of only a few ingredients, such as peppermint, strawberry leaves and ginger, but are still very tasty. Another alternative to coffee and black tea could be one of the grain-based beverages such as Pero or Postum (made from bran and molasses). If you want to ease a child off hot chocolate, switch to hot carob, which has no caffeine and no theobromine.

One question remains: what about decaffeinated coffee? Is it a healthful substitute for real coffee? The final answer appears to be out to lunch, for this reason: the solvent commonly used to extract caffeine from coffee beans is methylene chloride, a chemical suspected of causing cancer. Tests by a consumer organization, however, have revealed no detectable traces of that solvent in the final product. So the danger, if any, would appear to be slight. Our opinion is that if decaffeinated coffee represents a step in your evolution away from regular coffee, with its *known* health hazards, it does make a certain amount of sense. Eventually, and ideally, you should not be drinking any coffee at all—decaffeinated or otherwise.

SLEEP EASIER WITH A NATURAL NIGHTCAP

One out of every seven or eight people has a devil of a time getting to sleep at night. Not just once in a while, but regularly. That's the word we get from the growing number of sleep disorder clinics that have sprung up around the country. These clinics are finding that insomnia may result from a variety of causes and may be treated in a variety of ways. And for better or worse, diet may be involved.

But first, before we say anything at all about improving your diet to sleep better, we must say something about sleeping pills, because if we don't, and you go on taking them, you will probably find that your new diet cannot even make a dent in your insomnia. Why is that? "Some of the most important aggravators of insomnia are drugs used to treat the problem," explains Thomas D. Borkovec, Ph.D., professor of psychology at Pennsylvania State University. "Most of the sleep-inducing drugs lose effect and eventually disrupt the stages of sleep."

Studies conducted at Penn State indicate that sleeping pills can actually bring on chronic insomnia if used for more than two weeks. As the pills lose their effectiveness, and the drugs actually begin disturbing sleep, the user tends to increase the dosage, causing a spiral effect. Stop taking the pills suddenly after you've been on them for a while and you may find that your sweet dreams are taken over by nightmares. "Sleeping medications suppress the amount of REM [rapid eye movement] stage of sleep in which dreams occur," Dr. Borkovec explains. "When a person is taken off the drugs, a REM rebound results. The person has very vivid and often horrifying dreams and the experience is much like that of an alcoholic having delirium tremens. A person often will continue taking the sleeping medication just to avoid the rebounds, which are most severe the first or second night. They diminish over the next four or five days."

Now that we've got sleeping pills out of the way, let's look at the question of diet. A good place to start would be with people who believe that a little nightcap is just the ticket for dreamland. If you believe that, we're here to tell you that you should consider a different travel agency. Because while alcohol may indeed send you off to dreamland, it can also shorten your stay.

"Alcohol affects sleep very adversely and should be avoided at bedtime," says Charles Pollak, M.D., co-director of the Sleep-Wake Disorders Center of Montefiore Hospital Medical Center in Bronx, New York. "When alcohol is first taken, it acts as a sedative. But then it metabolizes during sleep, causing a withdrawal effect. The person is aroused by it and will not sleep restfully as a result."

While some people don't drink coffee because they think the caffeine will keep them awake, others believe they won't be able to get to sleep without it. In fact, coffee disrupts sleep, says Dr. Pollak. "People may think they tolerate it well, but the caffeine causes arousal and disturbs sleep patterns." The caffeine in tea and colas may have the same effect, he adds.

On the positive side of the beverage ledger, research indicates that camomile tea, an inexpensive herb available in most health food stores, may have definite sleep-inducing qualities. In one study, 12 hospital patients were given camomile tea while undergoing cardiac catheterization, a rather uncomfortable medical procedure. Of the 12 people, 10 fell into a deep sleep after drinking the tea. Although they could be aroused, they fell back asleep and remained sleeping throughout the 90-minute procedure, which surprised the investigators considerably (*Journal of Clinical Pharmacology,* November/December, 1973).

Perhaps an even more traditional nighttime beverage is warm milk. Now, certainly there's something that works psychologically, you might think—what could be more soothing to your frayed spirits at the end of the day? But in fact, there's more to it than psychology. And there's also a better drink than plain warm milk.

In England, researchers decided to test a number of reputed sleeping aids on 16 people. The people were given one of four different bedtime snacks. One was a flavored drink made from soy, egg and sugar. Another was warm milk. Then there was an English milk-cereal drink called Horlicks, which is served warm. Finally, there were placebo (dummy) pills, given, of course, to see what the effect would be of pure suggestion (plus, not giving the stomach anything to digest). Result? For those people who normally had no snack at all around bedtime, the best quality sleep was induced by the placebo pill—quite possibly because these people were not accustomed to having anything of substance in their bellies at bedtime. But among those people who normally *did* have a snack, the warm milk or Horlicks did the job better than the soy drink or the pills. And Horlicks was apparently the best of the lot, because there was less wakefulness interrupting the first six hours of sleep after drinking that beverage, compared to either warm milk alone or the soy drink (*Proceedings of the Nutrition Society,* May, 1977).

A possible explanation as to why the cereal and milk combination has real rest-inducing powers emerges from a look at a related sleep agent, L-tryptophan. L-tryptophan is a natural amino acid, a component of protein, which lately has been the subject of intense research by psychologists and psychiatrists. Apparently, it is a natural sedative of sorts. According to Harold L. Williams, Ph.D., of the University of Oklahoma Health Sciences Center, L-tryptophan is a precursor of serotonin, a sleep-inducing substance naturally found in the brain. "Our studies showed that people given an oral dose of tryptophan went to sleep faster and experienced an increase in slow wave or deep sleep," says Dr. Williams. "The small intestine has enzymes which aid in transporting food products through the intestinal wall into the bloodstream. These enzymes put L-tryptophan into the bloodstream very quickly."

Since tryptophan is found in protein foods, some researchers have suggested that eating high-protein foods like milk, cheese, eggs or meat would help a person to sleep. The research, however, challenges this idea. "The amount of L-tryptophan in foods is minimal," says Dr. Pollak. "A person would have to eat enormous quantities of meat to have an effect on sleep." And according to some researchers, even enormous quantities of high-protein foods would have no effect. That's because foods that are high in protein contain other amino acids in addition to L-tryptophan. These other amino acids actually compete with L-tryptophan for the same carrier to the brain, and the result is that precious little L-tryptophan ever reaches the brain in concentrations large enough to do anything special.

There's another way, though, in which we can boost the amount of L-tryptophan reaching the brain, explains Carol E. Leprohon, of the department of nutrition and food science at the University of Toronto. And interestingly, it is yet one more example of why a diet emphasizing the natural complex carbohydrates such as grains is generally better for health than a diet emphasizing protein foods like meat and eggs. When you eat high-carbohydrate foods like cereals or breads, Ms. Leprohon explains, "the carbohydrates stimulate insulin release into the system, and when insulin is added, the amount of other amino acids decreases in the blood, while the amount of L-tryptophan remains the same. L-tryptophan then has the advantage of getting to the brain." Although researchers are not certain just how long the process takes, Ms. Leprohon says that eating a high-carbohydrate snack about half-an-hour before bedtime should be effective in inducing a restful night's sleep.

EAT, DRINK AND BE MERRIER

Emotional turmoil is something all of us must experience, just as surely as a ship must experience stormy seas. Usually we can ride with the waves, but sometimes, just as a ship gets washed aground, we become immobilized on the shoals of fear, uncertainty, anxiety or depression. We need help to get our keels free, to get moving again with the tide.

That help may come from a number of sources. One is time. Just as the changing tide has refloated many a grounded ship, time alone somehow seems to heal a good many of our hurts. Family and friends are also important sources of help. There is also professional help, which may come from therapists trained in the art of healing words, or perhaps from therapists who prefer to daub psychic hurts with tranquilizers.

Then there is diet. If you haven't been acting yourself lately, diet is probably the first thing that would come into the mind of your mother or spouse. And the last that would come into the mind of your doctor. But somewhere in between those two extremes, there is a reasonable role for nutrition in times of emotional stress. We can't be very exact or systematic because obviously, we are all different. But let's begin by considering the importance of a nutrient that seems to pop up in case after case of mental and emotional problems: thiamine, or vitamin B_1.

A typical study identifying thiamine as a factor in emotional stress was carried out by investigators at the Nutrition Research Center, Institute of Medicine and Pharmacy, Bucharest, Rumania, who set out to examine a group of 65 patients admitted to a clinic because of neurotic symptoms. Neurosis, broadly speaking, is not exactly a dangerous illness, and neurotics are basically in touch with reality and able to function reasonably well. But they are plagued by such symptoms as anxiety, poor memory, confusion or hypochondria. Many people who are otherwise quite normal and healthy suffer from mild neurosis.

In a series of laboratory tests designed to compare the 65 patients with a control of 49 healthy individuals, the Rumanian researchers found that the neurotics excreted only half as much thiamine in their urine as the controls. That normally indicates a deficiency of thiamine. In addition, blood tests revealed an excess of pyruvate, an intermediate breakdown product which accumulates in the blood when dietary thiamine intake is deficient.

"These differences suggest that patients with neurosis exhibited biochemical evidences of thiamine deficiency," the authors point out. "When the intake of thiamine is reduced, mental symptoms appear resembling those of neurasthenia—intolerance of noise, inability to concentrate, memory defects, irritability, depression and other neurological manifestations. . . . Such a biochemical lesion could diminish the individual's ability to adapt to the multitude and rapidity of stimuli of modern lifestyles" (*Nutrition Reports International,* September, 1975).

The Rumanians, like most Americans, had a high-sugar intake as a result of their dependence on refined, processed foods. According to the authors, that aggravated their mental symptoms, because additional thiamine is used up as the body metabolizes sugar. "A consideration of the changes in food habits prevailing in many countries raises the question as to whether the increasing occurrence of neurosis may not arise from a thiamine-glucose imbalance," the researchers suggest. Intriguing, isn't it? As life becomes faster and more complicated, our diets have more sugar but less thiamine, exactly what we *don't* need if we want to cope.

A classic study of thiamine and its effect on behavior was described by Josef Brozek, Ph.D., at the Symposium on Nutrition and Behavior held at the University of Minnesota, April 27, 1956. Dr. Brozek, a professor in that university's School of Public Health, reported that large swings in mood and attitude were observed among 10 healthy male volunteers deprived of thiamine. Without the vitamin, the subjects became depressed. They lost their ability to concentrate, their alertness and feeling of well-being. They became more apprehensive, irritable, forgetful and nervous. Some complained of dizziness and headaches. They lost patience with each other and with the staff members conducting the study. Tempers flared. Supplements of thiamine were then added to the men's diet, said Dr. Brozek, "when it appeared that the deficiency had progressed as far as we considered safe." Within a few short days, "thiamine supplements restored appetite and brought about a dramatic change in the attitudes of the subjects."

While thiamine is probably of key importance in mental health, nearly all the B vitamins seem to be intimately involved in maintaining a positive and tranquil outlook on life. Niacin has been known for many years to be of prime importance in psychological health. Way back in 1947, Tom Spies, M.D., in his pioneering book, *Rehabilitation Through Better Nutrition* (W. B. Saunders), detailed the many mental problems that can accompany, not an out-and-out deficiency of niacin, but merely an inadequate intake. The list of symptoms he compiled reads like a passage out of a neurotic's diary: irritability, depression, memory loss, insomnia, nervousness, distractability, apprehension, morbid fears, mental confusion and forgetfulness.

Although you probably read about thiamine, riboflavin and niacin when you

Selected Good Sources of Major B Vitamins

	Thiamine (B₁) (milligrams)	Riboflavin (B₂) (milligrams)	Niacin (B₃) (milligrams)
Recommended Dietary Allowance	1.4 (men) 1.0 (women)	1.6 (men) 1.2 (women)	18 (men) 13 (women)
Therapeutic Requirement	5–10 (adults)	5–10 (adults)	100 (adults)

Food	Portion Size	Thiamine (B₁) (milligrams)	Riboflavin (B₂) (milligrams)	Niacin (B₃) (milligrams)
Beef liver	3 ounces	0.22	**3.56**	**14**
Brewer's yeast	1 tablespoon	**1.25**	**0.34**	3
Chicken dark meat	3 ounces	0.10	0.16	**4.5**
Chicken light meat	3 ounces	0.07	0.08	**10**
Buttermilk	¾ cup	0.075	**0.33**	0.15
Wheat germ toasted	¼ cup	0.44	0.20	1.2
Haddock	6 ounces	0.06	0.12	**5.4**
Yogurt	½ cup	0.5	**0.22**	0.1
Turkey light meat	3 ounces	0.04	0.12	**9.4**
Peanut butter	1 tablespoon	0.02	0.02	**2.4**

NOTE: Boldface numbers indicate especially high values.

were in school, chances are you didn't hear very much about pyridoxine, or vitamin B_6. But within the last 5 to 10 years, there has been an explosion of interest in this vitamin, due in no small part to popularization of the Pill. At last count, 10 million women in the United States were downing a daily dose of hormones to prevent pregnancy. And of those, about seven percent plummeted to the depths of depression as a direct result. For

Selected Good Sources of Vitamin B₆

Pyridoxine (B₆)

Recommended Dietary Allowance (micrograms)*	Therapeutic Requirement (micrograms)
2,000	2,000–25,000

Food	Portion Size	Micrograms
Banana	1 medium	560
Beef liver	3 ounces	560
Brewer's yeast	1 tablespoon	390
Cod	3½ ounces	340
Carrot		
raw	1 medium	140
Halibut	3½ ounces	110
Flounder	3½ ounces	100
Wheat germ		
toasted	1 tablespoon	74

*1,000 micrograms = 1 milligram.

years, physicians had recognized that *something* in birth control pills can cause irritability, anxiety, and even serious depression in some women. But they didn't know exactly what it was or how it worked. Now, many are convinced that it has to do with the Pill's depressing effect on the body's B vitamin stores, especially B₆, but also B₁₂ and folate. Writing in the British medical journal *Lancet* (April 28, 1973), doctors at St. Mary's Hospital Medical School in London reported that of 22 emotionally distraught women on the Pill, 11 were found to be severely deficient in pyridoxine. All the women were then treated with 20 milligrams of vitamin B₆ twice a day. And within two months' time, the dark moods of the vitamin-deficient women brightened significantly.

There are many other studies linking vitamin B_6 to women's moods, particularly when there is a lot of estrogen active in the body. A study of 15 depressed pregnant women showed that those with the deepest depression had the lowest blood levels of vitamin B_6 (*Acta Obstetrica et Gynecologica Scandinavica,* February, 1978). When 250 "depression-prone" women received oral contraceptives supplemented with B_6, 90 percent remained free of severe depression (*Ob. Gyn. News,* March 15, 1978). In another study, doctors measured the blood level of B_6 in 39 depressed women on the Pill and found that 19 had a severe deficiency. When they gave these women B_6, 16 improved in mood (*Lancet,* August 31, 1974).

We mentioned that folate is of notable importance to women during the reproductive years. But it's also important in maturity—so much so that it is safe to estimate that many elderly people believed to be "senile" are actually suffering from nothing more or less than a deficiency of the B vitamins, particularly folate. Folate (or folic acid) is found throughout the body, but it is especially concentrated in the fluid of the spinal column —the switchboard of the central nervous system. M. I. Botez, M.D., of the Clinical Research Institute in Montreal, has found that many signs of approaching senility may actually be caused by a folate deficiency "short-circuiting" the nervous system. Speaking to the annual meeting of the Royal College of Physicians and Surgeons of Canada, the neurologist reported that four of his psychiatric patients complained of fatigue, weight loss, insomnia and severe constipation. They also had cold, numb legs and poor reflexes. Testing them, Dr. Botez found they had low-blood levels of folate. He started them on supplements and injections of this vitamin and after three months, their subjective symptoms disappeared, they gradually put on weight, and their reflexes normalized. These improvements coincided with rises in the concentration of folate in their blood (*Clinical Psychiatry News,* April, 1976). These patients, who had been under psychiatric care for an extended period, and had been unresponsive to various medications taken before the study, did not know they were receiving folate, Dr. Botez told the meeting. So let's have no remarks about "the power of suggestion."

In Scotland, 10 elderly patients—5 of them actually diagnosed as senile—had nervous system disorders so severe that their spinal cords were thought to be degenerated. Upon closer investigation, they were found to be folate-deficient. *Folate treatment led to an improvement in mood in all patients.* The symptoms of two patients with severe mental illnesses were "dramatically resolved" (*British Medical Journal,* May 15, 1976).

One interesting sidelight is that in the Canadian study, patients had "restless leg syndrome." This syndrome is characterized by deep, ill-defined disagreeable sensations in the legs and an irresistible urge to move them. The problem vanished when the patients were treated with folate. (If you have this syndrome, cut out coffee, too.)

B_{12} is another vitamin that needs looking after when there is psychological stress or other symptoms in connection with a poor diet or aging. In a recent study at

Selected Good Sources of Folate and Vitamin B₁₂

Folate (Folacin, Folic Acid)				Vitamin B₁₂		
Recommended Dietary Allowance (micrograms)*		Therapeutic Requirement (micrograms)		Recommended Dietary Allowance (micrograms)		Therapeutic Requirement (micrograms)
400		1,000		3		4

Food	Portion Size	Micrograms		Food	Portion Size	Micrograms
Brewer's yeast	1 tablespoon	313		Brewer's yeast	content varies with product	
Black-eyed peas	½ cup	230		Beef liver	3 ounces	64
Beef liver	3 ounces	123		Tuna		
Orange juice	¾ cup	102		drained	½ cup	2.4
Romaine lettuce	1 cup	98		Sole	6 ounces	2
Cantaloupe	½ medium	82		Haddock	6 ounces	1
Beets				Whole milk	¾ cup	0.9
cooked	½ cup	67				
Brussels sprouts						
cooked	8 sprouts	56				
Broccoli						
cooked	½ cup	50				

* 1,000 micrograms = 1 milligram.

NOTE: *Adapted from* Human Nutrition, *McGraw-Hill Book Co., 1976, and "Folacin in Selected Foods,"* Journal of the American Dietetic Association, *February, 1977.*

the Geriatric Center in Arhus, Denmark, the blood of 273 elderly patients was tested for B₁₂. One out of every three had low serum levels for that vitamin. The B₁₂ levels increased in the patients during their stay in the therapy center, which offered a better diet than they had been getting at home. That is very important, because vitamin B₁₂ is essential to the function of the central nervous system. Even a slight deficiency can produce such symptoms as fatigue, irritability and numbness. And in more severe vitamin B₁₂ deficiencies, the symptoms of dementia, depression, confusion and paranoia are often mistaken for those of senility. *Clinical Psychiatry News* (March, 1976) reported one case in which a 35-year-old man was admitted to a Canadian hospital after an apparent suicide attempt. He was severely depressed and lacked sexual drive and motivation. He was also suffering from insomnia, memory impairment and generally regressed behavior. Testing at the hospital revealed a severe vitamin B_{12} deficiency. He was treated with a series of B_{12} shots for eight consecutive days, after which he was discharged with complete remission of his symptoms.

If you are confused by the similarity in symptoms caused by deficiencies of the various B vitamins, you are not alone. It's quite clear that our nutritionists and physicians have a great deal to learn about this area. A few things, however, strike us as being fairly clear. One is that many people have special nutritional vulnerabilities. We might compare it with the inborn tendency some people have for a hernia. Most surgeons believe that those who have hernias are born with a specific localized weakness which is just waiting, so to speak, for the right stress to turn it into a full-blown rupture. Give two people the same suitcase to lift in an awkward position, and the person with the vulnerability will have a hernia while the other one will just grunt. It's probably that way with nutrition and emotional ruptures, too. A poor diet that will have few if any noticeable effects on one person will make another seriously ill because of a vulnerability.

But there's more to it than that. Besides vulnerability, there is the matter of variability. Simply put, relative deficiencies of the same nutrient can and will lead to a bewildering variety of symptoms in different people. Someone who wants to wait until it all makes sense before doing anything about nutrition will probably wind up doing nothing. Or turning to tranquilizers to simply obscure the whole question.

In a practical sense, there is not much point in trying to separate the effects of the various B vitamin deficiencies unless you are a physician or a biochemist. Furthermore, most people who are deficient in one B vitamin are also more or less deficient in others, because they tend to be found in similar foods. Liver and other organ meats, fish and poultry, whole grains, beans, yeast, dark green leafy vegetables, nuts, seeds, and blackstrap molasses are all good sources of the Bs. These foods are very heavily represented in our recipes throughout this book, so if you are concerned about the health of your nervous system, you will have a lot to choose from.

NUTRITIONAL TRANQUILIZERS DOCTORS USE

Minerals are also important in the health of the nervous system. In one study, depressed patients had "significantly lower" blood levels of magnesium than healthy people (*Journal of Nervous and Mental Disease,* December, 1977). In another study, depressed patients who took the drug Lithium and improved had a rise in their magnesium levels, while the magnesium levels of those who took Lithium and didn't improve stayed much the same (*Lancet,* December 14, 1974). August F. Daro, M.D., a Chicago obstetrician and gynecologist, routinely gives all of his depressed patients calcium and magnesium. "Many depressed men and women are short on both minerals," he told us.

"I put them on a combination of 400 milligrams of calcium and 200 milligrams of magnesium a day. Calcium and magnesium especially take care of premenstrual depression."

As Dr. Daro remarks, calcium is also important in calming the nerves. That was demonstrated 10 years ago by psychiatrists at the Washington University School of Medicine. Ferris N. Pitts, M.D., and James N. McClure, M.D., worked with nine patients suffering from anxiety neurosis, and nine normal controls. The patients displayed a variety of symptoms: feelings of impending doom, fear of insanity, fear of heart attack, fear of smothering or choking to death, etc. The doctors found that by giving lactate, a normal chemical product of glucose metabolism, anxiety symptoms could be provoked in all nine patients, as well as in two of the normal controls. But when calcium was administered along with the lactate in subsequent tests, the anxiety symptoms generally did not occur (*New England Journal of Medicine,* December 21, 1967). It's worth pointing out that here again, we see the importance of individual difference: it wasn't just the *amount* of lactate involved, but the *vulnerability* of the individuals stressed by it, which made all the difference in this experiment.

Skim milk, yogurt, tofu, salmon with the bones in, soybeans and broccoli are all good sources of calcium. For magnesium, look to brown rice, nuts, peas, soybeans, dark green leafy vegetables, and whole grain products such as wheat germ.

The very special foods that you should be putting on your daily menu are those rich in many of the B vitamins *and* calcium and/or magnesium as well. These would include the dark green leafy vegetables, whole grains and wheat germ, broccoli, nuts, and blackstrap molasses. If, perhaps, you've wondered why so many people seem to have nutritionally related emotional problems, look over these lists and ask yourself how many people eat such foods regularly. Or at all.

There is another way that food interfaces with emotions and behavior, and that is through low blood sugar, or hypoglycemia. If your moods or energy levels seem to change rather drastically at different times of the day, we refer you to the section on "Low Blood Sugar (Hypoglycemia)."

There is, of course, a lot more to the relationship of food and emotions than pure biochemistry. The very act of preparing food is probably one of the more profound things that we do. And as we serve it to others, we are giving them some very important messages. Just imagine, for a moment, spending an hour or more carefully preparing a good meal for someone. Do you think that meal would likely be deficient in important nutrients? Doubtful. Maybe in one or two, but the next day, they'd be there. Now, consider a meal prepared not out of love, but habit and haste. Can you imagine that meal being deficient in B vitamins, and minerals? Can you imagine it being excessively high in sugar and other refined carbohydrates, which actually rob the body of the B vitamins? If you can, you can then understand the intimate back-and-forth relationship between good food and good feelings.

CALMING THE HYPERACTIVE CHILD WITH A BETTER DIET

Every normal, healthy child is hyperactive once in a while. So are adults, for that matter. But the truly hyperactive child in the medical sense is something else. His attention span is so short that classroom learning is practically impossible. Not only for him, but for classmates: a hyperactive child may be aggressive, cry or scream with little provocation, and throw frequent tantrums. But it's deeper than the ordinary "antisocial" kind of behavior. Tantrums may become seizures. There is frequently a kind of unnatural clumsiness, even for a boy at the awkward age. He may have an IQ of 140 and have trouble dressing himself. In a way, the hyperactive child is possessed—the trouble is, experts can't seem to agree on the name of his demon. But for thousands of parents, and at least some scientists, the demon is diet: the modern, junk-food diet so full of additives, preservatives, artificial flavors and colors, sugar and other unnatural ingredients. Remove them from the child's diet and you might at least get to first base with the child's behavior problem. If you stick with it, maybe second. And if you're lucky, all the way home.

The diet theory began in 1973 with Ben Feingold, M.D., an allergist and pediatrician from San Francisco, who believes that additives are a major cause of hyperactivity. In perhaps 50 percent of all cases, Dr. Feingold said, improvement will come about when the additives are removed, particularly food colors and flavors, BHA, BHT and MSG. And for some children, he said, it is necessary to avoid aspirin and foods chemically related to aspirin (the salicylate-containing foods and flavors, including lime, lemon and wintergreen flavors, berries, peaches, apricots, prunes, plums, grapes, oranges, cucumbers and tomatoes).

In the years since then, the Feingold thesis has been confirmed and disproved, attacked and defended. At one extreme are parents who have become active in the Feingold Association, a national organization composed of parents of hyperactive children. Most if not all of these parents report very positive, sometimes almost incredibly good results with the Feingold approach. At the other extreme are scientists (many associated with the food industry in one way or another) who seem unreasonably cynical. If you listen to the parents, the Feingold diet almost never fails. If you listen to the food industry's scientists, it almost never works. But let's try to see if there isn't some middle ground we can look to for help.

Arnold Brenner, M.D., a pediatrician from Randallstown, Maryland, put 32 of his hyperactive patients on the Feingold diet. But he didn't want them to get better. He had, in his own words, a "desire to disprove the Feingold hypothesis." Instead, he proved it. Eleven of the 32 children had an "excellent response": a dramatic decrease in hyperactivity, restlessness and distractability.

Eight other children "probably improved" as judged by their schoolteachers, parents and Dr. Brenner. In all, 19 of 32 got better (*Clinical Pediatrics,* July, 1977). When

Dr. Brenner checked up on the "excellent" children six months later, he found that 3 of them had gone off their diet "with marked deterioration in their school performance."

In another study, 31 hyperactive children were given allergy tests to measure their sensitivity to salicylates and artificial colors and flavors. Of those who *were* sensitive, 15 were put on the Feingold diet. Fourteen of these children, writes the author of the study, "responded with improved behavior in the areas of overactivity, distractability, impulsiveness and excitability. Sleep . . . problems were resolved partially or completely" (*Medical Journal of Australia,* August 14, 1976).

The New York Institute of Child Development in New York City also treats hyperactive children, but researchers there suspected that sugar might complicate the problem. And in fact, when they studied the blood sugar metabolism of 265 children enrolled at the institute, they found that 74 percent had definite abnormalities and difficulties in handling refined carbohydrates. When they put the children on a corrective diet that cut out all sugar and emphasized frequent feedings of natural foods, particularly those high in protein, they reported that after two to three weeks, the children were no longer hyperactive.

Another believer in demon sugar is Patricia Hardman, director of the Woodland Hall Academy in Maitland, Florida, a school for children with hyperactivity and learning disabilities. At her institution, says Mrs. Hardman, "sugar is eliminated from the diet of every child. If a child comes to school extremely depressed or complains that nothing is going right, or if he flies off the handle and can't be controlled, we ask what he's been eating. It's almost always the case that the night before he had ice cream or soda or some other food with a lot of sugar. We had one child who was tested for his IQ and scored 140. Two days later, he was tested and scored 100! It turned out that grandma had come for a visit, and that morning had made the child pancakes for breakfast. Of course they were smothered in sugar syrup. Well, we waited another three days—three days without sugar—and tested him again. Sure enough, he scored 140."

William G. Crook, M.D., agrees. "I think sugar is the number one cause of hyperactivity, and food coloring is the number two cause, especially red dye," he told us. "But if a child eats an M&M, it's hard to tell whether it's the sugar or the food coloring that makes him hyperactive. Then again, an allergy to chocolate may be the cause."

Dr. Crook, a pediatrician from Jackson, Tennessee, says that "allergic reactions to foods, food colors and dyes are one of the most common causes of hyperactivity in the patients I see." These allergic reactions, he adds, can also cause persistent stuffy nose, recurrent colds, fatigue, headaches, tummy aches, muscle aching and bed-wetting. "A food allergy will strike at a particular organ or part of the body," Dr. Crook explains. "It can upset digestion, clog the nose or inflame the brain. If the brain is involved, the child can become hyperactive." In a five-year study of 182 hyperactive children, Dr. Crook found that 75 percent were eating food that either caused or aggravated their problems. In this group, 38 were allergic to milk, 30 to corn, 28 to chocolate, 20 to eggs and 15 to wheat.

A similar study was conducted by Doris Rapp, M.D., an allergist at the Meyer Memorial Hospital in Buffalo, New York. Dr. Rapp tested 24 hyperactive children and found that over 70 percent showed evidence of having an allergy. Fifty percent of these children showed improvement in their hyperactivity in one week or less on a diet that excluded milk, eggs, wheat, corn, sugar, cocoa and food coloring (*Journal of Learning Disabilities,* June/July, 1978).

Most doctors, it must be said, would not go along with the idea that allergies are a major cause of the hyperactivity that afflicts an estimated 10 million American children. Nor, for that matter, do they accept Dr. Feingold's thesis. What *do* they believe? The consensus is probably that hyperactivity may arise from a number of ill-understood causes, and if there is a treatment that's best, it is probably Ritalin, or a similar drug, of the amphetamine family. These drugs are powerful stimulants, but they seem to work the opposite way on hyperactive children. Nor are they free of side effects. They can cause insomnia. They can make a child lose his appetite and lose weight. And they can stunt growth. What's more, Ritalin may only *appear* to calm down a hyperactive child. In reality, it could be turning him into a kind of robot. One investigator of children on Ritalin has claimed that "their responses are still increasing in rate, but the variety of the response is decreasing." In other words, the buzz saw in the child's brain is still spinning, but the drug has taken it out of gear. What's more, writes Barbara Sahakian, Ph.D., a researcher at the Massachusetts Institute of Technology, "Amphetamines decreased responding in novel situations and on novel tasks or in learning tasks where changes in behavior were necessary" (*New Scientist,* November, 1978).

All of which becomes terribly relevant when the medical establishment tells us there's "no proof" that diet can change hyperactivity. That it's not even worth trying. Because what that really means is: don't ask questions, just give the kid his downer.

Are we exaggerating? We honestly don't think so. We've been at meetings where health professionals, including dietitians, have tried to dissuade parents from trying dietary modification, even in cases where the hyperactive child has not responded to drugs. Apparently, such people feel it is better to suffer—yes, even better to let an innocent child suffer—than to try an alternative remedy not accepted by the establishment. Even when that remedy has been recommended by first-rate doctors and is perfectly safe.

But let's take the broad view and admit that with hyperactivity, as in most cases of nervous and emotional problems, diet is not the only environmental factor that may be involved. We like the attitude of Ray Wunderlich, M.D., a St. Petersburg, Florida, pediatrician and author of a book on hyperactivity, *Allergy, Brains and Children Coping* (Johnny Reads, 1973). Although Dr. Wunderlich believes that allergies to such foods as sugar, wheat, corn and milk are frequent causes of hyperactivity—particularly when the foods are highly processed instead of natural—he offers this further insight into the healing of a hyperactive child:

The family who feeds junk foods to their kid is a disordered family whose priorities aren't in order for bringing up a healthy child. Perhaps the parents are ill themselves, or have drifted along with the culture. In any case, making a concerted effort to put their child on a good diet will not only improve his physical health and possibly remove the cause of hyperactivity, but will also provide order and structure within the family unit and so make the disorderly child more orderly.

One final note: Dr. Feingold believes that if you are seriously trying his diet, it is imperative to be in touch with a local chapter of the Feingold Association. That's because so many additives that may cause problems are not listed on labels, thanks to loopholes in the law. If you are interested in taking this approach, therefore, you can write to: Feingold Association of the United States, 759 National Press Building, Washington, DC 20045.

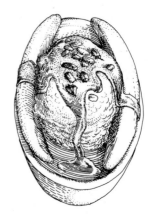

BREAKFASTS

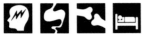

Banana Split Breakfast

Makes one serving
1 banana
½ cup (125 ml) ricotta cheese
1 teaspoon (5 ml) wheat germ
1 teaspoon (5 ml) bran
2 tablespoons (30 ml) Strawberry Topping
1 tablespoon (15 ml) chopped walnuts

A banana split for breakfast? That's good for the nerves? Yes —and for the soul, too!

Cut banana in half lengthwise, and place in a bowl, as with a banana split. Combine the ricotta cheese with the wheat germ and bran and place a "scoop" in the middle of the banana halves. Drizzle *Strawberry Topping* over ricotta and sprinkle with walnuts. Makes a calcium-rich treat.

Orange-Cinnamon Waffles

Makes two servings
1 cup (250 ml) whole wheat
   flour
1 teaspoon (5 ml) baking soda
¼ teaspoon (1 ml) cinnamon
1 egg
½ cup (125 ml) orange juice
½ cup (125 ml) buttermilk or
   yogurt
2 tablespoons (30 ml) soy oil

Orange-Cinnamon Waffles *will please many senses: they smell wonderful, taste delicious, and have a fine texture. Serve with some fresh, chopped orange sections or applesauce.*

Combine the dry ingredients in a medium mixing bowl. In a smaller bowl, beat the egg and add orange juice, buttermilk and oil. Add to the dry ingredients and stir just until combined.
Bake batter in a hot waffle iron and serve.

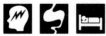

Whole Wheat Waffles

Makes four servings
1 cup (250 ml) whole wheat
   flour
¼ cup (60 ml) wheat germ
2 teaspoons (10 ml) baking
   soda
2 tablespoons (30 ml) corn oil
1½ cups (375 ml) buttermilk
1 egg, beaten

Combine dry ingredients in a medium bowl. Add oil and milk to egg, and toss lightly with dry ingredients until combined. Do not beat.
Heat waffle iron, and pour on batter. Serve with applesauce or fresh fruit topping at breakfast, or with *Creamed Fish and Pimiento* or *Mushrooms Stroganoff-Style with Toasted Cashews* as a light luncheon or supper dish.

Rice and Raisin Breakfast Cereal

Makes two servings
½ cup (125 ml) brown rice
1 cup (250 ml) water
¼ cup (60 ml) raisins
   dash cinnamon

Place ingredients in a heavy-bottom saucepan and bring to a boil over high heat. Reduce heat and simmer until most of the water is absorbed and "craters" are visible in the surface of the rice. This should take about 15 to 20 minutes. Cover and steam over very low heat for 5 to 10 more minutes, until the remaining water is absorbed and the rice is tender. Serve plain or with skim milk.

Wheat Pancakes

Makes two servings
1 cup (250 ml) whole wheat
flour
¼ cup (60 ml) bran
¼ cup (60 ml) wheat germ
1 teaspoon (5 ml) *Baking
Powder*
1 egg
1 tablespoon (15 ml) oil
1 tablespoon (15 ml) medium
unsulfured molasses
1½ cups (375 ml) skim milk

*Some of our taste-testers felt these were the best pancakes
they'd ever had. We can't guarantee you'll agree, but at least they're
super-healthful!*

Combine dry ingredients in a medium mixing bowl. In another
bowl, beat egg and add oil, molasses and milk. Add wet ingredients to
the flour mixture and stir just until combined. Cook on a hot, lightly
oiled griddle, turning when bubbles appear on the surface. Makes eight
pancakes.

Note: If there is batter left, add some raisins or raisins and sunflower
seeds to the batter, cook the pancakes, and store them in a refrigerator
or freezer. Served rewarmed in the oven, they are delicious with a thick
soup on a winter evening. They can also be reheated in a toaster.

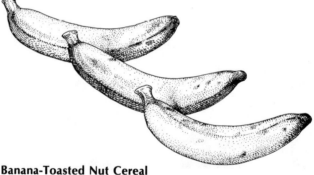

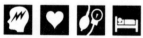

Banana-Toasted Nut Cereal

Makes one serving
2 tablespoons (30 ml) walnuts,
chopped and toasted
2 tablespoons (30 ml) raisins
(optional)
¾ cup (175 ml) water
⅓ cup (80 ml) rolled oats
½ banana, sliced
¼ teaspoon (1 ml) cinnamon

To toast walnuts, place the walnut meats in a heavy-bottom pan
over medium heat, stirring until they are browned. Set aside.

In a saucepan, combine raisins (if desired) and the water, bring
to a boil and stir in the oats. Cook until thickened. Remove from heat
and add walnuts, banana and cinnamon.

SOUPS

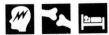

Salmon Bisque

Makes four servings
1 onion, chopped
2 tablespoons (30 ml) sunflower oil
2 tablespoons (30 ml) whole wheat flour
1 cup (250 ml) whole milk
15½ ounces (439 g) canned salmon, drained
1 cup (250 ml) *Chicken Stock* or *Vegetable Stock*
½ teaspoon (2 ml) thyme

Rich in calcium and B vitamins, this bisque also has four-star flavor.

Saute onion in oil until tender in a large skillet. Stir in whole wheat flour and cook over medium heat for two to three minutes. Add milk slowly, stirring after each addition, to prevent lumping. Simmer over medium heat until sauce begins to thicken.

Flake 1½ cups (375 ml) of salmon meat and set aside. Place remaining salmon with bones in a blender with the stock. Process on medium speed until smooth.

Stir flaked salmon, blended salmon and thyme into skillet with sauce, and heat through. Serve hot.

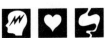

Noodle Soup

Makes three servings
2 cups (500 ml) *Chicken Stock* or *Vegetable Stock*
1½ teaspoons (7 ml) tamari
1 cup (250 ml) *High-Protein Noodles*

Bring stock and tamari to a boil. Add fresh noodles and return to the boil. Boil for about one minute, just until noodles are tender. Remove from heat and serve.

SALADS

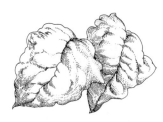

Spinach-Orange Salad

Makes two servings
spinach leaves
1 orange
1 tablespoon (15 ml) sesame tahini
1 tablespoon (15 ml) yogurt

A colorful and tasty salad that will brighten the table at any time of the year.

Wash enough spinach for two servings and set aside. Peel orange with a knife down to the pulp. Section the orange over a small dish which will catch the orange juice. On two salad plates, arrange the spinach leaves and decorate with orange sections. Squeeze the juice from the pulp left on the orange. Combine orange juice with tahini and yogurt. Shake in a jar or place in a blender on low speed until smooth. Serve dressing over the orange sections and spinach.

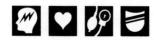

Fabulous Fruited Rice Salad with Yogurt Dressing

Makes four servings

One of our favorite salads—crunchy, juicy 'n' chewy.

Salad:
1½ cups (375 ml) cooked
        brown rice
   1 cup (250 ml) chopped
        pineapple
   1 pear, diced
   2 scallions, finely chopped
 ¼ cup (60 ml) walnuts, chopped
   2 tablespoons (30 ml) minced
        fresh parsley

Combine rice with fruit, scallions, walnuts and parsley. Combine dressing ingredients by shaking in a small jar with a lid or stirring vigorously in a bowl.

Toss salad ingredients with dressing until thoroughly coated. Chill and serve.

Dressing:
1 tablespoon (15 ml) safflower oil
1 tablespoon (15 ml) yogurt
1 teaspoon (5 ml) lemon juice
        dash freshly grated
        nutmeg

BREADS

Orange-Raisin Bread

Makes one loaf
2¾ cups (675 ml) whole wheat
        flour
   4 teaspoons (20 ml) *Baking
        Powder*
 ½ cup (125 ml) sunflower
        seeds
 ½ cup (125 ml) raisins
   1 tablespoon (15 ml) grated
        orange rind
   1 egg, slightly beaten
   1 cup (250 ml) orange juice
   1 tablespoon (15 ml) sesame
        tahini
 ½ cup (125 ml) yogurt
   2 tablespoons (30 ml) maple
        syrup

Makes a lovely breakfast bread, plain or spread with a little Yogurt Cream Cheese.

Combine dry ingredients in a large mixing bowl, including raisins and orange rind. In a separate bowl, combine remaining ingredients. Add wet to dry ingredients, mixing lightly until combined. Turn batter into a lightly oiled 8½ × 4½-inch (22 × 11-cm) bread pan. Bake in a preheated 325° F. (165° C.) oven for one hour, or until done.

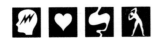

Brown Rice Bread

Makes two loaves
6 cups (1.5 l) whole wheat
 flour
2 cups (500 ml) cooked
 brown rice
1 cup (250 ml) soy flakes
1 tablespoon (15 ml) active
 dry yeast
2½ cups (625 ml) lukewarm
 water
1 teaspoon (5 ml) honey
1 tablespoon (15 ml) brewer's
 yeast
2 teaspoons (10 ml) caraway
 seeds
2 teaspoons (10 ml) kelp
 powder

Combine whole wheat flour, brown rice and soy flakes. Dissolve the yeast in ¼ cup (60 ml) of the lukewarm water and add the honey.

When the yeast is foamy, add to the flour mixture with two cups (500 ml) of the remaining lukewarm water and the brewer's yeast, caraway seeds and kelp. Mix well, adding additional lukewarm water if necessary to make a firm but soft dough.

Turn dough onto a floured surface and knead for about five minutes. Because of the rice, the dough may be slightly more crumbly than others.

Put the dough back into the bowl and cover. Allow to rise in a warm place until doubled in size, about 45 to 60 minutes.

Turn the dough back onto a floured surface and knead again for a few minutes. Divide dough in half and shape into two loaves. Lightly oil two 8½ × 4½-inch (22 × 11-cm) bread pans using equal parts of liquid lecithin and corn oil mixed together. Place loaves in pans and leave to rise until almost double. Bake loaves in the middle of a preheated 400° F. (200° C.) oven for 35 minutes or until the loaves sound hollow when tapped. Remove from pans and cool on baking rack.

MAIN DISHES

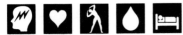

Makes four servings
3–4 medium tomatoes, coarsely
 chopped, or 2 cups
 (500 ml) cherry
 tomatoes
2 scallions
2 cloves garlic
2 tablespoons (30 ml) soy oil
2 teaspoons (10 ml) tamari
1 teaspoon (5 ml) basil
2 pounds (1 kg) fish fillets
 (cod, flounder,
 haddock, etc.)

Baked Fish Mediterranean

Hints of a sunshine coast steal through this easy-to-prepare dish along with the garlic, tomatoes and herbs.

Place the coarsely chopped tomatoes or whole cherry tomatoes in a blender with the scallions, garlic, oil, tamari and basil. Process on low, then medium speed until the sauce is smooth.

In an 8 × 8-inch (20 × 20-cm) casserole dish, place the fish fillets in a thick layer on the bottom, and pour the blended tomato sauce over them. Bake in a preheated 375° F. (190° C.) oven for 30 minutes, or just until the fish is cooked through.

Note: Any leftovers can be used in the recipe that follows: *Super Second-Day Chowder.* If you serve this baked fish with brown rice and carrots, plan to cook some extra amounts for the chowder.

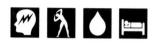

Makes four servings
1 cup (250 ml) skim milk
1 cup (250 ml) cooked
    brown rice
1 cup (250 ml) cooked
    carrots or other
    vegetable
1 cup (250 ml) cooked,
    flaked *Baked Fish
    Mediterranean*
½–¾ cup (125–175 ml) sauce
    from *Baked Fish
    Mediterranean*

Super Second-Day Chowder

For a quick-as-a-wink entree that is simple and delicious, you will have only yesterday's leftovers to thank.

In a large saucepan, combine the milk, rice, carrots, fish and sauce. Over medium heat, bring the chowder just to a boil, stirring frequently. Serve hot.

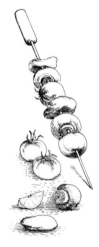

Makes two servings
⅓ cup (80 ml) water
3 tablespoons (45 ml) lemon
    juice
1 tablespoon (15 ml) tamari
1 clove garlic, crushed
½ teaspoon (2 ml) finely grated
    lemon rind
¼ teaspoon (1 ml) thyme
¼ teaspoon (1 ml) rosemary,
    crushed
¾ pound (340 g) chicken livers,
    halved
1 green or red sweet pepper
1 cup (250 ml) mushroom caps
1 cup (250 ml) cherry tomatoes

Chicken Liver Kebabs

Skewers present an array of vegetables in addition to tasty marinated livers.

Combine the water, lemon juice, tamari, garlic, lemon rind and herbs. Place the chicken livers in a shallow dish and pour marinade over top. Refrigerate several hours or overnight, basting occasionally with the marinade.

To prepare, halve the pepper and remove the seeds. Cut pepper into large pieces, about the size of the mushrooms. Lightly steam the pepper and mushrooms until they are only slightly tender.

On long metal skewers, arrange the tomatoes, pepper, mushrooms and liver alternately. Spoon a little of the marinade over each, then place under a hot broiler. Turn to cook both sides, and remove from broiler while livers are still slightly pink inside. Serve immediately.

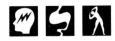

Split Pea Vegetable Soup

Makes six servings
1 cup (250 ml) dried split peas
4 cups (1 l) water
2 cups (500 ml) chopped
      tomatoes or cherry
      tomatoes
2 stalks celery, chopped
2 carrots, sliced
6 scallions, chopped, or ½ cup
      (125 ml) chopped onions
6 mushrooms, chopped
1 tablespoon (15 ml) tamari
½ teaspoon (2 ml) cumin
      powder

We couldn't call this plain ole split pea soup because of the terrific blend of vegetables swimming in its broth.

Place the split peas in the water in a large kettle. Puree the tomatoes on low speed in a blender and add to the peas with the other vegetables and the seasoning. Bring to a boil, reduce heat and simmer until split peas are tender, about 45 to 60 minutes. Serve hot.

Oriental Chicken Rolls

Makes two servings
1 whole chicken breast
4 scallions
4 cloves garlic, minced
2 teaspoons (10 ml) minced
      fresh ginger root
2 tablespoons (30 ml) tamari
2 tablespoons (30 ml) soy oil
¼ cup (60 ml) water
1 teaspoon (5 ml) ginger

While prepared here as a main dish, Oriental Chicken Rolls *also make unique cold hors d'oeuvres. Cool after baking, chill, then cut in thin slices.*

Chicken rolls must be started the day before they are to be served. Cut the flat breast muscle from the bone, saving the remaining meat and the bones for soup.

Cut the chicken breast in half and then slice each half in two pieces, crosswise. Cut tops from scallions so that they are each two inches (5 cm) long. Place one minced garlic clove, ½ teaspoon (2 ml) ginger root and one scallion on each breast piece. Roll up and tie securely with string. Marinate overnight in a mixture of tamari, oil, water and ginger.

When ready to bake, drain the chicken rolls saving the excess marinade. Place the breasts in a small casserole dish, spoon two tablespoons (30 ml) of the marinade over the chicken, cover and bake in a preheated 350° F. (175° C.) oven for 45 minutes. To serve, remove strings and place on a bed of cooked brown rice.

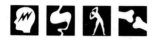

Split Pea Casserole

Makes six servings
3 cups (750 ml) cooked
    brown rice
1 tablespoon (15 ml) brewer's
    yeast
1 cup (250 ml) cottage cheese
3½ cups (875 ml) *Split Pea
    Vegetable Soup*
wheat germ

Made with leftover Split Pea Vegetable Soup, *this casserole is a quickie if you have cooked brown rice on hand. If you don't, plan to make double or triple the amount you use next time, and refrigerate or freeze the rest.*

Combine the rice, brewer's yeast and cottage cheese in the bottom of a large casserole dish. Pour on the soup and sprinkle with wheat germ. Place in a 350° F. (175° C.) oven about 30 minutes, until thoroughly heated.

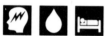

Pate Ring

Makes eight servings
2 cups (500 ml) sliced
    mushrooms (about ½
    pound [225 g])
1 medium onion, chopped
1 teaspoon (5 ml) corn oil
1 cup (250 ml) chicken livers
4 cups (1 l) dry whole grain
    bread, diced
½ cup (125 ml) chopped green
    peppers
1 cup (250 ml) chopped celery
2 eggs, beaten
½ cup (125 ml) walnuts,
    chopped
¼ cup (60 ml) chopped fresh
    parsley
½ teaspoon (2 ml) paprika
1 teaspoon (5 ml) crushed
    tarragon
⅛ teaspoon (0.5 ml) freshly
    grated nutmeg

Saute mushrooms and onion in oil, adding a few drops of water as needed to prevent scorching. When onions are translucent, add chicken livers and stir until redness disappears, and insides are pink. Do not overcook. Chop livers fine.

In a large bowl, combine livers with bread cubes and add remaining ingredients. When ingredients are combined, place in a lightly oiled Bundt pan or ring mold and bake in a preheated 350° F. (175° C.) oven about 45 minutes, until browned.

To serve, fill center with boiled peas and glaze *Pate Ring* with *Good Gravy.* Serve extra gravy on the side; you will want to double recipe for gravy in this case. Or fill center with creamed vegetables, using *Cauliflower White Sauce.*

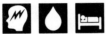

Makes four servings

2 cups (500 ml) cooked,
    cubed turkey breast
2 stalks celery, finely chopped
1 medium onion, finely
    chopped
1 sweet red pepper, finely
    chopped
2 tablespoons (30 ml) olive oil
1½ cups (375 ml) *Chicken
    Stock* or *Turkey Stock*
2 tablespoons (30 ml) minced
    fresh parsley
4 cups (1 l) cooked brown
    rice

Turkey with Vegetables on Brown Rice

Cube turkey breast, which has been roasted or poached without skin, and set aside.

Saute celery, onion and pepper in the oil until soft. Stir in turkey meat and stock. Heat through. Add the parsley and serve over brown rice.

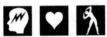

Makes two servings

8 ounces (225 g) tofu, cubed
¾ cup (175 ml) *V-7 Juice*
    dash cayenne pepper
2 tablespoons lemon juice
1 tablespoon (15 ml) oil
1 teaspoon (5 ml) tamari
2½ cups (625 ml) sliced
    mushrooms (about ½
    pound [225 g])
5 scallions, sliced
1 cup (250 ml) cooked brown
    rice
¼ cup (60 ml) coarsely
    chopped fresh parsley

Red Flannel Tofu

Marinate the tofu in the *V-7 Juice,* cayenne and lemon juice for at least one hour. Heat oil and tamari in a wok. When beginning to sizzle, add mushrooms and cook several minutes. Add scallions and cook two or three more minutes. Then add tofu mixture. When steaming, add rice and stir until mixture is very hot. Serve immediately. A green salad and whole wheat bread or *Pita Bread* make a good accompaniment.

Tuna Casserole

Makes six servings

2 teaspoons (10 ml) corn oil
2 cups (500 ml) sliced
    mushrooms
1 onion, chopped
1 stalk celery, chopped
1 clove garlic, crushed
2 tablespoons (30 ml) basil
½ teaspoon (2 ml) thyme
4 cups (1 l) cooked brown rice
6½ ounces (184 g) water-packed
    tuna, drained
½ pound (225 g) poached fish
    fillets, flaked
½ cup (125 ml) grated mild,
    hard cheese (longhorn or
    mild cheddar)
    Cauliflower White Sauce I
    or *II*
2 tablespoons (30 ml) grated
    Parmesan cheese

Heat the oil in a large skillet, and saute mushrooms, onion, celery, garlic and herbs until vegetables are tender.

In a large mixing bowl, combine the rice, tuna, fish and the mushroom mixture. Place in a deep casserole dish and sprinkle with the grated cheese. Cover with *Cauliflower White Sauce,* and sprinkle with Parmesan.

Bake in a preheated 350° F. (175° C.) oven 30 to 45 minutes, until hot and bubbly.

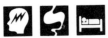

Spinach-Rice Casserole

Makes four servings

1 cup (250 ml) brown rice
2 cups (500 ml) water
1 pound (450 g) spinach (5–6
    quarts [5–6 l] unpacked)
2 eggs, beaten
½ cup (125 ml) yogurt
1 clove garlic, crushed
    dash freshly grated nutmeg
¼ cup (60 ml) grated Parmesan
    cheese
¼ cup (60 ml) walnuts, chopped
1 tablespoon (15 ml) sesame
    seeds
    dash cayenne pepper
1 teaspoon (5 ml) tamari
½ teaspoon (2 ml) oregano
¼ cup (60 ml) wheat germ

Cook rice in water. Thoroughly wash spinach and chop fine. In a medium bowl, combine eggs with yogurt and remaining ingredients, except wheat germ. Toss spinach, rice and egg mixture to combine in a large bowl, and place in a lightly oiled casserole. Top with the wheat germ. Bake in a 350° F. (175° C.) oven for 35 minutes.

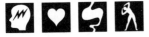

Confetti Rice 'n' Beans

Makes six servings

1 onion, chopped
1 green pepper, chopped
1 tablespoon (15 ml) soy oil
1 cup (250 ml) brown rice
1 tablespoon (15 ml) sesame
    seeds
2½ cups (625 ml) water
1 cup (250 ml) cooked beans
2 cups (500 ml) tomato puree
1 cup (250 ml) fresh or frozen
    corn
1 teaspoon (5 ml) tamari
1 teaspoon (5 ml) basil
½ teaspoon (2 ml) marjoram
½ teaspoon (2 ml) thyme
    dash cayenne pepper

In a heavy skillet, saute onion and green pepper in oil. When the onion is translucent, stir in rice and sesame seeds. Stir over medium heat for 2 to 3 minutes. Add water and cover pan for 35 minutes, until rice is nearly tender. Add beans, tomato puree, corn, tamari and spices. Cook 15 to 20 minutes. Serve hot.

A good accompaniment is corn bread and a crisp salad.

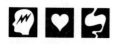

SIDE DISHES

High-Protein Noodles

Makes two cups (500 ml)
¾ cup (175 ml) whole wheat
    flour
2 tablespoons (30 ml) soy flour
1 teaspoon (5 ml) brewer's
    yeast
¼ teaspoon (1 ml) kelp powder
½ cup (125 ml) yogurt

Mix together the flours, brewer's yeast and kelp powder in a medium bowl. Place the mixture in a mound on a sturdy work surface. With your fingers, form a "well" or large indentation in the center of the mound of flour. Place the yogurt in the well.

With a fork, beat the yogurt lightly, pulling in a little of the flour mixture as you work. Try to keep the yogurt in the center of the flour so it does not run over the work surface. When most of the flour is incorporated into the yogurt, begin to knead the dough with your hands until all of the flour is used. Set the dough aside, under the overturned mixing bowl. Clean off the work surface and your hands, then lightly flour the work surface and begin to knead the dough again. Flatten the dough slightly, then lift the far edge of the circle of dough, fold toward you, and push down into the remaining dough with the heel of your hand. Repeat, turning the dough as you work. The dough should be kneaded about 8 to 10 minutes, until it is smooth.

Divide the kneaded ball of dough in two, and cover the one half with the inverted mixing bowl. Sprinkle flour on the work surface, and flatten the other half with the heels of your hands. Form a flattened circle with the dough.

With a lightly floured rolling pin, begin in the center of the circle and begin to roll out toward the edges. Turn the dough as you work, so that it will be round. Continue rolling and stretching the dough until it is about ⅛ inch (3 mm) thick, almost translucent. Work quickly so that the dough does not dry out.

When it is rolled as thin as you can get it, let it rest on a lightly floured surface, covered loosely with a towel. Roll the remaining ball of dough.

When the rolled dough has rested 8 to 10 minutes, turn it over and cover again with the towel. After about 20 minutes, it will have lost its shiny surface and become slightly dry to the touch. You can lightly dust the surface of the rolled dough, if you wish, for you will be rolling the dough up and do not want it to stick together.

The dough should be rolled like a jellyroll. With a sharp knife, cut "slices" off the roll as wide as you desire the noodles. Separate the noodles as soon as they are cut by lifting them up with the tips of the fingers and very gently shaking them loose.

The noodles can be cooked in a large amount of boiling water immediately, or they can be left to dry on a lightly floured surface until they are leathery. (Time will depend upon the temperature of the room and the humidity.) The noodles can be frozen at this stage, after being placed in an airtight plastic bag. They can also be refrigerated up to a week.

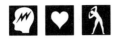

Baked Vegetable Rice

Makes six servings

3 cups (750 ml) cooked brown
  rice
2 cups (500 ml) finely chopped
  leeks
1 stalk celery, finely chopped
1 cup (250 ml) cottage cheese
2 tablespoons (30 ml) chopped
  fresh parsley
2 teaspoons (10 ml) basil
½ teaspoon (2 ml) oregano
½ teaspoon (2 ml) marjoram
¼ teaspoon (1 ml) cumin
  powder

Toss together the rice, vegetables, cheese and herbs in a large bowl. Place in a lightly oiled, shallow 8 × 8-inch (20 × 20-cm) baking pan. Bake rice mixture, covered, in a preheated 350° F. (175° C.) oven for one hour.

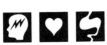

Toasted Brown Rice Stuffing

Makes about two cups
½ cup (125 ml) brown rice
1½ cups (375 ml) *Chicken
    Stock* or *Vegetable
    Stock*
1 teaspoon (5 ml) tamari
2 teaspoons (10 ml) corn oil
1 tablespoon (15 ml) finely
    chopped onions
1 tablespoon (15 ml) finely
    chopped celery
1 tablespoon (15 ml) minced
    fresh parsley
1 cup (250 ml) dry whole
    grain bread crumbs
1 egg, beaten
2–3 tablespoons (30–45 ml)
    buttermilk (optional)
½ teaspoon (2 ml) basil
½ teaspoon (2 ml) thyme
    pinch marjoram
    pinch rosemary, crumbled

Spread the uncooked rice in a shallow baking pan and place in a preheated 400° F. (200° C.) oven until light brown. Stir to prevent burning. Set aside, and turn down oven to 350° F. (175° C.).

Place toasted rice in a saucepan with stock and tamari, cover, and simmer over low heat until broth is absorbed.

In a skillet, heat the oil, and saute the onions, celery and parsley until tender, adding a few drops of water, if necessary, to prevent scorching.

When vegetables are done, toss them with bread crumbs, rice, egg, buttermilk (if the mixture seems too dry), and seasonings.

Stuffing can be used to fill chicken breasts before roasting, or can be placed in a small casserole dish, covered, and baked for about 20 minutes at 350° F. (175° C.).

MISCELLANEOUS

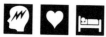

Banana Hors d'Oeuvres

Makes four to six servings
¼ cup (60 ml) yogurt
¼ teaspoon (1 ml) chili powder
½ teaspoon (2 ml) turmeric
½ teaspoon (2 ml) ginger
2 cloves garlic, crushed
2 bananas
  wheat germ

Unusual hors d'oeuvres which can also be served as a vegetable with a main course such as Savory Chicken Curry.

Combine yogurt with the spices and garlic. Peel bananas and cut diagonally into thick slices. Place bananas and yogurt into dish and marinate bananas for at least two hours, preferably four. Roll the slices in wheat germ and bake in a preheated 350° F. (175° C.) oven for 20 minutes. Serve warm with toothpicks.

Sesame Tofu Dip

Makes ¾ cup (175 ml)
¼ cup (60 ml) lemon juice
2 tablespoons (30 ml) sesame
  seeds
1 clove garlic
2 scallions
1 tablespoon (15 ml) soy oil
8 ounces (225 g) tofu
2 tablespoons (30 ml) sesame
  tahini
¼ cup (60 ml) fresh parsley
¼ teaspoon (1 ml) paprika

Combine the lemon juice and sesame seeds in a blender and process on medium speed until the seeds are pulverized. Add the garlic, scallions and oil. Add half the tofu, and process on low speed until combined; repeat with remaining tofu along with the tahini. Add the parsley and paprika and process on medium speed until smooth. Chill and serve with *Pita Bread,* crackers or with raw fresh vegetables.

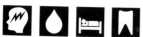

Mark's Trail Mix

Makes one cup (250 ml)
½ cup (125 ml) raisins
¼ cup (60 ml) sunflower seeds
¼ cup (60 ml) chopped walnuts

You don't have to take a hike to enjoy this energy-giving, nutrient-rich snack.

Combine all ingredients. Store in a tightly covered jar in the refrigerator.

Raisin Chews

Makes one dozen
3 tablespoons (45 ml)
    *Yogurt Cream
    Cheese*
1 teaspoon (5 ml) brewer's
    yeast
2 tablespoons (30 ml)
    peanut butter
1 teaspoon (5 ml) honey
1 teaspoon (5 ml)
    blackstrap molasses
12–24 raisins
    wheat germ

Combine all ingredients except raisins and wheat germ.

Form small balls, placing one or two raisins in the center of each, and roll in wheat germ. Serve as a confection.

BEVERAGES

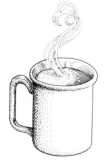

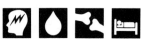

Peanut Butter Toddy

Makes one serving
3 tablespoons (45 ml) peanut
    butter
1 tablespoon (15 ml) medium
    unsulfured molasses
½ teaspoon (2 ml) brewer's
    yeast
1 cup (250 ml) skim milk

A hot, delicious peanut butter drink loaded with protein, potassium, calcium, iron and B vitamins.

Place peanut butter, molasses and brewer's yeast in small saucepan and stir in a small amount of milk. Over low heat, combine ingredients until smooth. Add remaining milk, and continue stirring until hot, but not boiling. Serve in warmed mug with a spoon.

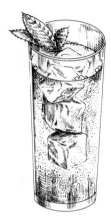

Summer Drink on the Green

Makes two servings
½ cup (125 ml) packed spinach
½ cup (125 ml) apple juice
1 banana
1 tablespoon (15 ml) sesame
      tahini
2 ice cubes
   mint sprigs or lemon slices
      (garnish)

Place all ingredients in a blender and whip until frothy. Makes about 1½ cups (375 ml).

For a garnish, try a sprig of mint or place a lemon slice on the edge of the glass.

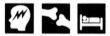

Banana-Strawberry Drink

Makes one large serving
1 cup (250 ml) skim milk
1 small or ½ large banana
2 strawberries
1 teaspoon (5 ml) brewer's yeast
1 teaspoon (5 ml) medium
      unsulfured molasses
1 teaspoon (5 ml) peanut butter
2 ice cubes

Place all ingredients in a blender and process on medium speed until smooth. Serve immediately.

Clove Tea

Makes one serving
3–4 whole cloves
   1 cup (250 ml) water

Before preparing your favorite herbal tea, flavor the water with cloves.

Place the cloves in the water in a small saucepan. Bring to a boil. Remove cloves, then prepare tea as usual.

Variation: Add a cinnamon stick, or substitute one for the cloves.

Hot Carob Drink

Makes two servings
1 tablespoon (15 ml) carob
    powder
½ cup (125 ml) water
2 teaspoons (10 ml) honey
1½ cups (375 ml) skim milk
½ teaspoon (2 ml) *Vanilla
    Extract*
dash cinnamon

Combine carob, water and honey in a saucepan and bring to a boil. Reduce heat and simmer one to two minutes. Pour in milk and heat, but do not boil. Remove from heat. Stir in vanilla and a dash of cinnamon. Warm two mugs by rinsing with boiling water. Fill with hot beverage and serve.

Warm Golden Milk

Makes two servings
¼ teaspoon (60 ml) turmeric
4 whole cardamom seeds
½ cup (125 ml) water
1 cup (250 ml) whole milk
honey

A sophisticated, deeply soothing nightcap.

Boil turmeric and cardamom seeds in water in a small saucepan for eight minutes. Meanwhile, in another pan, bring milk just to the boiling point; turn off heat. Add turmeric mixture, remove cardamom seeds, and serve with honey to taste.

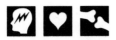

Carob Yogurt Frosty

Makes one serving
½ cup (125 ml) yogurt
¼ cup (60 ml) cold water
2 or 3 ice cubes
1 tablespoon (15 ml) *Carob
    Syrup*
½ banana

Process in blender on medium speed until creamy.

DESSERTS

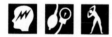

Sweet Potato Cheesecake

Makes 10 servings
1 pound (450 g) tofu
1 egg
¼ cup (60 ml) maple syrup
1 teaspoon (5 ml) finely grated
  orange rind
1 teaspoon (5 ml) *Vanilla
  Extract*
1 egg white
1 cup (250 ml) cooked sweet
  potatoes, with skins
½ cup (125 ml) yogurt
½ cup (125 ml) cottage cheese
2 tablespoons (30 ml) orange
  juice
¼ cup (60 ml) walnuts, chopped
¼ cup (60 ml) wheat germ
¼ cup (60 ml) bran
  orange slices

Combine one-half of the tofu, the egg, maple syrup, orange rind and vanilla in a blender on low speed. Place in a large bowl. Blend the remaining tofu with the egg white, and mix with the first tofu mixture. Then blend sweet potatoes, yogurt, cottage cheese and juice. Combine with the tofu mixture, stirring in the nuts by hand.

Lightly oil a 9-inch (23-cm) springform pan and sprinkle with the wheat germ and bran. Pour the cheesecake batter into the pan and place in a preheated 350° F. (175° C.) oven. Bake 35 to 40 minutes, until the cheesecake is firm. Turn off the heat, open the oven door and allow cheesecake to cool a bit before removing. Place in refrigerator when cheesecake reaches room temperature, and chill for at least six hours before serving.

To serve, loosen sides of cake from the pan, remove rim and garnish cheesecake with orange slices.

Banana-Rice Cream

Makes two servings
1 cup (250 ml) soft, cooked
  brown rice
1 banana
1 tablespoon (15 ml) gelatin
½ cup (125 ml) cold water
1 tablespoon (15 ml) honey
½ teaspoon (2 ml) finely grated
  lemon rind
½ teaspoon (2 ml) *Vanilla
  Extract*
½ cup (125 ml) buttermilk
  sliced fruit

Rice and bananas are both good sources of vitamin B$_6$.

Place rice and banana in a blender. Dissolve the gelatin in the water and add to the rice and banana mixture with all of the remaining ingredients except fruit. Process on medium speed until very smooth. Place mixture in two one-cup (250 ml) dessert dishes. Chill until firm. Serve with fresh fruit topping.

Note: For softer cooked rice, add 2½ cups (625 ml) of water for each cup of raw rice when preparing boiled brown rice. Or, add ¼ to ½ cup (60 to 125 ml) of water to 1 cup (250 ml) of regular cooked rice and heat over low flame, stirring often, until water is absorbed and rice is soft.

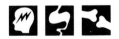

Makes eight servings

Filling:

1 quart (1 l) skim milk
¼ cup (60 ml) honey
1-inch (2.5-cm) piece
　　vanilla bean or 1
　　teaspoon *Vanilla*
　　Extract
⅔ cup (150 ml) brown
　　rice
2 eggs, separated
2 tablespoons (30 ml)
　　honey

Crust:

¼ cup (60 ml) skim milk
2 teaspoons (10 ml)
　　active dry yeast
2 teaspoons (10 ml)
　　honey
¼ cup (60 ml) lukewarm
　　water
1 tablespoon (15 ml) corn
　　oil
1¼–1½ cups (300–375 ml)
　　whole wheat flour

Brown Rice Pie

Based on a traditional Dutch recipe, Rijstevlaai.

To make the filling, combine the milk, honey, vanilla and rice in a heavy-bottom saucepan and bring to a boil over medium heat. Turn down heat and simmer about 40 to 45 minutes. The rice should be nearly tender and there should be a little milk left in the pan.

While the rice is cooking, prepare the crust. Scald the milk and set it aside to cool. Dissolve the yeast with the honey in the lukewarm water in a medium bowl. Combine the yeast mixture with the oil and lukewarm milk. Stir in enough flour to make a soft dough. Do not knead. Set aside to rise about 20 minutes.

To complete the rice filling, remove the rice from the stove when it is done cooking and take out the vanilla bean, if used. In a small bowl, beat the egg yolks with the honey. Whip the egg whites with a whisk or eggbeater in a medium bowl until stiff. When the rice mixture has cooled somewhat, stir some of the rice into the egg yolks, then add the yolks to the remaining rice mixture. Fold in the stiffly beaten egg whites.

When the dough has risen, roll out and place dough in a 9-inch (23-cm) pie plate. Trim the dough to fit, and flute the edges. Prick bottom of pie shell with a fork, and fill with the rice mixture. Bake in a preheated 400° F. (200° C.) oven for 30 minutes, or until the top is well browned.

Note: Excess dough can be rolled flat and wrapped around banana slices, then baked until brown: a tasty, nutritious snack!

Chapter 5

Slenderizing Naturally

Reaching and maintaining a healthful weight is one of the very best things you can do for your total well-being.

If you fatigue easily, slenderizing will replace energy-sapping flab with new vigor and vitality.

If you have heart disease, slenderizing will take a load off your strained heart, almost certainly lower your blood fats, improve any angina and make it easier for you to get the exercise you need.

If you have high blood pressure, slenderizing will help bring it down.

If you have adult (maturity-onset) diabetes, slenderizing will tend to normalize your blood sugar and in some cases make it unnecessary to take drugs.

If you have arthritis, slenderizing will take strain off your joints. If you have a tendency to develop gout, slenderizing will help prevent the formation of painful crystals.

And, if you have none of those ailments, slenderizing could help protect you against all of them.

Getting your weight back to normal can also help avoid the need for surgery in such cases as hernia, gallstones and obstructed coronary vessels. If surgery is unavoidable, slenderizing will make it easier for the surgeon to do a faster, cleaner job, and enable you to heal your incision much faster and more comfortably.

If your self-image is tarnished and pitted, slenderizing will replace it with bright new confidence and optimism. You will feel better, look younger, and people will pay you such gratifying compliments that you'll swear it's a Cinderella story come true. Who would have guessed such beauty lay hidden beneath that flab?

You're convinced, you say? You didn't even *need* convincing? Well, then, let's stop wasting time and get down to work. Because that's what losing weight is. Only it's *not* the kind of work you probably think it is, so our very first job is to clear our minds of misconceptions and learn the new rules of natural weight control.

New Rule #1. What you put into your shopping basket is more important than what you put on your dinner plate.

That doesn't seem to make sense, but think about it a minute. Most "diets"—and our approach is most definitely *not* a diet—concentrate almost entirely on exactly how much of which foods you are supposed to eat. But how you are supposed to feel *satisfied* with such small amounts, they never tell you! The result is that after a week or two on one of those melt-your-fat-so-fast-you'll-have-to-mop-up-the-floor diets, you feel so deprived you just can't stand it. So you start rummaging through your shelves and refrigerator like the secret police looking for stolen microfilm. And what do you find? According to our own weight loss police, it's probably cupcakes, Oreos, pretzels, potato chips, ice cream, cake or pie. Most likely, several of the above. And you eat them so fast you hardly taste them. And you may not *stop* eating until your stomach hurts.

Sometimes, it's not quite that dramatic. At suppertime, you put on your plate only what your diet tells you to eat. An hour or two later, when you're watching TV, you get an irresistible urge to snack—which doesn't seem quite so unreasonable at that point because you ate such a small dinner. So you gulp down 300 calories or more in a big dish of ice cream.

Face it. Willpower is not your strong suit. Regardless of what you plan and hope to eat, so long as your kitchen is forever stocked with irresistible goodies, you will be forever overweight.

It's a lot easier to make rational decisions at the market than when you're standing in front of your own refrigerator looking at a big wedge of cheesecake. So take advantage of that fact and begin thinking a little more while you shop.

If you don't buy it, you won't eat it. But we aren't going to give you a long list of no-nos because we've found that people vary a lot in their weaknesses, just as they do in their strengths. A very simple, but very effective technique to use when shopping is to strictly avoid buying those items which you know are *irresistible* to you personally. Foods which you know you abuse. The list may be extensive or quite small. It could be just ice cream, or even a certain flavor of ice cream. Maybe it's a brownie mix. Corn chips. Or perhaps something that seems relatively wholesome but is loaded with fat and calories, like potato salad, lunchmeat, or cheese spreads. Perhaps you can't control your intake of something that may even enjoy the status of a health food, like nuts or dried fruits.

And when you pass by that item on the supermarket shelf, tell yourself this: *I'm not really depriving myself by passing this by. With me, eating this item is a habit, a compulsion. I don't eat it because I'm hungry or my stomach needs it. I eat it because my nerves crave it. And there are better ways to satisfy and calm my nerves than ingesting food mindlessly.*

New Rule #2. The more natural foods you put into your shopping basket, the easier it will be for you to lose weight permanently.

The unnatural additives you want to avoid here are fat and sugar. In that order. Ounce for ounce, fat has more than twice as many calories as sugar. A tablespoon of sugar has about 50 calories, but a tablespoon of oil has 120. An enormous number of processed foods contain large amounts of added fat, often in the form of "vegetable oil" —which usually means coconut oil, the worst kind for your health. Shortening is used in many baked goods. Cold cuts and sausage products such as hot dogs are not only made from fatty meat, but contain added animal fat as well. When you eat a hamburger at McDonald's, you're not only getting beef fat from the burger, but pig fat from the bun, in which it's used for flavoring.

Sugar or a similar refined carbohydrate is almost always found in processed foods. Two of the worst examples we can think of—because they're disguised as "natural"—are commercial fruit-flavored yogurt and commercial granola. A carton of *plain* yogurt has about 150 calories. The fruit-flavored variety usually has between 260 and 280. The fact is, there is so little real fruit added to these items that nearly all the caloric difference comes from plain sugar, about six or seven teaspoons per cup! And commercial granola is no better. One popular variety is sweetened with brown sugar, honey, chopped dates and raisins (both of the latter are high in natural sugar). If they put all those different sources of sugar together, they would weigh more than the main ingredient of the granola, which is rolled oats. But if they did that, they would have to list sugar as the very first ingredient and that wouldn't be good for the image of granola as a "natural" food.

The simplest way to get away from this saturation of calories is to stick with the most natural foods possible. If you like granola, for instance, use any of our recipes for muesli, which have no added oil and no sweeteners. If you want meat, get natural meat, not cold cuts or sausages, which often have added fat. If you want fish, get natural fish—not fish sticks. If you want fruit, get natural fruit—not the kind canned in sugar water. *Every step toward natural is a step toward slenderness.*

New Rule #3. To lose weight without hunger pangs, bulk up on the natural carbohydrates.

Bulk up on carbohydrates? Did we really say that? No! We said *natural* carbohydrates. Despite all the badmouthing carbohydrates and starches have gotten recently during the craze of high-protein crash diets, the natural carbohydrate foods are your best bet for getting your weight under control.

Here's why the confusion. There are *two different kinds* of carbohydrate food. One kind consists of whole foods, rich in starch, fiber, protein, vitamins and minerals. We call them the natural carbohydrates, but they've also been labeled the "honest carbohydrates," while scientists refer to them as *complex* carbohydrates. They all have substantial amounts of starch, and include grains, such as wheat, corn, rice, oats, barley and rye, as well as potatoes, beans, lentils and peas.

The other kind of carbohydrate food—which isn't really a food at all, but a food *extract*—is not much more than sugar: white sugar, brown sugar, date sugar, corn syrup, molasses, maple syrup and honey. In the last two instances, the extracting is done mainly by nature, but all are classified as *simple* carbohydrates because they are basically sugar rather than starch. More obviously, they contain no fiber or protein and no meaningful amounts of vitamins or minerals, except in the unusual case of blackstrap molasses.

There is a world of difference between the way your body handles these two kinds of carbohydrate foods. The *complex* carbohydrates let us know that we've eaten something substantial. They are digested slowly and absorbed gradually, producing relatively moderate fluctuations in blood sugar levels. In addition, they come complete with nutrients essential for their own metabolism. By comparison, *simple* carbohydrates don't fill us up. They are quickly absorbed into our bloodstreams causing a sudden surge in blood sugar levels. Then, an hour or two later, when our blood sugar plummets to very low levels, we find ourselves fighting off fatigue by eating—*again.*

The fibrous bulk of the complex carbohydrates not only fills us up, but actually reduces the calories we are able to absorb from our food. A study carried out by the U. S. Department of Agriculture in cooperation with the University of Maryland reveals that when you eat a diet just *moderately* high in fiber, your body absorbs about five percent fewer calories than when you eat a typically low-fiber diet. That five percent reduction will mean, on the average, about 100 fewer calories absorbed and turned into fat-power each day. No whole grain products were used in this high-fiber diet, however, because the purpose of the study was to see if a *moderate* increase of fiber would have any effect. Our guess is that if you follow a truly high-fiber diet, the kind presented in this book, the number of calories you save yourself each day could easily reach 150. And that means losing about 10 pounds over a period of months—while still eating the same number of calories you'd consume on a typical low-fiber diet built around eggs, milk, cheese, meat, juices and white bread.

New Rule #4. To help extinguish the smoldering fires of appetite, drink plenty of water.

Water is neither carbohydrate nor protein; vitamin nor mineral. Yet, it's one of the most important things in our diet.

Often we eat something that has a high water content—like ice cream or pie —simply because our mouths and throats are dry. Drink some good spring water instead.

Most of us have gotten into the habit of drinking soda or juice or beer because they seem more interesting than water. In fact, we estimate that many people with a weight problem could easily lose 10 or 20 pounds without cutting out any real food from their diets. All they'd have to do is replace drinks loaded with calories with plain water. And water, remember, is the most effective thirst quencher in the business.

New Rule #5. Make sure your environment is not hazardous to your weight.

Now that we've talked a little about what you eat, let's take a look at *how* you eat. In fact, let's take a look around your *house.* Is there any food in the living room? Bowls of candy, nuts, even fruit? Why subject yourself to constant temptation? Put them away.

Now take a look in your kitchen. Are there cookies sitting on the counter? Rolls, cakes, leftovers? No? Good! Now open that refrigerator. What are the first things you see? If they are things you don't want to eat, put them way in the back. Better yet, put them in the trash can. But if you can't, for one reason or another, at least make sure they're in a place where you won't "accidentally" see them and get an irresistible impulse to put them in your mouth every time you open the refrigerator.

New Rule #6. Plan your meals. Don't let supper become an accident.

Often in trying to lose weight, we force ourselves to stop thinking about food. But it's one thing not to be *obsessed* with food and quite another to ignore it. Eventually, your hunger will get the better of you and drive you into the kitchen to search out this and that and everything else that looks halfway edible. And the longer you delay your meal, the hungrier you are, and the more likely you are to eat junk food, because junk food seldom needs any preparation other than being stripped of its cellophane wrapper.

If things aren't that bad in your house, you can still do yourself a favor by planning ahead not only *what* you want to eat, but how *much* of it should be prepared. Don't try to cook *less* than you think is reasonable, but don't cook a whole lot more, either. Otherwise, the temptation to "get rid of those leftovers" may be more than you can cope with.

Here is another technique. If you *have* cooked more than you plan to eat on that particular evening, don't take all of it to the table. Leave it on the stove to cool, or if you can, cover it immediately and stash it away in the refrigerator.

As soon as you are done eating, clear everything from the table. If you have a habit of "cleaning up" other people's plates, clear yourself away from the table, too. Get busy doing something in another part of the house—the workshop, your bedroom, the den. Be aware of the fact that we all feel much fuller and more satisfied half-an-hour after we're done eating than we do when we're still at the table. It takes that long for the "fullness" message to get through to our appetite center. Don't spend that half-an-hour nibbling on leftovers.

New Rule #7. Fill up on real food, not fat.

Before you start worrying too much about the fat content of cheese, whole milk and meat, consider the fat content of fat itself. Oil, shortening, butter. Many people can't cook without it. Or *think* they can't. The result is that perfectly nutritious low-calorie vegetables get coated with 100 extra calories for every tablespoon of butter used. Every tablespoon of oil that's used to fry or saute—or even used in a salad—adds 120 calories. The calories in a piece of bread are increased fully 50 percent by a single pat of butter.

Precious little of that fat is really necessary to make food palatable. For sauteing, we use the steam-stir method described earlier in the section "Getting It All Together." What we do is simply substitute water or a zesty mixture of fat-free liquid and herbs, and cook the food a little more slowly, so it turns out juicy, tender, and free of added fat. If you eat bread with your meal, dip it in these liquids to moisten it, rather than spread on butter. (Margarine, by the way, has the same number of calories as butter.) On salads, use skim milk yogurt mixed with vegetable juices and some herbs and spices instead of oil.

Once you've learned these simple techniques, you can become a little more conscious of foods that contain large amounts of fat. The worst are probably mayonnaise, tartar sauce, and sour cream. If you put one pat of butter and two heaping tablespoons of sour cream on a medium baked potato, you're getting more calories from what's *on* the potato than what's *in* it. Substitute yogurt for sour cream and you slash the calories by an amazing 75 percent! For dishes that seem to demand mayonnaise, use our delicious *Tofu Mayonnaise* (see *Index*) instead and get all the good taste while saving almost 90 percent of the calories. Go from whole milk to low-fat milk and save about 50 calories per cup. Go all the way to skim milk and save 70 calories—all from eliminating fat.

In case you have any lingering doubts about the caloric importance of natural carbohydrates vs. fat, think about this: a single four-ounce stick of butter or margarine contains more calories than 10 pieces of whole grain bread or five baked potatoes.

New Rule #8. Plan your snacks.

Don't try to kid yourself into thinking you're never going to have another snack as long as you live. We all get the munchies sometimes. The important thing is to be *ready.* Because if there's nothing there that fills the bill, there's no telling where your wandering eyes are going to go or what your hands are going to grab. So have a *reasonable* snack on hand, like some good crisp apples or oranges, and tell yourself that these items will be your snacks when you get the urge. Raw carrots or wedges of cabbage are also good snacks. Stay away from nuts and dried fruits; it's too easy to eat too many of them.

New Rule #9. Don't convict yourself of homicide for eating an ice cream cone.

Once in a while, you're bound to goof up. It may be at someone else's house, or at a big party, or maybe you're just shopping when you pass an ice cream stand and the next thing you know, you've ordered a double decker. Fret not. A snack like that only has the caloric power to put an ounce or two on you and most likely, you'll adjust for that little increase by being a little less hungry at your next meal.

So don't get angry at yourself. Don't feel guilty. *The less emotional you are about your eating, the easier it will be for you to eat rationally.*

If you are in doubt about occasional indulgences, ask yourself: *Did I just hit a pothole? Or am I stuck in a ditch?* If you just ran over a pothole, forget it and keep rolling along. If you feel you're stuck in a ditch and need help to pull yourself out, we immodestly recommend a book called *Lose Weight Naturally* by Mark Bricklin (Rodale Press, 1979).

New Rule # 10. The ultimate secret: take it easy.

That could be the most important rule of all. Nearly everyone believes the faster they take weight off, the better they're doing. Actually, the exact opposite is true. Every knowledgeable medical person who has experience in weight reducing knows that the faster weight comes off, the faster it goes back on. At the end of every crash diet is a head-on collision with old eating habits. *No matter how much weight you have lost, if you go back to eating the way you did before, you will wind up weighing exactly what you did before you went through all that agony.*

But if you take it easy, if you lose no more than one or two pounds a week, you will be giving your eating habits an honest chance to change. This is a *learning process* we're talking about, not a pain endurance contest. It takes time to learn something new. Habits, especially, change only gradually. The important thing is not what you weigh a month from now, but what you weigh for the rest of your life. So give yourself a chance to succeed. Take it easy.

BREAKFASTS

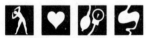

Raisin Breakfast Rice

Makes two servings
3 cups (750 ml) water
½ cup (125 ml) brown rice
¼ cup (60 ml) millet
½ unpeeled apple, chopped
2 tablespoons (30 ml) raisins
¼ teaspoon (1 ml) cinnamon

Combine ingredients in a medium saucepan and bring to a boil over moderate heat. Stir, reduce heat, and simmer with lid on for 25 to 30 minutes, until water is absorbed and rice is tender. Do not stir.

Serve as is, or with a little orange juice or skim milk.

French Toast

Makes four servings
1 egg
2 egg whites
2 tablespoons (30 ml) skim milk
½ teaspoon (2 ml) *Vanilla
    Extract*
¼ teaspoon (1 ml) cinnamon
4 large slices whole grain bread

Makes a delicious breakfast, especially with dark breads such as pumpernickel. The recipe works best with breads that are slightly stale.

Beat egg and egg whites together in a shallow bowl with a whisk or a fork. Add the milk, vanilla and cinnamon.

Heat a skillet brushed with oil. Dip slices of bread into egg mixture, coating both sides, and place in a skillet, turning when bottom is browned. *French Toast* can also be grilled under a broiler.

Serve it hot topped with applesauce or a combination of fresh fruits such as sliced bananas, melons and strawberries.

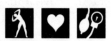

Fruited Yogurt Muesli

Makes one serving
⅓ cup (80 ml) rolled oats
⅔ cup (150 ml) water
3 tablespoons (45 ml) yogurt
1 teaspoon (5 ml) honey
1 tangerine
½ unpeeled apple, chopped

Soak oats in water overnight, or let stand 45 to 60 minutes in the morning. Stir in yogurt, honey, tangerine sections with membrane removed, and apple.

Variation: Use an orange, grapefruit, peach, pineapple, grapes or strawberries in place of the tangerine. Substitute pear for apple.

SOUPS

Minestrone

Makes eight servings

½ cup (125 ml) dried white
   beans
2 teaspoons (10 ml) sesame oil
1 cup (250 ml) diced zucchini
1 cup (250 ml) diced carrots
1 cup (250 ml) diced potatoes
⅓ cup (80 ml) thinly sliced
   celery
2 tablespoons (30 ml) finely
   chopped onions
½ cup (125 ml) finely chopped
   leeks
2 cups (500 ml) chopped, ripe
   tomatoes or drained
   Italian plum tomatoes
4 cups (1 l) *Chicken Stock,*
   Vegetable Stock,
   reserved vegetable water
   or combination
1 bay leaf
1 teaspoon (5 ml) kelp powder
1 teaspoon (5 ml) minced fresh
   parsley
½ cup (125 ml) brown rice
1 cup (250 ml) fresh or frozen
   peas
   grated Parmesan cheese

Soak the beans overnight and cook until barely tender (see *Index,* "Cooking Beans"). In the oil in a large skillet or saucepan, saute the zucchini, carrots, potatoes and celery for 2 to 3 minutes, and set aside. In the same saucepan or skillet, steam-stir the onions and leeks in a small amount of water for 5 minutes, until soft and lightly browned. Stir in the tomatoes, the vegetables, stock, bay leaf, kelp and parsley. Bring to a boil over high heat, then reduce heat and simmer, partially covered, for 20 minutes. Remove bay leaf and add the drained rice. Simmer 25 to 30 minutes more, adding peas during the last 5 to 10 minutes of cooking. To serve, garnish lightly with grated Parmesan cheese.

Note: To vary leftover soup, add tomato puree and leftover *Savory Chicken Curry* or *Pate Ring* and serve as a sauce over pasta. Season with oregano, basil and garlic to taste.

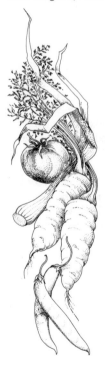

Oven Split Pea Soup

Makes four servings
2 onions, chopped
2 stalks celery, chopped
1 bay leaf
1 cup (250 ml) dried split peas
1 teaspoon (5 ml) basil
1 teaspoon (5 ml) thyme
½ teaspoon (2 ml) kelp powder
¼ teaspoon (1 ml) celery seed
⅛ teaspoon (0.5 ml) dried hot
      red pepper flakes
1 carrot, sliced
½ cup (125 ml) minced parsley
1 clove garlic, minced
2 large tomatoes, chopped
3 cups (750 ml) water

A good dish to make when you are using the oven for other baking chores. If you will not be using the oven for the full 1½ to 2 hours, the soup can be finished in a pot on top of the stove.

Place ingredients in the order given in a two-quart (2 l) casserole dish. Cover and bake in a preheated 350° F. (175° C.) oven for 1½ to 2 hours, stirring once, after 1 hour, during baking. Remove from oven; place two cups (500 ml) of soup in a blender and process on medium speed until smooth. Stir into the rest of the soup. Serve hot.

Thick Cream of Corn Soup

Makes four servings
½ sweet red pepper, chopped
3 scallions, chopped
1 teaspoon (5 ml) corn oil
2 teaspoons (10 ml) whole
      wheat flour
1 cup (250 ml) skim milk
1½ cups (375 ml) fresh or
      frozen corn
2 teaspoons (10 ml) tamari
1 egg white

In a heavy-bottom pan, saute the pepper and scallions until tender in the oil. Add a few drops of water, if necessary, to prevent sticking. When the scallions are tender, add the flour and stir over low heat for one or two minutes. Stir in milk slowly to prevent lumps from forming, and stir until mixture begins to thicken. Remove pan from heat while preparing corn. Place 1 cup (250 ml) of corn and the tamari in a blender, and process until smooth. Stir blenderized corn and remaining ½ cup (125 ml) of corn into milk mixture, and return pan to a low heat. Heat through.

Beat egg white until stiff with an eggbeater, and fold into corn soup just before serving.

Chicken Soup Chinese-Style

Makes two servings
2 cups (500 ml) *Chicken Stock*
½ cup (125 ml) shredded
carrots
½ cup (125 ml) sliced
mushrooms
½ cup (125 ml) fresh
High-Protein Noodles
1 teaspoon (5 ml) tamari
1 egg white, beaten

Bring the stock to a boil in a medium saucepan, add the carrots and mushrooms and simmer until they are tender, about 15 minutes. Stir in the fresh noodles (these are homemade noodles that have not been dried) and cook another 1 or 2 minutes, until tender.

Stir in tamari; then, while whipping the soup rapidly, add the egg white. When the egg is cooked, turn off heat and serve.

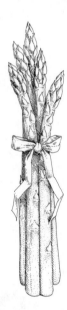

SALADS

Asparagus Vinaigrette with *Pimiento*

Makes four servings
4 cups (1 l) water
12–16 spears asparagus
¼ cup (60 ml) *Vinaigrette
Dressing*
lettuce leaves
4 slices *Pimiento*

Bring the water to a boil in a large skillet. Meanwhile, clean the asparagus and cut off the tough lower section of the stems.

Place the asparagus in the boiling water for about 10 minutes, just until crisp-tender. Immediately remove the spears from the boiling water and place in ice water or run under cold water from the faucet until cooled. Spread spears on a kitchen towel placed over a cooling rack. The spears should not touch.

When the asparagus is thoroughly cooled, place in a long, narrow dish and pour on the *Vinaigrette Dressing.* Place spears in the refrigerator to marinate three to four hours.

When ready to serve, place lettuce leaves on salad plates, arrange three to four spears per serving on the lettuce, and place a "belt" of *Pimiento* two-thirds of the way down the stalks. Serve chilled.

Pineapple, Grape and Almond Salad

Makes two servings
¾ cup (175 ml) chopped
   pineapple
¾ cup (175 ml) red grapes,
   halved
2 tablespoons (30 ml) slivered
   Blanched Almonds,
   toasted
2 tablespoons (30 ml) yogurt
   spinach leaves

A salad that scores high in nutrition and taste appeal.

Combine the pineapple, grapes and almonds in a medium bowl and toss with the yogurt. Divide between two plates on beds of spinach leaves. Serve chilled.

Minted Fruit Salad

Makes four servings
1 cup (250 ml) pineapple cubes
1 tablespoon (15 ml) chopped
   fresh mint
½ cantaloupe
½ unpeeled apple
½ pear
½ cup (125 ml) seedless grapes
   yogurt
   mint sprigs (garnish)

Combine pineapple cubes and mint in a large bowl. Use a melon baller or cut cantaloupe into cubes, chop apple and pear halves, and slice grapes in half. Combine fruits, toss with yogurt to taste, and chill before serving. Garnish with fresh mint sprigs.

Ceviche Salad

Makes eight servings
½ pound (225 g) haddock fillets
   lime or lemon juice
   spinach leaves
   red onion slices (garnish)

This South American specialty is a change-of-pace salad for a low-calorie luncheon or as an unusual appetizer for dinner.

Place fillets in a shallow glass dish and cover with lime or lemon juice, or a combination of both. Refrigerate the fish for five to six hours, turning once or twice during that time. The acid will "cook" the fish, leaving it flaky and white, with a delicious taste.

For each serving, place spinach leaves on a salad plate, place thin slices of ceviche on top, and garnish with thinly sliced onion rings.

Picnic Potato Salad

Makes four servings
4–5 medium potatoes
⅓ cup (80 ml) soy oil
1 tablespoon (15 ml) cider or
  malt vinegar
2 teaspoons (10 ml) honey
½ teaspoon (2 ml) dry mustard
½ teaspoon (2 ml) basil
¼ teaspoon (1 ml) thyme
¼ teaspoon (1 ml) spearmint
  leaves
dash marjoram
dash cayenne pepper

Because there are no eggs or mayonnaise in this potato salad, it can safely be left outdoors without refrigeration until hungry picnickers enjoy it.

Wash, but do not peel, potatoes. Cube and place in a large saucepan in cold water to cover. Bring to a boil, reduce heat and simmer until tender. Drain and place potatoes in a large bowl.

Mix the remaining ingredients thoroughly. Slowly spoon the oil and herb mixture over the hot potatoes. (Use spearmint tea if no dry spearmint is on hand.) Let stand at room temperature. When the potatoes have cooled, toss with the dressing and refrigerate.

Variation: Add ½ cup (125 ml) chopped celery, ½ cup (125 ml) chopped scallions, or 2 tablespoons (30 ml) minced fresh parsley to the potato salad. Leftover cooked peas or chopped, cooked broccoli can be a colorful addition.

Autumn Roots Salad

Makes six servings
1½ cups (375 ml) cubed celery
  root (celeriac)
1 cup (250 ml) cubed
  Jerusalem artichokes
1 cup (250 ml) peeled and
  cubed kohlrabi
Vinaigrette Dressing

A nice example of a seasonal approach to salads. You may have to visit a farmer's market to get some of the ingredients.

To peel the celery root, cut first in slices, then remove fibrous outer layer. Cube the root and steam or blanch for one or two minutes, until crisp-tender. Place in a medium bowl. Scrub and cube the Jerusalem artichokes (sometimes called sunchokes) and steam or blanch one to two minutes until crisp-tender. Drain and add to celery root.

Again, steam or blanch kohlrabi cubes for one to two minutes until crisp-tender. Drain and add to other vegetables. While still warm, toss with *Vinaigrette Dressing.* Chill salad thoroughly before serving.

Note: Autumn Roots Salad can also be served warm. Try it too, served hot with *Whole Wheat White Sauce.*

Zesty Zucchini Salad

Makes four servings
2 medium zucchini
2 tablespoons (30 ml) corn oil
2 tablespoons (30 ml) cider
    vinegar
2 teaspoons (10 ml) tamari
½ teaspoon (2 ml) dried hot red
    pepper flakes
¼ teaspoon (1 ml) walnuts,
    chopped

If you like hot food, this one's for you!

Cut the zucchini in half across, then cut into thin "fingers." (The zucchini you use should be about seven or eight inches [18 or 20 cm] long.) Steam just until tender.

Combine the remaining ingredients and pour over the zucchini. Cool, then chill thoroughly before serving. Toss with the marinade occasionally so zucchini is well flavored.

Fresh Tomato Salad

Makes four servings
2 cups (500 ml) cherry
    tomatoes, chopped
¼ cup (60 ml) watercress, finely
    chopped
1 tablespoon (15 ml) minced
    fresh parsley
¼ cup (60 ml) cottage cheese
2 tablespoons (30 ml)
    buttermilk
dash freshly grated nutmeg
lettuce leaves
parsley sprigs (garnish)

Chop cherry tomatoes, and partially drain. Toss with watercress and parsley.

In a blender, combine cottage cheese and buttermilk and process on low or medium speed until smooth. Pour over tomatoes, dust with a little nutmeg, and stir to combine. Serve in salad bowls lined with lettuce leaves and garnish with parsley sprigs.

Cucumber and Yogurt Salad

Makes six servings
3 medium cucumbers
1½ cups (375 ml) yogurt
1 tablespoon (15 ml) lemon
    juice
½ teaspoon (2 ml) chili
    powder
⅛ teaspoon (0.5 ml) cumin
    powder
2 teaspoons (10 ml) minced
    fresh flat-leaf parsley

A traditional Indian dish, very cooling on a hot day or served beside a spicy main course dish.

Shred cucumbers, combine with remaining ingredients and chill to allow flavors to blend. Makes three cups (750 ml).

Note: The cucumbers can be cubed or sliced rather than shredded.

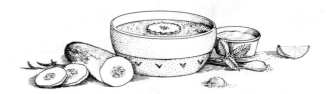

Creamy Salad Dressing

Makes 2 ½ cups (625 ml)
1 medium cucumber, peeled
1 cup (250 ml) yogurt
1 scallion
2 tablespoons (30 ml) fresh mint
1 tablespoon (15 ml) lemon
    juice
1 tablespoon (15 ml) sesame
    tahini

Combine ingredients in a blender and process on medium speed until smooth.

Tomato-Tahini Dressing

Makes ¾ cup (175 ml)
¾ cup (175 ml) yogurt
1 tablespoon (15 ml) sesame
    tahini
1 tablespoon (15 ml) tomato
    paste
1 teaspoon (5 ml) tamari
1 teaspoon (5 ml) mild vinegar

Stir ingredients together in a small bowl until well blended. Serve chilled over tossed salad or in tuna, macaroni or chicken salads.

Quick Tahini-Yogurt Dressing

Makes ⅓ cup (80 ml)
2 tablespoons (30 ml) sesame
    tahini
¼ cup (60 ml) yogurt

Shake ingredients together in a covered jar until well blended. Serve on tossed salad.

Sesame-Fruit Dressing

Makes ¼ cup (60 ml)
2 tablespoons (30 ml) apple
    juice
1 tablespoon (15 ml) sesame
    tahini
1 tablespoon (15 ml) yogurt
    dash cinnamon

Combine ingredients in a covered jar or blender. Shake or blend on medium speed until combined.

BREAD

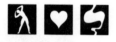

Creamy Double-Corn Bread

Makes eight servings
1 cup (250 ml) whole grain
    cornmeal
1 cup (250 ml) whole wheat
    flour
2 teaspoons (10 ml) *Baking
    Powder*
1 cup (250 ml) fresh or frozen
    corn
1 cup (250 ml) buttermilk
2 eggs, beaten

Combine the dry ingredients in a large mixing bowl. In a blender, process corn on low speed until creamy. In a medium bowl, stir corn into buttermilk and eggs. Add corn mixture to the dry ingredients, stirring until smooth. Place the batter in a lightly oiled 8 × 8-inch (20 × 20-cm) baking pan and place in a preheated 375° F. (190° C.) oven for 30 minutes.

MAIN DISHES

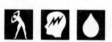

Fish Fillets Florida

Makes two servings
¾ pound (340 g) fish fillets
    (such as haddock or
    flounder)
½ cup (125 ml) orange juice
1 orange
1 tablespoon (15 ml) minced
    fresh parsley

In a large skillet, poach fish fillets over medium heat in the orange juice, turning when nearly cooked through, about four to five minutes.

Peel and section orange, removing seeds. After turning fish fillets, place orange sections diagonally over the top of each fillet. Cover pan and heat through. Sprinkle with parsley and serve with the pan juices.

Note: This dish can be served over cooked brown rice.

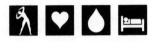

Baked Cod or Haddock in Parchment Paper

Makes four servings
2 pounds (1 kg) haddock or
    cod
½ teaspoon (2 ml) corn oil
1 cup (250 ml) sliced carrots or
    radishes
4 sliced scallions
2 tablespoons (30 ml) sesame
    seeds

Sauce:
1 tablespoon (15 ml) lemon
    juice
2 teaspoons (10 ml) tamari
1 teaspoon (5 ml) water
    1-inch (2.5-cm) piece fresh
        ginger root
1 teaspoon (5 ml) curry

John F. Carafoli, who designed this book, lives on Cape Cod and enjoys preparing the local fish and shellfish. Here's one of his favorite recipes.

Wash and dry the fish. Cut into four pieces. Cut a piece of parchment paper twice the size of the portions of fish you are going to wrap. Lightly oil the paper. Lay the carrots or radishes on the paper. On top place one piece of fish. Sprinkle sauce over the fish. Place a sliced scallion on top. Sprinkle with sesame seeds and wrap, crimping edges to seal.

Place on a cookie sheet. In a 375° F. (190° C.) preheated oven, bake for 14 minutes. Serve. Let each person unwrap his or her own portion.

Note: If parchment paper is not available, aluminum foil may be used.

Variation: Substitute finely sliced broccoli or cabbage for the above vegetables.

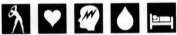

Creamed Fish and *Pimiento*

Makes four servings
½ stalk celery, chopped
½ small onion, chopped
1 tablespoon (15 ml) corn oil
2 tablespoons (30 ml) whole
    wheat flour
1½ cups (375 ml) skim milk
1 pound (450 g) fish fillets,
    cubed
2 tablespoons (30 ml) finely
    chopped *Pimiento*

Saute the chopped celery and onion in the oil until the onion is translucent. Stir in the whole wheat flour, and continue stirring over low heat for one or two minutes.

Remove the pan from the heat, and stir in the milk slowly, to prevent lumping. Return the pan to medium heat and stir until the sauce begins to thicken.

Add the fish and *Pimiento.* Cover and simmer over low heat for about 10 minutes, until the fish is cooked. Delicious over *Rice Waffles,* or try it with boiled potatoes.

Eggplant Pizza

Makes four servings
1 large eggplant
2 teaspoons (10 ml) corn oil
1 teaspoon (5 ml) oregano, crumbled
½ teaspoon (2 ml) basil, crumbled
¼ teaspoon (1 ml) thyme, crumbled
½–¾ cup (125–175 ml) tomato sauce
¼ cup (60 ml) grated low-fat Swiss or mozzarella cheese
1 tablespoon (15 ml) grated Parmesan cheese

Cut off the top and stem end of the eggplant. Cut the eggplant in round slices about ½ inch (1 cm) thick. Meanwhile, bring a large pot of water to the boil. Drop half the eggplant into the boiling water, blanch for about two minutes, and remove with a slotted spoon. Repeat this with the remaining eggplant.

Place the blanched eggplant slices on a lightly oiled baking sheet, brush tops with the two teaspoons (10 ml) of corn oil, and dust with herbs. Cover with aluminum foil. Place baking sheet in a preheated 375° F. (190° C.) oven for 15 to 20 minutes, until the eggplant slices are easily pierced, but not mushy.

When you are ready to serve, spread the eggplant slices with tomato sauce (see *Index* for several choices to keep on hand) and sprinkle with the cheese. Broil until the cheese is melted. Serve hot.

Mushroom Pasta Sauce

Makes four servings
½ cup (125 ml) shredded carrots
1 medium Spanish onion, finely chopped
1 stalk celery, finely chopped
2 cups (500 ml) sliced mushrooms
1 teaspoon (5 ml) basil
1 teaspoon (5 ml) oregano
⅔ cup (150 ml) tomato paste
¾ cup (175 ml) water

Combine carrots, onion and celery in a heavy-bottom saucepan. Add a few tablespoons (50 ml) of water and steam-stir over medium heat until the vegetables are limp, but not browned. Add the mushrooms and continue cooking, adding a little water as needed, until the vegetables are very soft. Stir in the seasonings, tomato paste and water, and simmer for 30 minutes. Add additional water if sauce is thicker than desired.

Serve over whole wheat pasta.

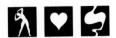

Makes four to six servings

Crust:

2½ cups (625 ml) cold water
1½ cups (375 ml) whole grain
    cornmeal
2 teaspoons (10 ml) chili
    powder
½ teaspoon (2 ml) cumin
    powder
1 teaspoon (5 ml) tamari

Filling:

1 cup (250 ml) cooked
    kidney, pinto or black
    beans
1 cup (250 ml) cooked
    soybeans
1 stalk celery, chopped
1 green pepper, chopped
1 medium onion, chopped
2 cloves garlic, minced
2 tablespoons (30 ml) tomato
    paste
2 tablespoons (30 ml) chili
    powder
2 teaspoons (10 ml) cumin
    powder
½ teaspoon (2 ml) cumin seed
1 tablespoon (15 ml) lemon
    juice
3 tablespoons (45 ml) water
½ cup (125 ml) fresh or frozen
    corn
    dash cayenne pepper
    alfalfa sprouts (garnish)

Tamale Pie

Combine water, cornmeal, chili powder, cumin powder and tamari in a heavy saucepan and stir over medium heat until the mixture thickens and comes to a boil. Lightly oil an 8 × 8-inch (20 × 20-cm) casserole dish, and place two-thirds of the cornmeal mixture on the bottom and halfway up the sides of the dish. Set aside the remaining cornmeal mixture.

Process the beans together in a blender on low speed or with a food mill until thoroughly mashed. In a large skillet, steam-stir the celery, pepper and onion in a small amount of water until the onion is translucent; add the garlic toward the end of cooking. Add the beans and the remaining ingredients, except sprouts, and stir over medium heat for five to eight minutes. Stir frequently, or the beans will stick.

Pour the bean mixture over the cornmeal layer in the casserole dish. Spread remaining cornmeal mixture over beans. Bake in a preheated 350° F. (175° C.) oven 30 minutes. Top each serving with fresh alfalfa sprouts.

Makes one serving
1 cup (250 ml) sliced
    mushrooms
4 tablespoons (60 ml) water
¼ teaspoon (1 ml) basil
1 slice whole grain bread
½ teaspoon (2 ml) tamari
2 tablespoons (30 ml) water
3 tablespoons (45 ml) shredded
    Swiss cheese

Broiled Mushrooms on Toast

In a small skillet, steam-stir the mushrooms in two tablespoons (30 ml) of water until water has evaporated and mushrooms are tender.

Toast bread and place on a small, shallow ovenproof pan or plate. Top with mushrooms. Pour over tamari mixed with the remaining two tablespoons (30 ml) of water. Top with the cheese. Broil until cheese is melted. Serve hot.

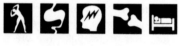

Makes two servings
1 cup (250 ml) whole
    wheat macaroni
1 cup (250 ml) fresh or
    frozen peas
¾ cup (175 ml) ricotta
    cheese
½–¾ cup (125–175 ml) boiling
    water, reserved from
    cooking macaroni
1 tablespoon (15 ml) grated
    Parmesan cheese

Macaroni with Ricotta

Place macaroni in a large saucepan half-filled with boiling water, and cook until tender yet firm. Reserve ¾ cup (175 ml) of the boiling water, and then drain macaroni. Cook peas only one to two minutes in a little water, until crisp-tender.

In a blender, combine ½ cup (125 ml) of boiling water with the ricotta. Blend on low speed until smooth, adding a little more water, if necessary, to get a thick, saucelike consistency.

In a serving bowl, toss the hot macaroni and the peas with the ricotta "sauce" and sprinkle with freshly grated Parmesan.

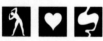

Makes six servings
1 cup (250 ml) whole grain
    cornmeal
1 egg, beaten
2 cups (500 ml) buttermilk
1 teaspoon (5 ml) baking soda
4 cups *Lentil Stew, Chili Beans,*
    or *Oven-Baked Lentils*

Corn Pone

Place the cornmeal and egg in a medium bowl. In the buttermilk, dissolve the baking soda and add to the cornmeal and egg mixture; combine.

Place four cups (1 l) of *Lentil Stew, Chili Beans,* or *Oven-Baked Lentils* in the bottom of a lightly oiled 8 × 8-inch (20 × 20-cm) casserole dish, and carefully spoon the cornmeal mixture over top. Bake in a preheated 450° F. (230° C.) oven for 30 minutes, or until the corn bread topping begins to brown and pull away from the sides of the dish.

SIDE DISHES

Basil Mushrooms

Makes one serving
1 cup (250 ml) mushrooms
2 tablespoons (30 ml) water
½ teaspoon (2 ml) tamari
¼ teaspoon (1 ml) dried basil
1 tablespoon (15 ml) chopped
    fresh basil

Brush dirt from mushrooms and slice. Combine water, tamari and basil and pour over mushrooms in a heavy skillet. Steam-stir until water has evaporated and mushrooms are tender.

Note: If desired, you can make a larger batch and freeze a portion to use later.

Variation: For *Basil Mushrooms and Peas,* stir one cup (250 ml) of fresh or frozen peas and an additional tablespoon (15 ml) of water into the mushrooms after they have begun to simmer. Cook just until peas are crisp-tender.

Quick Minted Tomatoes

Makes four servings
1 teaspoon (5 ml) sesame oil
1 clove garlic, minced
2 cups (500 ml) cherry
    tomatoes
1 tablespoon (15 ml) finely
    chopped fresh mint
¼ cup (60 ml) yogurt
¼ teaspoon (1 ml) coriander

Heat oil in a skillet and add garlic, stirring to keep the garlic from scorching. Reduce heat and add tomatoes and mint. Cover tomatoes, stirring frequently, until tomatoes are cooked, 5 to 10 minutes. Stir in the yogurt and coriander and serve while hot. Makes about two cups (500 ml).

Curried Green Tomatoes

Makes four servings
1 tablespoon (15 ml) corn oil
2 tablespoons (30 ml) finely
    chopped onions
1 teaspoon (5 ml) curry
1 teaspoon (5 ml) brewer's yeast
2 cups (500 ml) cubed green
    tomatoes

Saute the onion in oil until it begins to soften. Add the remaining ingredients and stir over low heat until the tomatoes are crisp-tender, about 10 minutes. Serve hot.

Curry is quite compatible with green tomatoes. Leftovers are a nice addition to vegetable soup. Stir in just a minute or two before serving the soup.

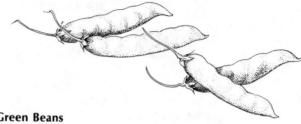

Italian Green Beans

Makes two servings
2 cups (500 ml) sliced green
    beans
½ cup (125 ml) tomato sauce

    Steam green beans just until crisp-tender. Combine in a medium saucepan with tomato sauce. Heat through and serve promptly.

Note: This recipe is delicious with *Stockpot Tomato Sauce, Mediterranean Tomato Sauce,* or your own tomato puree.

Sesame Green Beans

Makes four servings
2 cups (500 ml) sliced green
    beans
1 tablespoon (15 ml) sesame
    seeds
½ teaspoon (2 ml) honey
¼ teaspoon (1 ml) tamari

A surprise ending for beans—no mystery, they're delicious!

    Cook green beans in a small amount of boiling water just until crisp-tender. Drain, saving the water for soups. Combine the sesame seeds, honey and tamari and toss with the green beans in a serving dish.

Boiled New Potatoes

Makes two servings
6 small new potatoes
    boiling water to cover

    Drop the potatoes into boiling water and cook covered 20 to 30 minutes, until tender. At this point the skins can be removed, though they are quite delicious left intact.

    Serve with chopped mint, chives or parsley, or mix some yogurt with freshly grated horseradish and serve on the side.

Makes four servings
4 baking potatoes
1½ cups (375 ml) cherry
     tomatoes or 2 medium
     tomatoes
½ green pepper, finely
     chopped
3 tablespoons (45 ml) yogurt
     dash cayenne pepper

Stuffed Potatoes Mexican-Style

It's important to find new ways to enjoy baked potatoes without slabs of butter.

Punch potatoes once with a fork or knife and bake them in a preheated 400° F. (200° C.) oven for 45 to 60 minutes, until soft. Meanwhile, chop tomatoes, and add to green pepper.

In a saucepan with a few tablespoons (50 ml) of water, steam the tomatoes and pepper until the pepper is tender. Remove from heat. Stir in yogurt when tomato mixture has cooled slightly.

Remove potatoes from the oven. Cut an "X" in each potato, extending across the entire top. Pull potatoes open slightly, and spoon tomato mixture into opening. Serve hot. (If necessary, place under the broiler for a moment to warm sauce.)

Makes four servings
3 medium potatoes
2 stalks broccoli, sliced

Potatoes and Broccoli

Wash potatoes and cut, unpeeled, in large cubes. In a large saucepan, place potatoes in cold water to cover and bring to a boil. Meanwhile, slice the broccoli stems and separate the florets into a size similar to the potato cubes. When potatoes are boiling, add broccoli and cover, steaming until both potatoes and broccoli are just tender.

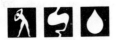

Makes three servings
2 cups (500 ml) cubed potatoes
     (about 3 medium)
1 teaspoon (5 ml) tamari
2 tablespoons (30 ml) mild
     vinegar
1 tablespoon (15 ml) sesame
     tahini
½ cup (125 ml) finely chopped
     green peppers
¼ cup (60 ml) finely chopped
     scallions
2 tablespoons (30 ml) yogurt

Green Pepper-Potato Salad

Cube the potatoes, with skins intact, and place them in a medium saucepan with enough water to cover. Bring to a boil and simmer until tender, about 10 minutes.

Meanwhile, in a small saucepan, bring tamari and vinegar to a boil. Add tahini, stirring until dissolved. When potatoes are tender, drain and place in medium mixing bowl with green peppers and scallions. Pour hot tahini dressing over all, tossing to combine. Add yogurt and toss again. Chill before serving. Makes 2½ cups (625 ml).

Braised Fennel

Makes four servings
2 bulbs fennel
¼ cup (60 ml) *Chicken Stock*
   or *Vegetable Stock*
¼ teaspoon (1 ml) tamari
   pinch thyme

The slightly anise flavor of this vegetable makes it a surprising and pleasing addition to the dinner menu. It is a fine complement to fish.

Cut any tough outer stems from the fennel bulbs. Cut the fennel bulbs in quarters and place in a heavy-bottom saucepan or skillet. Add half of the stock along with tamari.

Over low heat, braise the fennel slowly, turning occasionally, until it is tender. Add remaining stock when necessary to prevent scorching. Cooking time may be 30 to 45 minutes, depending on the bulbs.

When the fennel is tender, sprinkle with a tiny pinch of dried thyme, crushed between the fingers. Serve hot.

Herbed Frying Peppers

Makes two servings
2–3 large frying peppers, cut in
      strips
  ¼ cup (60 ml) *Chicken Stock*
  ½ clove garlic, minced
  ½ teaspoon (2 ml) oregano
  ½ teaspoon (2 ml) tamari

Heat a heavy pan or skillet, without oil, and add the peppers. Cook, stirring, over a fairly high heat until the peppers start to blister and turn dark brown at places. Add chicken stock and remaining ingredients and simmer until peppers are tender. These are good hot or cold.

Summer Squash and Tomato

Makes two servings
1 yellow summer squash, sliced
1 large tomato, chopped
½ teaspoon (2 ml) basil

A quick-cooking summer vegetable dish which makes a colorful addition to a dinner menu.

Steam-stir squash in a medium skillet with a few drops of water.

When it begins to get tender, add tomato and basil, and cook over low heat another minute or two.

Herbed Zucchini

Makes three servings
2 cups (500 ml) cubed zucchini
½ teaspoon (2 ml) basil
½ clove garlic, minced
1 tablespoon (15 ml) minced
    fresh parsley

Place zucchini with remaining ingredients in a saucepan or skillet. Add just enough water to prevent sticking, and steam, stirring frequently, until zucchini is tender.

Mulled Cucumber

Makes two servings
1 large cucumber
2 cups (500 ml) boiling water
2 tablespoons (30 ml) yogurt
    freshly grated nutmeg
    fresh parsley (garnish)

A sophisticated, delicately colored, low-calorie side dish.

Peel, halve lengthwise and seed cucumber. Slice into "half-moons." Place in saucepan with boiling water and cook until tender. Drain. Toss with yogurt and freshly grated nutmeg to taste. Serve hot.

Garnish, if desired, with fresh parsley, or chop a teaspoon (5 ml) of parsley and mix with yogurt before tossing with cucumber slices.

Oven-Braised Celery

Makes four servings
1 head celery (about 10 stalks)
1 teaspoon (5 ml) tamari
¼ cup (60 ml) water
2 tablespoons (30 ml) finely
    chopped onions

Place celery stalks in medium baking pan with cover. Combine tamari, water and chopped onions. Pour over celery. Bake, covered, in a preheated 375° F. (190° C.) oven for one hour.

Red Beets in the Pink

Makes four servings
2 cups (500 ml) cooked, sliced
    or cubed beets
2 tablespoons (30 ml) yogurt
    dash freshly grated nutmeg

Drain beets, adding yogurt while they are still hot from cooking. Add freshly grated nutmeg, toss and serve. Or, cool, add yogurt and nutmeg, and chill before serving.

Steamed Celery Root

Makes four servings
1 medium celery root (celeriac)

Here's something slightly exotic yet very simple to prepare. Buy celery root at your local farmer's market in season.

Cut the celery root in thick slices and peel. Cube and steam until tender.

The celery root can be served hot, with *Whole Wheat White Sauce* or cold, tossed with *Curried Tofu Mayonnaise.*

MISCELLANEOUS

Artichokes with Tofu Dip

Makes four servings
4 large artichokes
1 teaspoon (5 ml) corn oil
Tofu Garden Dip

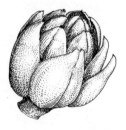

An exotic vegetable, leafy and spiny, the artichoke can be served hot or cold.

Bring a large kettle of water to the boil. While the water is heating, cut off the artichoke stems one inch (2.5-cm) from the base and remove the small bottom leaves. Wash the artichokes, and cut off the tips of the leaves, if desired (a kitchen scissors is best for this). Place the artichokes in the boiling water, add the oil, cover and boil gently 35 to 45 minutes, or until the base can be pierced easily with a fork.

When they are done cooking, lift out the artichokes and turn them upside down to drain. If they are to be served hot, prepare dip ahead of time and serve immediately. If cold, cool the artichokes, then chill until ready to serve with the dip.

Variation: Artichokes hot or cold are also tasty served with *Curried Tofu Mayonnaise.*

Tofu Garden Dip

Makes one cup (250 ml)
¾ cup (175 ml) crumbled tofu
2 tablespoons (30 ml) cider
    vinegar
1 tablespoon (15 ml) soy oil
1 teaspoon (5 ml) Dijon-style
    mustard
1 teaspoon (5 ml) lemon juice
½ teaspoon (2 ml) tamari
¼ cup (60 ml) packed spinach
    leaves
1 tablespoon (15 ml) fresh
    parsley
1 tablespoon (15 ml) fresh
    watercress or scallion
    tops
½ clove garlic (optional)

Place ingredients in a blender and process on low speed until smooth, stopping the blender to scrape down the sides of the container as necessary.

Curried Tofu Mayonnaise

Makes one cup (250 ml)
1 cup (250 ml) crumbled tofu
2 tablespoons (30 ml) cider
    vinegar
1 tablespoon (15 ml) soy oil
1 teaspoon (5 ml) Dijon-style
    mustard
1 teaspoon (5 ml) lemon juice
½ teaspoon (2 ml) tamari
1½ teaspoons (7 ml) curry

Place the ingredients in a blender and process on low speed until smooth.

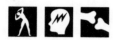

Makes eight servings

10 ounces (280 g) unpacked
       spinach
 2 teaspoons (10 ml) tamari
 8 cloves garlic
¼ cup (60 ml) fresh basil or 1
       tablespoon (15 ml) dried
       basil
12 ounces (340 g) tofu
 3 tablespoons (45 ml) sesame
       tahini

Makes two cups (500 ml)

1 large ripe tomato
1 small onion
⅔ cup (150 ml) tomato paste
1 tablespoon (15 ml) olive oil
2 teaspoons (10 ml) oregano
1 clove garlic

Makes one cup (250 ml)

 1 clove garlic
 2 tablespoons (30 ml) corn oil
 2 tablespoons (30 ml) whole
       wheat flour
 1 tablespoon (15 ml) brewer's
       yeast
½ teaspoon (2 ml) kelp powder
 1 teaspoon (5 ml) carob
       powder
 1 cup (250 ml) water
 1 teaspoon (5 ml) tamari
 2 tablespoons (30 ml) yogurt

Spinach Sauce

Wash spinach, leaving stems on leaves. Place spinach, tamari, garlic and basil in large saucepan. Steam-stir in water that has clung to the washed leaves until spinach is wilted. Add a tablespoon or two (15–30 ml) of water, if necessary, to prevent sticking to pan. Remove from heat and place in blender with tofu and tahini. Process on low speed. Return to saucepan and heat, stirring, but do not allow sauce to boil. Serve hot over whole wheat spaghetti or noodles, or cubed, boiled potatoes.

For a colorful dish, combine ⅓ cup (80 ml) cooked green beans and ⅓ cup (80 ml) cubed, boiled potato for each serving of spaghetti, and toss with *Spinach Sauce.* Sauce can be frozen for future use. Makes about 2½ cups (625 ml).

Quick Pizza Sauce

Combine the ingredients in a blender and process on medium speed until smooth. This sauce can be used as is, spread on whole wheat pizza dough, or can be used over pasta, thinned with a little vegetable broth or tomato juice if desired.

If the sauce will not be cooked further, as with pizza, simmer on top of the stove for 15 minutes or so.

Good Gravy

Cut garlic clove and rub raw edge inside skillet or saucepan. Place oil in pan, and over medium heat stir in flour, brewer's yeast, kelp and carob powders. Stir for two to three minutes over medium heat. Add water very slowly, stirring constantly to prevent lumping. Add tamari. Simmer, stirring, until thickened. Remove from heat and add yogurt. Place in a blender or whip to thoroughly combine yogurt and gravy. Serve hot over boiled or mashed potatoes, with rice or baked chicken.

Note: For a party dish, glaze *Pate Ring* with *Good Gravy* and fill center with cooked vegetables.

Whole Wheat-Cornmeal Pie Crust

Makes one 9-inch (23-cm) pie crust
¾ cup (175 ml) whole wheat pastry flour
¼ cup (60 ml) whole grain cornmeal
¼ cup (60 ml) corn oil
2 tablespoons (30 ml) water

Combine the ingredients in the bottom of a 9-inch (23-cm) pie plate. Toss with a fork until ingredients are combined.

Press the dough along the bottom and sides of the pie plate, fill, and bake as needed.

Hot Peach Pancake Sauce

Makes 1⅔ cups (400 ml)
2 large or 3 medium peaches
2 tablespoons (30 ml) apple juice
2 tablespoons (30 ml) maple syrup

A luscious topping that's a lot more healthful than plain syrup.

Wash, but do not peel peaches. Remove pits. Place one peach in a blender with apple juice and maple syrup and process on low speed until smooth. Cube remaining peach and place in a saucepan with blended ingredients. Bring just up to the boil and serve hot.

Blueberry Sauce

Makes 1½ cups (375 ml)
1½ cups (375 ml) blueberries
¼ cup (60 ml) apple juice
1 tablespoon (15 ml) maple syrup
1 bay leaf
dash freshly grated nutmeg

Adds delightful taste and color when served hot over pancakes.

Place ½ cup (125 ml) of the blueberries with the apple juice in a blender and process on medium speed until smooth. Pour into a saucepan with remaining blueberries and other ingredients. Bring to a boil, then simmer for five minutes. Remove bay leaf and serve hot over pancakes. Sauce can also be chilled and served over fresh fruit salad or on toasted fruit breads.

Apple Pancake Sauce

Makes 1¼ cups (300 ml)
2 cups (500 ml) chopped,
   unpeeled apples
¼ cup (60 ml) apple juice
2 tablespoons (30 ml) maple
   syrup

If you're easing into health foods, use a little more syrup at first and gradually cut down as the new taste grows on you.

Place ingredients in a blender and process on medium speed until smooth. If a thinner consistency is desired, add a little more apple juice. Serve at room temperature over whole wheat pancakes.

BEVERAGES

Sparkling Apple Juice

Makes one serving
½ cup (125 ml) apple juice
½ cup (125 ml) sparkling
   mineral water

Combine ingredients and serve over ice. This is a nice, not-too-sweet summer refresher.

Apple-Grapefruit Drink

Makes one serving
½ cup (125 ml) apple juice
½ cup (125 ml) grapefruit juice
   ice
   fresh mint (garnish)

A good summer thirst-quencher that is neither too sweet nor too sour. And has a lot less calories than soda.

Combine juices in a glass with ice cubes. Garnish with mint sprigs.

DESSERTS

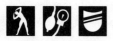

Peaches 'n' Pear Sauce

Makes two servings
3 large ripe peaches
1 ripe pear
   dash cinnamon

Chill fruit. Place washed and seeded peaches and pear, with skins, in a blender and process on low speed until smooth. Serve as a dessert sauce with, for example, *Banana Pound Cake.*

Apple Delight

Makes eight servings
4 cups (1 l) chopped unpeeled
 apples
½ cup (125 ml) apple cider
¼ cup (60 ml) honey
1 teaspoon (5 ml) *Vanilla
 Extract*
1 teaspoon (5 ml) cinnamon
⅛ teaspoon (0.5 ml) cloves
⅛ teaspoon (0.5 ml) freshly
 grated nutmeg
½ cup (125 ml) whole wheat
 flour
⅔ cup (150 ml) skim milk
2 eggs, beaten

In a deep oven casserole dish, toss the apples with the remaining ingredients. When thoroughly combined, place casserole in a cold oven and turn on heat to 375° F. (190° C.).

Remove from oven after 45 to 50 minutes, or when apple mixture is golden and the apples are tender.

Seed Cake Supreme

Makes one loaf
½ cup (125 ml) currants
 juice of ½ orange
2¼ cups (550 ml) whole wheat
 pastry flour
1½ teaspoons (7 ml) *Baking
 Powder*
½ teaspoon (2 ml) baking soda
1 tablespoon (15 ml) poppy
 seeds
1 tablespoon (15 ml) caraway
 seeds
1 tablespoon (15 ml) finely
 grated lemon rind
2 eggs, beaten
1 cup (250 ml) buttermilk
¼ cup (60 ml) honey
¼ cup (60 ml) corn oil
1 teaspoon (5 ml) *Vanilla
 Extract*

This loaf cake has an unusual, but decidedly delicious flavor. Some like the cake even better the second day, when the flavors have a chance to blend.

Begin this cake at least an hour-and-a-half before you plan to bake it, as you must soak the currants in the orange juice until they begin to get plump. To hasten the process, you might simmer them in the orange juice over a low flame. In a large mixing bowl, combine the dry ingredients, including lemon rind. In a separate bowl, add the soaked currants to the eggs, and beat in the remaining items. Stir the egg mixture into the dry ingredients until combined. Place batter in a lightly oiled 8½ × 4½-inch (22 × 11-cm) bread pan. Bake in a preheated 350° F. (175° C.) oven about 45 minutes, until a cake tester or toothpick comes out clean.

Chapter 6

The Anti-Cancer Diet

The ideas most of us have about the causes of cancer are pretty primitive. That is not entirely our fault, since major new insights have been gained in just the last 10 years or so.

The old view (probably still held by most people) is that cancer is a kind of lightning bolt, albeit a lightning bolt that strikes an astonishingly large number of people. You either get hit or you don't. As to why some people get hit and others don't, the answer is probably equal parts of heredity, fate, and varying exposure to thousands of chemicals in a world polluted by technology. Getting through life without getting cancer is like running across the wrong end of the shooting gallery. Good luck.

Such was the old view. Today, most scientists who study cancer regard it as a kind of constant challenge to the body's immune system rather than an irresistible bolt out of the blue. Cancer might even be compared to common forms of infectious bacteria which can frequently be found on our skin and inside our bodies, but which only begin multiplying and causing symptoms when something goes wrong with our bodily defenses. Scientists today speak of an extremely sophisticated bodily defense system which normally protects us against all kinds of invaders, *including* cancer.

Nutrition is one of the most important factors determining whether that defense system wins or loses the battle. "Diet," says Gio B. Gori, Ph.D., of the National Cancer Institute, "is an important factor in the causation of various forms of cancer . . . [evidence suggests] it is correlated with more than half of all cancers in women and at least one-third of all cancers in men" (*Food Technology,* December, 1979). Harry Demopoulos, M.D., of the New York University Medical Center, attributes no less than 45 percent of *all* cancer deaths to "disordered nutrition"—primarily too much food, too much fat, and deficiencies in fiber and vitamin A.

While new research is pointing to the importance of nutrition, it is also taking away some of the emphasis that was previously placed upon environmental hazards such as air and water pollution and food additives. That kind of pollution, which is sometimes impossible to avoid—from industry, maybe even your own job—probably causes no more than about five percent of all cancer deaths, Dr. Demopoulos estimates. It's *personal* environment that counts most—the everyday habits we call life-style. Most important of all is smoking. Not smoking probably does more to help prevent cancer than anything you or any government agency could do. Not smoking even makes you much less vulnerable to *other* toxic factors in the environment, including industrial pollution.

Other than smoking, most of the other important habits that can either encourage or discourage cancer involve nutrition in one form or another—foods, beverages, amounts, even the way your food is cooked. If you get this part of your life-style right, and don't smoke, either, you're way ahead of the game.

Still, you may find it difficult to believe that nutrition could play such an important role in causing or preventing cancer. That's because all of us tend to make the assumption that if something causes cancer, it must be because it contains an extremely toxic substance. Or conversely, if it prevents cancer, it must contain a chemical that demolishes cancer cells. And surely foods do not have such properties. But both assumptions are not quite correct. For the most part, it seems, foods associated with an increased risk of cancer are believed to do their mischief *not* by directly damaging the body, but by changing body chemistry. Specifically, certain hormones and bile acids (needed to digest fats) seem to be increased by these foods. And—here's the part we really don't understand—too-high levels of these hormones, bile acids and perhaps other substances encourage bacterial or biochemical actions which indirectly lead to cancer initiation. Possibly, the shift of balance in our hormones and other body juices simply makes it more difficult for our natural immunity system to do its job.

By the same token, anti-cancer foods do not directly attack cancer cells, but rather help create a kind of internal environment that promotes the most effective possible performance by the immune system.

Perhaps the major exception to these general principles is alcohol. Heavy drinking—something on the order of more than two or three drinks a day, day-in, day-out—is considered a definite risk for cancer at a number of sites in the digestive tract from the mouth down. The damage is probably quite direct. And it may not be the alcohol alone that is the villain, but also the accompanying chemicals that give each brew its particular taste. Called congeners, these chemicals vary dramatically in amount in the different alcoholic beverages people drink around the world, and these differences are believed to be directly related to widely varying rates of mouth and throat cancer. Heavy smoking combined with heavy drinking is one of the more popular ways people in our society give themselves cancer.

TOO MUCH FAT OILS THE DOOR FOR CANCER

Next to cigarette smoke and an unending stream of booze, many scientists agree the part of the diet that should be watched most carefully is the familiar enemy: fat. The evidence was convincing enough to lead the National Cancer Institute to recommend that Americans consume less fat to lessen the danger of cancer. And that includes unsaturated fats like margarine and corn oil, as well as the saturated ones like butterfat and lard.

Just as in the case of heart disease, what aroused the investigators' suspicions was the striking correlation between the amounts of fat eaten by various peoples and their susceptibility to certain cancers. A good example of this is seen in the work of G. Hems, of the Department of Community Medicine in Aberdeen, Scotland, who tabulated the breast cancer rates in 41 countries and related them to local diets. "It was concluded that variations of breast cancer rates between countries arose predominantly from differences in diet," he wrote in the *British Journal of Cancer* (vol. 37, no. 6, 1978). And one place where the shadow of suspicion fell most darkly was consumption of fats. Other studies have confirmed that the disease is less common in poor and developing nations, where rich foods are rarely on the menu, than in the wealthier countries of the West. Breast cancer increases among Japanese immigrants who give up their low-fat diet for our high-fat fare. And among the Seventh-day Adventists, breast cancer mortality rates are only one-half to two-thirds that of Americans in general. Many members of this religious group are vegetarians, whose saturated fat and cholesterol intake is bound to be well below average.

The link between fat and breast cancer, scientists speculate, may be those hormones we talked about before. Studies have related the development of the disease to abnormal levels of prolactin, estrogens and androgens. Production of these hormones apparently goes up when we eat a fat-rich diet. The sensitivity of hormone levels to diet has been shown clearly in at least two studies. In South Africa, native black women suffer very little from breast cancer, while white women fall prey to the disease much more frequently. Their diets are remarkably different, too: the native diet is mostly vegetables and very low in fat—less than 20 percent of total calories—while the whites consume a typical Western diet in which fats provide 40 percent of calories. Peter Hill, Ph.D., of the American Health Foundation, measured the hormone levels in groups of black and white women, and found that the black women had lower levels of a number of hormones, including prolactin. He put the black women on a Western diet for periods of six weeks to two months, then measured their hormones again. Now, he found, the proportions of the various hormones had changed significantly: they began to resemble the hormone profile of white women. And these new hormone levels—including the rise in prolactin—are ones that have been associated with increased rates of breast cancer (*Federation Proceedings,* March 1, 1979).

Dr. Hill conducted a similar study with South African and North American men. Rural, vegetarian, black South African men have a far lower rate of prostate cancer than North American men—and their diet has about half the fat of the diet consumed in America. Testing their urine, Dr. Hill found that the South Africans excrete considerably less androgens and estrogens than their American counterparts. For three weeks, Dr. Hill had his subjects switch diets: the Americans ate low-fat, vegetarian food, and the Africans ate rich American fare. Even in this short time, he found, a change in diet meant a switch in hormone profiles, too. There was a marked increase in androgen and estrogen excretion among the Africans, while that of the Americans decreased to the point where it resembled the hormone levels of the low-risk group.

"This study is a preliminary indication that a low-fat diet is one of the factors which can lower the risk of prostatic cancer," Dr. Hill told us. "By reducing total calorie intake, and substituting fruit and vegetable calories for animal calories, a high-risk prostatic cancer group was switched to a low-risk one."

It is important to remember that in these studies of diet and cancer, what are generally measured are *total* fats. In other words, replacing saturated fats with polyunsaturated fats may cut down on the risks of heart disease, but it seems to offer no protection against cancer.

In fact, some research suggests that large amounts of polyunsaturated fats may be even more dangerous where cancer is concerned. The statistics gathered by researchers at the University of Maryland point to one kind of fat, in particular, as worth being wary about—those containing *trans* fatty acids. *Trans* fatty acids don't occur naturally in vegetables, but are produced when polyunsaturated oils are partially hydrogenated—when they are processed with hydrogen to make them more solid or to give them longer shelf life. Many kinds of margarine, salad oil, mayonnaise and snack foods contain significant amounts of these subtances. Possibly, researchers speculate, these unnatural *trans* fatty acids change cell membranes, allowing carcinogens (cancer-causing substances) to pass through more easily.

OUR BEEF WITH BEEF

If you are not a smoker (and therefore not likely to develop lung cancer), the form of cancer you are most vulnerable to is cancer of the colon. Unfortunately, it is not only common, but quite deadly. Yet, there is very good reason to believe that we can, by making certain changes in our diets, significantly increase our protection against this particular form of malignancy. The reason for optimism is that there are very powerful indications that the incidence of bowel cancer is linked to certain dietary habits. But, by making the appropriate changes, we can put ourselves on the good side of the odds.

Medical epidemiologists are people who make it their business to study the relationship between various illnesses and the context in which they occur. And, in a nutshell, they tell us that colon cancer rates are higher in the United States, Canada and western Europe than in less developed African, Asian and Latin American countries— where very little animal protein is consumed. New Zealand, Australia, Argentina and Uruguay (all beef-eating countries) also have high incidence rates of bowel cancer. Also, groups of people who migrate from a country like Poland—where the colon cancer rate is traditionally low—to the United States or Australia, wind up with the higher incidence of their adopted land after a number of years.

At first, researchers were hard-pressed to identify any one factor in the diet of Western nations that might be responsible. All these countries are relatively affluent. As a result, diets tend to be high in saturated fat, sugar, white flour, beef and other animal protein, and low in natural fiber or roughage. But as John W. Berg, M.D., and Margaret A. Howell, Ph.D., told a conference on cancer in Bal Harbour, Florida, in 1973, closer investigation points directly at beef. In fact, according to Dr. Berg, "there is now substantial evidence that beef consumption is a key factor in determining bowel-cancer incidence."

The two National Cancer Institute researchers cited the example of Scotland, which has "reclaimed her usual distinction of having the world's highest death rate from bowel cancer." The highest rates occur in the rural beef-raising counties centered around Aberdeen. "Moreover, while the Scots consume less meat than any part of England, they eat 19 percent more beef than the English and have a 19 percent higher mortality rate from bowel cancer," the doctors reported.

In a very important study conducted jointly by American and Japanese cancer specialists, it was found that Japanese living in Hawaii, in a kind of transition from Eastern to Western culture and diet, had varying degrees of bowel cancer. The more Westernized their diet, the higher the degree of bowel cancer. The study suggests that of all Western foods, beef has the most dramatic correlation with bowel cancer.

Dr. Berg and his associates point out that the same trend—although on a lesser scale, is evident among various population groups in the United States. Bowel cancer rates are lower in the South and among blacks, for example. These populations eat more pork and chicken than beef. And people living in cities may risk a higher rate of colon cancer than those living on farms. "Beef coming to urban markets from feeding lots has a substantial fat content," the researchers say. "While the same comment would now hold true for beef supplied to rural populations through normal commercial channels, much of the beef used by farm populations in the past must have come from local slaughter of young cattle with a low fat content closely resembling that in veal." Finally, the researchers point out that Seventh-day Adventists, many of whom do not eat *any meat,* have a death rate from intestinal cancer 20 percent below that expected. Summing up their findings, the scientists declare "We have found . . . no populations with a high beef intake and a low rate of bowel cancer" (*Journal of the National Cancer Institute,* December 1973). A few years later, in another related study, Dr. Margaret Howell declared "Beef or cattle meat is probably the most suspect of the meats. . . . The evidence suggests that meat, particularly beef, is a food associated with the development of malignancies of the large bowel" (*Journal of Chronic Diseases,* vol. 28, 1975). The last word is not yet in on this question, and there remains doubt in some circles as to whether beef is really worse than any other source of animal protein and fat. A wise course of action, then, would be to minimize not just beef, but *all* fatty meats, such as we have done throughout this book.

Some investigators suspect that sugar, as well as fat, may contribute to the kind of internal environment that encourages cancer. G. Hems of Aberdeen, whose work we mentioned before in relation to fat and breast cancer, found that when comparing breast cancer rate and diet in 41 countries, consumption of refined sugar was a very powerful indicator. The more sugar, the more breast cancer (*British Journal of Cancer,* June, 1978). What's more, researchers have reported that when diets high in sugar are fed to one group of laboratory animals, and diets high in the complex carbohydrates (such as wheat, rice and potatoes) fed to another, the rats fed the sugar diets developed significantly more mammary tumors after being exposed to a cancer-causing chemical (*Nutrition and Cancer,* Spring, 1979). This link between sugar and cancer is relatively new and still controversial. Sugar has so many other undesirable qualities, however, that if the cancer link turns out to be true, it would only be one more reason to avoid the stuff.

Perhaps it has not escaped your attention that fat and sugar, besides being *suspected* of contributing to cancer, are also *known* to contribute mightily to overweight, because they are such concentrated forms of calories. And that in itself could be very important in protecting against cancer. "Of all dietary modifications," Dr. Gori of the National Cancer Institute says, "caloric restriction has had the most regular influence on tumor formation. With few exceptions, caloric restriction generally inhibits tumor formation." There is no better way to cut down on unnecessary calories than cutting back on both fat and sugar.

If cutting meat out of your diet is unsettling, compromise by cutting out preserved meats such as bacon, hot dogs and sausages. Besides containing lots of fat, these meats also contain nitrates or nitrites, which the body converts to nitrosamines, chemicals believed capable of causing cancer. Bacon is probably the worst of the lot, because it is cooked at high temperatures, which increases the production of nitrosamines, and also contains lots of salt, which does the same. Saccharin is another food additive worth avoiding. The most recent research indicates that while occasional use may not be harmful, heavy use is associated with an increased risk of bladder cancer. For that reason, we take a very dim view of the strategy of using saccharin in a reducing diet. Finally, the frying of meats, particularly when the meat is well done, can create chemical compounds believed capable of causing cancer. For that reason, we do virtually no frying at all in our book, instead using the steam-stir method. Actually, many foods, when exposed to high temperature for long periods of time, will begin to break down and form suspicious compounds. So as a general rule, try to eat as many foods as possible that can be enjoyed raw. When you do cook, try to use steaming, boiling or baking. Don't barbeque over direct flames. If you broil something, don't eat any parts that are burned.

So far we have given you a handful of negatives. Alcohol. Fat of all kinds, but especially animal fat and margarine fat. Beef, and meat in general. Gluttony. To a somewhat lesser extent, sugar, food additives and frying. Avoid habitual use or practice of these sins (smoking, too) and you have a powerful shield against cancer. But you can do even more. You can, in effect, give yourself a sword against cancer as well, by taking certain *positive* steps at the same time.

POSITIVE PROTECTION BEGINS WITH VITAMIN A

Your first positive step toward cancer protection might well be making sure that your diet is adequate in vitamin A. It's long been recognized that vitamin A is essential in maintaining the healthful condition of cells covering all the body's internal and external surfaces. These cells, making up the epithelium, cover all the major organs of the body and line its various passageways. Scientists know there is a significant relationship between the effects of vitamin A on the cells of the epithelium and the development of cancer in those tissues. And cancer in those tissues—which are found in the bronchial tubes and throat, stomach, intestine, uterus, kidney, bladder, testes, prostate and the skin —accounts for more than half of all cancers in both men and women.

Michael B. Sporn, M.D., of the National Cancer Institute, a leading authority on the vitamin A-cancer connection, explained to us that an important factor in vitamin A's cancer-preventing potential may be its control of a process called cell differentiation. Differentiation is the process that makes the cell what it is, a specialized worker in the body. But when the cell fails to mature properly and *de*-differentiates, the cell enters the primitive state and "its behavior becomes similar to that of a cancer cell," in Dr. Sporn's words. There is also the hormone connection. "Many of the body's hormones are involved in the proper maturation of cells, and vitamin A has the same hormonelike effects, but unlike a hormone, it cannot be manufactured in the body. The body must get its vitamin A from outside sources. . . ."

Animal studies have shown that vitamin A deficiency increases the risk of lung, bladder and colon cancer, all cancers of epithelial tissue. Scientists at the Massachusetts Institute of Technology reported an increased incidence of colon cancer in vitamin A-deficient animals exposed to cancer-causing chemicals—even in animals only marginally deficient in the vitamin, and exhibiting none of the common signs of vitamin A deficiency (*Cancer*, November, 1977).

"In our studies," the scientists reported, "the vitamin A levels have been only marginal, as opposed to acutely deficient, and the recognized clinical or histologic [microscopic] evidence for acute deficiency was not observed. Thus, with some segments of our United States population subject to marginal vitamin A deficits, we should consider the potential for tumor induction without obvious evidence for nutritional deficit." In other words, it's possible that a slight deficiency of vitamin A, not enough to cause a symptom like dry, bumpy skin, could be opening the door to something far more serious.

Many laboratory experiments suggest that when animals are subjected to chemical toxins designed to mimic the possible effect of the cancer-causing substances we encounter in everyday life, they are much less likely to develop cancer if their diets are at least adequate in vitamin A. But what about human beings? Curiously, we have indirect evidence that vitamin A may work the very same way—in this case, protecting smokers against the potent chemicals in cigarette smoke. When scientists compared the prior food intake of 292 men with lung cancer to 801 noncancer patients, they found that the lung cancer patients had tended to consume fewer vitamin A-rich foods than those men untouched by cancer. And the statistical association between high vitamin A and lower cancer risk was most pronounced among the men who smoked most heavily (*Journal of the National Cancer Institute,* June, 1979). These results confirm an earlier report from Norway. In that study, over 8,000 men were questioned about diet and smoking habits. Again, as intake of vitamin A rose, the incidence of lung cancer tended to decline (*International Journal of Cancer,* April, 1975). Vitamin A appeared to protect against lung cancer at all levels of cigarette smoking, and for all age groups. Protection of course is not complete, and heavy smokers in the high vitamin A group still faced a greater risk of developing lung cancer than nonsmokers. But it does mean that smokers (and quite possibly ex-smokers and those who live with smokers or near industrial pollution) would do especially well to pay attention to vitamin A in their diet.

It's possible that vitamin A protects against more than just lung cancer. The prostate contains epithelial tissue, just as the lungs do, and evidence from Japan suggests that that organ, too, may be protected by vitamin A. A 10-year study of over 100,000 Japanese men aged 40 and over revealed a substantially lower death rate from prostate cancer among men who ate green and yellow vegetables each day (*ICRDB Cancergram,* January, 1979). Japanese scientists theorize that it's the vitamin A in these vegetables that may be responsible for their cancer-preventing effects. Interestingly, the incidence of prostate cancer is lower and the consumption of vegetables higher among Japanese than Americans. Also, the prostate cancer rate is lower for American vegetarians than it is for meat eaters.

Everything we've talked about so far points to a central role for vitamin A in cancer *prevention.* There is little evidence to suggest that vitamin A might be an effective cancer treatment, a fact we wish to emphasize. But prevention is, after all, even more important. "No human population at risk for development of cancer should be allowed to remain in a vitamin A deficient state," Dr. Sporn wrote in *Nutrition Reviews* (April, 1977). Whether or not you are "at risk" for cancer is something only you can decide, based on family history, smoking habits, previous experience with cancer and so forth. But that is an extremely conservative viewpoint. A more aggressive attitude is: Why should *anyone* be deficient in vitamin A? But many are, even Dr. Sporn admits. That is particularly true in certain groups of people, including those who don't eat vegetables or milk, which are both important sources of vitamin A in the American diet.

The foods we prefer for vitamin A are liver (extraordinarily rich), as well as yellow fruits and vegetables like carrots, sweet potatoes, apricots, pumpkins and cantaloupes. Dark green leafy vegetables like spinach, dandelion greens, turnip greens and kale are also excellent sources of vitamin A.

VITAMIN C HELPS PROTECT US, TOO

When we were discussing additives that might cause cancer, we mentioned the nitrates and the nitrites used in preserved meats and pointed out that they can be converted to nitrosamines in the body. It is these nitrosamines which can cause cancer, scientists believe. But many scientists believe that vitamin C can block this dangerous reaction. While numerous studies have demonstrated that in animals, the evidence in humans is less conclusive although it too suggests that vitamin C can be protective. Scientists at the Ontario Cancer Institute in Toronto, for instance, found that the stools of normal individuals eating a typical Western diet *routinely* contained mutagens, which can damage the genetic material of cells. Mutagens are also believed to be potentially cancer-causing. Further testing showed that the mutagens in the stools were probably nitrosamines or nitrosamides. And when scientists fed one subject 4,000 milligrams of vitamin C a day over a two-week period, the levels of both the mutagens *and* the nitrosamines in his stools dropped dramatically *(Environmental Aspects of N-Nitroso Compounds,* International Agency for Research on Cancer, 1978). In somewhat simpler terms, we were told "there is strong evidence that people who are not getting enough fresh fruit or vegetables are more likely to get stomach cancer," by Sidney Mirvish, Ph.D., of the Eppley Institute for Research in Cancer in Omaha, Nebraska. "That's further evidence of the effects of ascorbic acid [vitamin C]."

John H. Weisburger, Ph.D., of the American Health Foundation in Valhalla, New York, believes that a greater intake of fruits and vegetables rich in vitamin C may explain the declining rate of stomach cancer in the United States, and the stabilization of the stomach cancer rate in Japan. In studies at the foundation, nitrite-rich raw fish, an important part of the traditional Japanese diet, was put through a simulated digestive system in the laboratory. The fish developed a high mutagenic potential, which was subsequently eliminated by the addition of vitamin C *(Science,* May 27, 1977).

According to Dr. Weisburger, the development of rapid transportation and refrigeration has led to increased consumption of fruits and vegetables in the United States and Japan. And the Westernization of the Japanese diet has lessened the consumption of nitrite-treated fish and pickled foods in that country. Both those developments, he believes, have caused drops in the rate of stomach cancer. "If all this information is correct," he told a scientific conference, "we should be able to prevent gastric cancer from childhood onward by ensuring that we have adequate vitamin C with each meal" (*Medical Tribune,* September 27, 1978).

A certain amount of theoretical work suggests that vitamin C might be able to help prevent cancers throughout the body, largely because of its general effect in boosting the immune system. During the late 1970s, this point of view was vigorously put forth by Linus Pauling, Ph.D., who together with Scottish surgeon Dr. Ewan Cameron, published a book called *Cancer and Vitamin C* (The Linus Pauling Institute of Science and Medicine, 1979).

For medical scientists and cancer specialists, the vitamin C question will doubtless continue to be a subject of debate. For us, however, it is perfectly reasonable to merely say that there are *many* reasons why we should make sure our diets contain plenty of vitamin C—for the sake of our immune systems, for strong cartilage and joints, healthy gums and so on. The possibility that it helps prevent cancer is just *one* of many reasons we should be getting plenty of vitamin C. All citrus fruits and melons are excellent sources of this vitamin; so are broccoli, brussels sprouts, cabbage, cauliflower, sweet peppers, fruits in general, tomatoes and dark green leafy vegetables.

FIBER PROTECTS THE BOWELS

Many cancer researchers believe that a high-fiber diet helps protect against cancer of the colon. One theory is that by increasing the bulk of the stools, and possibly by sponging up bile acid and other substances, fiber may reduce the concentration of chemicals that can promote cancer in the colon. By causing stools to move through the bowel much more quickly, fiber may also protect us by cutting in half the amount of time that fecal matter and degraded bile acids are in contact with the intestinal lining. Generally speaking, societies eating a high-fiber diet have a low incidence of colon cancer, although this interpretation is made somewhat difficult by the fact that these societies are usually also eating a low-fat diet. But still, the protection seems real. In a study of two Scandinavian populations, the group with a higher intake of dietary fiber had a lower incidence of colon cancer (*Lancet,* July 30, 1977). In Finland, the low incidence of colon cancer in spite of a high dietary fat intake has been attributed to high intake of dietary fiber. One researcher suggests that the highest risk of all is faced by people with a high intake of fat and a low intake of fiber.

Finding fiber in the marketplace by now should be no mystery to you. Look for it in all whole grain products, carrots, peas, potatoes, all kinds of beans and to a lesser extent, in just about all vegetables and fruits. Nuts and seeds are also good sources of fiber but they should be eaten in moderation because they are relatively high in calories.

SELENIUM—AN IMPORTANT TRACE MINERAL

Few people have heard about it yet, but there is a new mineral that the National Academy of Sciences has deemed essential to health—selenium. Selenium is classified as a trace element, which means it's needed only in very small amounts. While most minerals are measured in milligrams, selenium is measured in micrograms, amounts one thousand times smaller than a milligram. Yet, those very small amounts of selenium could be very important in cancer prevention, some scientists are saying.

A study conducted by Gerhard N. Schrauzer, Ph.D., of the University of California at San Diego, discovered that as levels of selenium in the blood rise, breast cancer rates fall. Analyzing data from 17 countries, Dr. Schrauzer discovered selenium levels in blood from blood banks in Japan, Taiwan, Thailand, the Philippines, Puerto Rico and Costa Rica were over three times as high as in samples from European countries and the United States. And the breast cancer mortality rate in Europe and the United States is correspondingly two to five times higher than in Asia and Latin America. North Americans are lucky to get half the amount of selenium that apparently boosts resistance to cancer. The average amount of selenium eaten by Americans is in the vicinity of 100 micrograms daily, while studies around the world suggest that as selenium intake approaches 300 micrograms a day, it appears to increase protection against certain types of cancer.

The human evidence so far is quite indirect, but in the laboratory, Dr. Schrauzer and others have run some very interesting experiments. In one animal study designed to serve as a model for human cancer development, Dr. Schrauzer added selenium to the drinking water of a group of mice that are bred with a high genetic predisposition toward breast cancer. After 16 months, 82 percent of the unsupplemented mice had developed tumors. But only 10 percent of those that received selenium developed tumors. What's more, their tumors grew more slowly and the mice survived from one to three months longer than those that received no selenium (*Annals of Clinical and Laboratory Science,* November/December, 1974). More recently, a study by Maryce M. Jacobs, Ph.D., of the Eppley Institute for Research in Cancer, sought to support the growing evidence that selenium may help prevent cancer of the colon and liver. Dr. Jacobs and her associate gave rats chemicals known to induce tumors of the colon and liver. At the same time, she fed groups of animals a continuous supplement of selenium in their drinking water. Four months later, 64 percent of the unsupplemented animals had developed tumors. But only 31 percent of the animals that received selenium showed signs of cancer. The survival rate of the supplemented animals was also excellent: 13 out of 15 were alive at the conclusion of the study. Discussing these results, Dr. Jacobs anticipates that selenium may have potential as a cancer preventive agent for humans as soon as the proper dosages can be determined (*Biological Trace Element Research,* March, 1979). Dr. Schrauzer suggests that it makes sense to add selenium to your diet now, recommending "anywhere from 100 to 250 micrograms of supplemental selenium a day," preferably in the form of a special high-selenium yeast. As for diet, Dr. Schrauzer suggests "more seafood, more cereal and bread products and a decrease in meat, fat and especially sugar." There is one exception though, to the advice to cut back on meat: liver, which along with kidney, happens to be the richest selenium source of all.

Interestingly, foods rich in selenium fall very nicely into the general pattern of natural low-fat, high-nutrition foods. Just as in the case of vitamin C, there is no need to eat exotic foods to get the selenium we want.

SPECIAL VEGETABLES AND OTHER FRIENDS

While vegetables in general may be considered anti-cancer foods in the sense that they're low in fat and many have good amounts of vitamins A and C, there are a few vegetables, belonging to the Brassica genus, that may well have special protective powers. A team of researchers headed by Saxon Graham, Ph.D., conducted dietary interviews with hundreds of men and women suffering from colon or rectal cancer and then compared their diets with those of people not suffering from the diseases (*Journal of the National Cancer Institute,* September, 1978). Those who didn't have cancer, the researchers found, tended to have eaten more cabbage (and cabbage dishes like sauerkraut and coleslaw), more brussels sprouts, and more broccoli. And it doesn't appear that this association is purely chance, because a number of animal studies suggest that *something* in these vegetables is an active defender against cancer. The researchers cite several other studies in this area. In one study rats were fed cabbage, broccoli and brussels sprouts in powder form; the powder increased a chemical reaction in the rats' intestines that can prevent tumors. In another study, scientists fed rats substances called indoles, found in these three vegetables—and again, the cancer-fighting chemical reaction increased. In a third study, two groups of animals were exposed to cancer-causing substances. One group was then fed indoles—and developed far less cancer.

It is also possible that chlorophyll, found in many vegetables, has protective properties. Chiu-Nan Lai, Ph.D., from the M.D. Anderson Hospital and Tumor Institute in Houston, told us she believes that the key anti-cancer property found in many vegetables is chlorophyll. "Brussels sprouts, broccoli, spinach and leafy lettuce are rich in chlorophyll," says Dr. Lai. "My laboratory research has demonstrated that extracts of chlorophyll from those vegetables definitely lower the mutagenic activity of known cancer-causing agents. Tomatoes, cucumbers, celery and other low-chlorophyll vegetables produced less of an antimutagenic effect."

Sprouts can also be credited with being more than merely nutritious and low in calories. Researchers at the University of Texas System Cancer Center in Houston reported in *Nutrition and Cancer* (Fall, 1978) that they have found an anti-cancer effect in sprouts of wheat, mung beans and lentils. It's likely that other forms of sprouts (such as alfalfa, sunflower and soy) have a similar effect. The doctors who did the sprout research have suggested that it could be the chlorophyll in the sprouts that is the active protective agent.

The two other foods that may have some degree of anti-cancer potential are yogurt and soybeans. One bacteria found in yogurt, *Lactobacillus acidophilus,* inhibits the enzymes that activate carcinogens in the bowel (*Journal of the National Cancer Institute,* February, 1980). Soybeans, as well as lima beans and possibly other seed foods, contain substances called protease inhibitors, which have an antitumor effect, according to the National Cancer Institute. When these foods are cooked at very high temperatures for long periods of time, the protease inhibitor tends to disappear, but normal cooking or roasting leaves some of the protective effect intact.

If you have been with us from the beginning, it may seem as though just about everything in the world either causes or prevents cancer. But if you stop and think about it for a minute, the cancer promoters and cancer defenders form themselves very nearly into two quite distinct camps. Cancer *promoters* are typified by the foods served at fast-food stands. Meat fried at high temperature, lots of fat or sugar added to everything, little or no fiber and no vegetables at all except possibly potatoes (which are french fried to death). Cancer *defenders* are typified by what you would be eating if your diet consisted entirely of the food you raised in your own garden or foraged in the woods. High in vitamins A and C from fruits and vegetables; lots of fiber, lots of chlorophyll-rich greens. Another way to look at the division between the promoters and defenders of cancer might be to say that the promoter foods are those given to us by modern technology and food processing, while the defender foods are the foods we lived on from the time of the Garden of Eden to the 19th century. In other words, in moving toward an anti-cancer diet, we are not following a fad, but rather turning away from a fad—the fad of "factory food" which has been in existence for only 100 years, and is suspected of contributing to many chronic diseases other than cancer, such as heart disease, diverticulosis and gallbladder disease.

Finally, we freely admit that the information presented here, as well as our opinions, are controversial and subject to constant revision as new findings are made. However, lest anyone think that the very idea of a diet designed to minimize the chances of getting cancer is just too farfetched, we would like to quote two sentences from a recent issue of the respected journal *Preventive Medicine* (March, 1980). The lines conclude an article entitled "Nutrition and Cancer" written by A. B. Miller of the National Cancer Institute of Canada, with the assistance of six internationally recognized experts in the field of cancer cause and prevention:

> *In conclusion, there would seem to be sufficient evidence to propose modifying the diet of Western countries to reduce total fat and increase dietary fiber on the lines of the prudent diet, and to introduce certain protective factors, such as an increase in green vegetables and vitamin C. Although further research is required, such measures are unlikely to be hazardous and can be advocated with a strong hope for benefits in the population.*

SOUPS

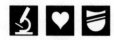

Carrot-Apricot Soup

Makes four servings
⅓ cup (80 ml) dried apricots
⅔ cup (150 ml) apple juice
8–10 carrots, thinly sliced
2½ cups (625 ml) *Chicken Stock* •
1 medium onion
3 cloves garlic
1 teaspoon (5 ml) tamari
1 teaspoon (5 ml) finely minced fresh parsley
1 teaspoon (5 ml) finely minced fresh dillweed
1 tablespoon (15 ml) sesame tahini
1 tablespoon (15 ml) yogurt
1 cup (250 ml) cooked soybeans

Simmer dried apricots in apple juice until plump, 5 to 8 minutes. In another saucepan, combine carrots, broth, onion, garlic, tamari and herbs. Bring to a boil and simmer until carrots are tender, about 15 minutes. Place apricot mixture and half of carrot mixture in a blender with tahini and yogurt. Process on low speed until smooth. Combine puree with remaining carrot mixture and stir in soybeans. Serve hot.

Variation: For a soup that is less sweet-tasting, substitute broth or water for unsweetened apple juice. *Vegetable Stock* or *Garlic Broth* may be substituted for the *Chicken Stock*. Try cooked chick-peas instead of soybeans.

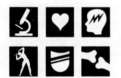

Green Zinger Soup

Makes two cups (500 ml)
1½ cups (375 ml) yogurt
1 cup (250 ml) chopped spinach
2 scallions, chopped
¼ cup (60 ml) chopped parsley
1½ teaspoons (7 ml) lemon juice
1 teaspoon (5 ml) tamari
1 clove garlic, mashed
paprika (garnish)

Barbara decided to see what she could do with some extra spinach one night and the result had so much taste and character we had to include it here. Full of vitamins, minerals and healing factors, and a fine soup for company.

Put the yogurt in a blender and then slowly add the other ingredients, with the blender on medium speed, until they are reduced to soup. Some of the spinach will be totally pulverized, while much of it will still be in small bits.

The combination of spinach, parsley and scallions gives real zing to this soup. If it's *too* zingy for you after you taste it, try adding a little more yogurt.

Finally, garnish each bowl with a sprinkle of paprika. (A good alternative would be a single cross-sectional slice of sweet red pepper.)

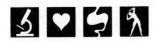

Creamy Borscht

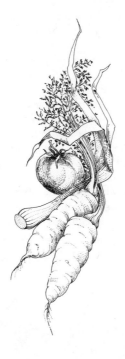

Makes 10 servings
4 cups (1 l) water
3 cups (750 ml) shredded
    cabbage
2 medium beets, peeled and
    cubed
1 medium onion, chopped
1 medium carrot, diced
5 cloves garlic
2 bay leaves
1 tomato, chopped
2 tablespoons (30 ml) lemon
    juice
1 tablespoon (15 ml) tamari
½ cup (125 ml) *Yogurt Cream
    Cheese*
2 tablespoons (30 ml) sesame
    tahini

In a soup kettle, combine water, cabbage, beets, onion, carrot, garlic and bay leaves. Bring to a boil, cover, and simmer 30 minutes. Add tomato, lemon juice and tamari, and simmer 15 minutes more. Remove bay leaves.

Place *Yogurt Cream Cheese* and tahini in bottom of blender. Add half of the soup and blend until smooth. Combine with remaining soup. Serve hot or cold.

Creamy Borscht is such a lovely color, it can be served in a tureen to highlight a buffet table or placed in small, individual bowls to add color to a dinner setting.

Note: Soup can be frozen for later use.

SALADS

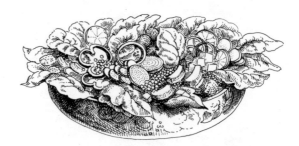

Antipasto Alla Salute!

*Makes four generous
servings*

¾ cup (175 ml) cooked
    chick-peas with cooking
    liquid, chilled
6½ ounces (184 g) unsalted
    water-packed tuna,
    drained
1 cup (250 ml) cubed Swiss or
    other firm cheese
¼ cup (60 ml) chilled
    *Mushrooms
    Italian-Style*
½ pound (225 g) spinach or 1
    head romaine lettuce
4 artichoke hearts, quartered
1 large sweet red pepper,
    thinly sliced in rings
1 large red onion, thinly sliced
1 large carrot, thinly sliced
1 lemon, very thinly sliced
4 cloves garlic, sliced or
    mashed
½ cup (125 ml) broccoli florets
¼ cup (60 ml) red wine
    vinegar
1 tablespoon (15 ml) olive oil
1 teaspoon (5 ml) of your
    favorite mixed herbs
    (such as thyme,
    oregano, sage,
    rosemary, marjoram,
    basil)

A festive salad brimming with virtually every known vitamin and mineral, as well as special healing factors.

Our aim here was to create an antipasto with the color, taste and variety of the traditional Italian version but without the fatty, preservative-laden meats, the high-salt anchovies and olives, and eggs. In doing that, we came up with a salad so nutritious that it makes a fine meal in itself, too.

You can prepare this antipasto two different ways. The first way is to simply combine all the ingredients in a large bowl and serve. The alternative way, which you might want to try when you're in a creative mood or some special company is coming, involves dividing the ingredients into two categories: those that will be simply tossed together and those that will be spread on top in concentric circles or some other design. We leave it to you to decide which ingredients you want to highlight and how. When we served this antipasto, we made the tuna the center of attention, but then mixed it in with all the other ingredients as we served it to our guests.

Depending on how much liquid you have in your salad from various ingredients, you can adjust the amount of oil added. As for the artichoke hearts, you can, if you wish, steam artichokes for about 20 minutes and remove the hearts or simply buy a small jar of them, preferably unsalted. The interesting thing about the thinly sliced lemons is that you can eat them whole, skin and all. If you have a lot of oranges on hand, you can also cut some of them in thin slices.

Mushrooms Italian-Style

Makes four servings
¼ cup (60 ml) water
1 tablespoon (15 ml) lemon
     juice
1 tablespoon (15 ml) sunflower
     oil
2 teaspoons (10 ml) tamari
½ teaspoon (2 ml) thyme
½ teaspoon (2 ml) basil
1 clove garlic, minced
5 cups (1.25 l) sliced
     mushrooms (about 1
     pound [450 g])
1 tablespoon (15 ml) minced
     fresh parsley

In a saucepan, combine water, lemon juice, oil, tamari, thyme, basil and garlic. Add mushrooms, stir and cover. Cook slowly until mushrooms are tender and water evaporates, about 20 minutes.

Add parsley during the last minute or two of cooking. Serve over chicken or poached fish, or as a vegetable side dish.

Note: Try chilled mushrooms served alone or tossed into salads.

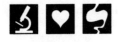

Brussels Sprout Salad with Buttermilk Vinaigrette Dressing

This is an unusual and tasty salad.

Makes four servings
2 cups (500 ml) brussels sprouts
1 carrot, shredded
1 unpeeled apple, chopped
¼ cup (60 ml) walnuts, chopped

Dressing:
2 tablespoons (30 ml) mild
     vinegar
1 tablespoon (15 ml) buttermilk
½ teaspoon (2 ml) Dijon-style
     mustard
¼ cup (60 ml) soy or sunflower
     oil

For salad, wash brussels sprouts and remove discolored outer leaves. With a very sharp knife on a cutting board, thinly slice sprouts. Combine brussels sprouts, carrot, apple and walnuts.

For dressing, in a blender combine vinegar, buttermilk and mustard. Process until combined. Add oil gradually, until mixture is thick.

Add enough dressing just to moisten salad, and toss. Reserve leftover dressing for tossed salads.

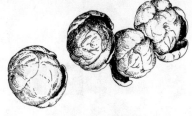

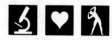

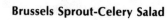

Brussels Sprout-Celery Salad

Makes four servings
2 cups (500 ml) brussels sprouts
1 cup (250 ml) chopped celery
1 unpeeled apple, chopped
Vinaigrette Dressing

A good, crunchy salad from winter fruit and vegetables.

Wash brussels sprouts and remove discolored outer leaves. With a very sharp knife on a cutting board, thinly slice sprouts.

Combine ingredients and toss with enough *Vinaigrette Dressing* to moisten. Serve immediately.

Variation: Add ½ cup (125 ml) of raisins and two tablespoons (30 ml) of chopped walnuts for a brussels sprout salad Waldorf-style.

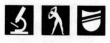

Broccoli with Cashews

Makes four to six servings
3 cups (750 ml) broccoli florets
3 tablespoons (45 ml) soy or
    sunflower oil
3 tablespoons (45 ml) lemon
    juice
1 teaspoon (5 ml) marjoram
1 teaspoon (5 ml) tamari
2 tablespoons (30 ml) cashew
    pieces, toasted

A vibrant cold salad sparkling with taste.

Steam the broccoli florets just until tender, yet crisp. Combine the oil, lemon juice, marjoram and tamari. Pour this marinade over the broccoli and allow to cool. Chill thoroughly. To serve, sprinkle with cashews.

Note: Save the broccoli stems for a combination vegetable dish, soup or casserole.

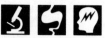

Very Orange Salad

Makes four servings
2 cups (500 ml) shredded
    carrots
1 orange, chopped
¼ cup (60 ml) orange juice
2 tablespoons (30 ml) yogurt
2 tablespoons (30 ml) raisins
    (optional)
dash freshly grated nutmeg
spinach or lettuce leaves

Oranges and carrots give this salad its color and healthy doses of vitamins A and C.

Combine the carrots and chopped orange sections. Mix the orange juice with the yogurt and pour over the carrot and orange combination. Add raisins, if desired. Sprinkle with a dash of nutmeg and toss to combine. Chill. Serve on spinach or lettuce leaves.

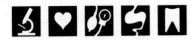

Makes six servings
1 medium unpeeled apple,
    cubed
¼ cup (60 ml) pitted dates,
    diced
¼ cup (60 ml) walnuts, chopped
½ cup (125 ml) alfalfa sprouts
¼ medium head cabbage, thinly
    shredded (about ½
    pound [225 g])
Sesame-Fruit Dressing or
    Tofu Mayonnaise

Cabbage-Apple-Date Salad

This change-of-pace salad has two tasty surprises: dates and crunchy walnuts.

Place apple, dates, walnuts and sprouts with cabbage in a large bowl. Toss with *Sesame-Fruit Dressing* or *Tofu Mayonnaise*.

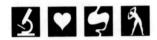

Makes six servings
2 cups (500 ml) whole wheat
    macaroni
½ bunch broccoli
2 stalks celery with tops
1 bunch scallions (about 4)
    juice of 1 lemon
⅓ cup (80 ml) chopped parsley
2 tablespoons (30 ml) corn oil
¼ cup (60 ml) cider vinegar
1 teaspoon (5 ml) Dijon-style
    mustard
2 teaspoons (10 ml) tamari
2 tablespoons (30 ml) yogurt
¼ teaspoon (1 ml) dillweed
¼ teaspoon (1 ml) cayenne
    pepper
2 cloves garlic, minced

Liz's Macaroni and Vegetable Salad

Here is something different that is terrific for picnics—a crunchy macaroni salad without mayonnaise.

Cook the macaroni in water until firm, but not soft. Be careful not to overcook it or the salad will become mushy. As soon as it is done, drain and rinse macaroni with cold water. Remove tough lower areas from the broccoli. Chop or slice the vegetables, and mix all ingredients together in a large bowl. You may want to adjust the amount of yogurt to get the consistency that seems best to you.

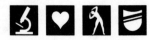

Makes four servings
3 cups (750 ml) packed spinach
    leaves
4 romaine lettuce leaves
6 mushrooms
½ cup (125 ml) sliced Jerusalem
    artichokes
1 teaspoon (5 ml) sesame seeds
Vinaigrette Dressing

Tossed Salad Vinaigrette

Thoroughly wash spinach in a large amount of water to remove grit. Set aside to drain. Wash lettuce. Break up into bite-size pieces. Remove stems from spinach and tear into pieces. Add to romaine in a salad bowl.

Wipe mushrooms with a damp cloth or wash, if necessary. Slice and add to spinach and lettuce. Add artichokes.

Toast sesame seeds in a small iron skillet over low heat. Stir to prevent scorching. Do not add oil. Add sesame seeds to salad and toss with *Vinaigrette Dressing*.

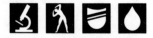

Makes four servings
½ cup (125 ml) young
    dandelion greens
2 cups (500 ml) packed lettuce
    or spinach leaves
½ cup (125 ml) alfalfa sprouts
¼ cup (60 ml) mung bean
    and/or sunflower seed
    sprouts
Creamy Garlic Dressing

Spring Dandelion Salad

Spruced up with sprouts, this green salad makes good use of dandelions as soon as they appear in the spring.

Early dandelion greens, picked before the plants have flowered, are essential. Older, larger plants produce a very bitter leaf. Be certain to wash the greens thoroughly in several changes of water. Chop and add to the salad bowl along with lettuce and sprouts. Toss with dressing and serve.

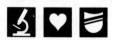

Makes three servings
1 cup (250 ml) sliced
    mushrooms
½ cup (125 ml) shredded
    carrots
¼ cup (60 ml) alfalfa sprouts
¼ cup (60 ml) cooked
    chick-peas
2 tablespoons (30 ml) chopped
    cashews, toasted
Creamy Garlic Dressing

Mushroom-Cashew Salad

Combine the mushrooms, carrots, sprouts, chick-peas and cashews. Toss with enough dressing to coat and chill before serving.

Mushroom Salad

Makes four servings

2½ cups (625 ml) thinly sliced
    mushrooms (about ½
    pound [225 g])
2 teaspoons (10 ml) lemon
    juice
¼ cup (60 ml) sliced scallion
    greens
½ cup (125 ml) alfalfa sprouts
2 teaspoons (10 ml) sesame
    seeds, toasted
2 tablespoons (30 ml) yogurt
2 teaspoons (10 ml) sesame
    oil
lettuce or spinach leaves

Toss fresh mushrooms with lemon juice. Combine remaining ingredients except for leafy greens, and toss to combine. Serve on lettuce or spinach leaves.

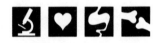

Coleslaw with Yogurt Dressing

Makes four servings

1 cup (250 ml) shredded
    cabbage
1 cup (250 ml) shredded sweet
    potatoes or carrots
1 tablespoon (15 ml) sunflower
    seeds
Yogurt Dressing for Coleslaw

Combine cabbage and sweet potatoes in bowl. Toss with sunflower seeds and *Yogurt Dressing for Coleslaw.* Makes two cups.

Yogurt Dressing for Coleslaw

Makes ½ cup (125 ml)

½ cup (125 ml) *Yogurt Cream
    Cheese*
1 tablespoon (15 ml) cider
    vinegar
1 teaspoon (5 ml) honey

Combine ingredients and stir together until blended. Makes enough dressing for two cups (500 ml) of coleslaw.

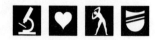

Makes four servings
1½ cups (375 ml) cooked
    brown rice
1 sliced orange
¼ cup (60 ml) chopped
    walnuts
¾ cup (175 ml) alfalfa sprouts
2 tablespoons (30 ml) wheat
    germ
4 tablespoons (60 ml) grated
    Parmesan cheese
1 green pepper, finely sliced
½ cup (125 ml) shredded
    carrots
½ cup (125 ml) chopped
    endive
⅓ cup (80 ml) sliced scallions
1 teaspoon (5 ml) sunflower
    oil
¼ cup (60 ml) *Black Magic
    Sauce*

Cold Orange-Rice Salad

Our taste-testers said: "Very zippy . . . very colorful . . . loved texture . . . unique taste!"

The rice can be warm or cold, whichever is convenient. Combine all ingredients in a large salad bowl, tossing well.

You may want to add additional *Black Magic Sauce* or herbs to this dish.

Note: As a main dish, this will serve two.

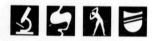

Makes four servings
3 parsnips, shredded
2 carrots, shredded
1 medium sweet potato,
    shredded
Creamy Garlic Dressing

Shredded Vegetable Salad

Do not peel the scrubbed vegetables before shredding. Toss with enough *Creamy Garlic Dressing* to moisten.

MAIN DISHES

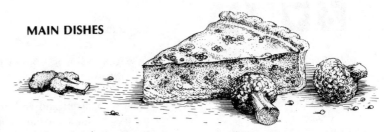

Broccoli-Cheese Quiche

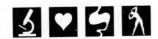

Makes six servings
1 cup (250 ml) broccoli florets
1 cup (250 ml) cottage cheese
¼ cup (60 ml) buttermilk
2 eggs, beaten
2 scallions, minced
    dash freshly grated nutmeg
9-inch (23-cm) unbaked
    No-Roll Pie Crust

Steam broccoli for three to four minutes, just until crisp-tender. Rinse with cold water, drain and set aside.

Combine the cottage cheese and buttermilk in a blender on low speed. To make a smooth mixture without a blender, the cottage cheese can be pressed through a sieve. Place the cheese mixture in a mixing bowl and add the eggs, scallions and nutmeg.

Pour cheese mixture into pie shell. Arrange broccoli florets on top, pressing down into the cheese mixture.

Bake in a preheated 400° F. (200° C.) oven 20 minutes. Reduce heat to 350° F. (175° C.) and continue baking 10 to 15 minutes more. The quiche should be puffed and browned. Serve hot or cold.

Mushroom-Tofu Delight

Makes two servings
8 ounces (225 g) tofu, cubed
½ cup (125 ml) *Black Magic Sauce*
2½ cups (625 ml) halved
    mushrooms (about ½
    pound [225 g])
4 sweet red peppers, sliced
¼ cup (60 ml) thinly sliced
    carrots
¼ cup (60 ml) shredded
    carrots
3 tablespoons (45 ml)
    chopped fresh parsley
½ cup (125 ml) sprouted lentils

One of the easiest and nicest ways to get acquainted with tofu.

Marinate the tofu for about two hours in the *Black Magic Sauce.* Pour enough of the sauce into a wok or skillet on high heat in order to steam-stir the mushrooms and peppers. When mushrooms are slightly tender, add the tofu and the remainder of the liquid. Cook for several minutes, stirring briskly, until the ingredients are hot. Add carrots and parsley and cook for one more minute. Finally, add the sprouts, continue stirring briskly for another 30 seconds and serve immediately.

To complement the protein in the tofu and the lentils, serve with some whole wheat bread.

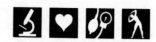

Makes eight servings
2 cups (500 ml) cooked
   soybeans
3–4 slices whole grain bread,
   crumbled
1 tablespoon (15 ml) chopped
   fresh parsley
1 tablespoon (15 ml) of your
   favorite mixed herbs
   (such as thyme,
   oregano, sage,
   rosemary, marjoram,
   basil)
1 clove garlic, crushed
1 egg
2 tablespoons (30 ml) tomato
   juice

Soy Spaghetti Balls

Imagine enjoying a hearty spaghetti dinner without worrying about saturated fat, cholesterol and lack of fiber. Dig in!

Mash soybeans and add bread. Stir in herbs, garlic, egg and tomato juice and mash mixture until thoroughly combined. Shape into balls and place on a lightly greased cookie sheet. Bake in a 425° F. (220° C.) oven for 30 to 45 minutes while preparing your favorite spaghetti sauce. Makes about 24 balls.

When serving, place whole wheat spaghetti on plate, arrange three or four spaghetti balls on spaghetti, and cover with tomato sauce. Remaining spaghetti balls can be added to soup later in the week, or frozen for the next spaghetti dinner.

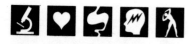

Makes two servings
8 ounces (225 g) tofu
½ cup (125 ml) *Black Magic
   Sauce*
1 teaspoon (5 ml) sunflower oil
2 cups (500 ml) shredded
   cabbage
1 cup (250 ml) shredded
   carrots
1 cup (250 ml) cherry tomatoes
4 tablespoons (60 ml) slivered
   almonds
½ cup (125 ml) freshly shelled
   peas
½ cup (125 ml) alfalfa sprouts
1 cup (250 ml) cooked brown
   rice

Rainbow Rice

An intriguing medley of tastes and textures.

Marinate the tofu in the *Black Magic Sauce* for 30 minutes or longer. Pour remaining sauce into a hot wok or skillet along with the oil. When the mixture begins to steam vigorously, add the cabbage, carrots, tomatoes, almonds and the marinated tofu. Stir together briskly. When the mixture begins to steam again, add the peas and continue stirring for about one minute. Now, add the sprouts, stir for another 30 seconds and serve over the rice.

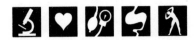

Makes eight servings

Filling:

    1 medium onion, chopped
    1 cup (250 ml) chopped
        cabbage
    1 cup (250 ml) diced carrots
    1 cup (250 ml) fresh or frozen
        peas
    1 cup (250 ml) fresh or frozen
        corn
    1 teaspoon (5 ml) chili
        powder
    ¼ teaspoon (1 ml) thyme
    1 tablespoon (15 ml)
        sunflower oil
    1 tablespoon (15 ml) whole
        wheat flour
    ½ cup (125 ml) skim milk
    1 egg, beaten

Crust:

    1 cup (250 ml) whole wheat
        pastry flour
    ¼ cup (60 ml) sunflower oil
    2 tablespoons (30 ml)
        buttermilk

Topping:

    2–3 tablespoons (30–45 ml)
            soft whole grain
            bread crumbs
    2 tablespoons (30 ml) grated
            Parmesan cheese

Baked Vegetable Pie

Place onion, cabbage and carrots in a saucepan or lightly oiled skillet and steam-stir in a few tablespoons (50 ml) of water to prevent scorching. When vegetables are crisp-tender, stir in peas, corn and seasonings. Cover and set aside.

In a small saucepan or skillet, warm oil and stir in flour. Stir over medium heat for a few minutes, until flour is golden brown. Stir in milk slowly, to prevent lumping. Combine sauce with vegetable mixture, along with egg.

For crust, place flour, oil and buttermilk in a 9-inch (23-cm) pie plate. Toss with a fork until combined, then press along bottom and sides with fingers.

Place filling in unbaked crust. Combine bread crumbs and Parmesan cheese for topping, and sprinkle over filling.

Bake pie in a preheated 350° F. (175° C.) oven about 20 to 25 minutes, until firm. Serve hot or at room temperature.

Note: Pie can be made ahead of time and refrigerated, then baked before serving. If pie is chilled, baking time may be slightly longer. Also, pie can be reheated after baking.

SIDE DISHES

Carrots Piquant

Makes four servings
8–10 carrots (about 1 pound
        [450 g])
2 teaspoons (10 ml) sesame
        oil
1 tablespoon (15 ml) minced
        fresh ginger root
4 cloves garlic, minced
2 teaspoons (10 ml) sesame
        seeds
2 teaspoons (10 ml) poppy
        seeds
½ teaspoon (2 ml) turmeric
1 teaspoon (5 ml) cumin
        powder
2 teaspoons (10 ml)
        coriander
½ teaspoon (2 ml) chili
        powder

One of our all-time favorite carrot recipes, subtle and surprising. We might mention versatile, too, because leftover carrots can be tossed with yogurt and chilled, then served on greens as a salad.

Wash and cut the carrots in long, thin strips. In a large skillet, saute the carrots in oil until nearly tender, adding a little water, if needed, to prevent scorching. Remove carrots from the pan. Place ginger, garlic, sesame and poppy seeds in the skillet and stir over medium heat until golden, again adding water if needed. Stir in the turmeric, cumin, coriander, chili powder and carrots, and fry together for two or three minutes. Serve hot.

Variation: Substitute parsnips, potatoes or turnips for all or part of the carrots.

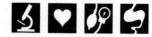

Kohlrabi and Carrots

Makes four servings
1 cup (250 ml) peeled and
        cubed kohlrabi
1 cup (250 ml) sliced carrots
Whole Wheat White Sauce or
        yogurt

In a saucepan, place the kohlrabi and carrots in water to cover, and bring to a boil. Reduce heat and simmer until the vegetables are tender, about 15 minutes.

Serve with *Whole Wheat White Sauce* or toss with a little yogurt. Serve hot.

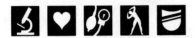

Makes four servings
2 large stalks broccoli
½ sweet red pepper

Steamed Broccoli and Red Peppers

Cut off ends from the broccoli stalks; peel away any tough skin from the main stems. Slice stems and separate stalks into individual florets.

Seed sweet red pepper half and slice in lengthwise strips. Cut strips in two. Combine the broccoli and red pepper in a steamer or colander over boiling water. Steam, covered, just until crisp-tender. The broccoli should remain a bright green. Serve hot.

This combination is a colorful and tasty vegetable dish to serve with fish.

Note: Leftovers give a lift to vegetable soup or tomato sauce for pasta. Add the steamed vegetables just before serving, and heat them through.

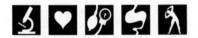

Makes four servings
2 cups (500 ml) chopped
     broccoli
2 cups (500 ml) chopped
     cauliflower
1 large or 2 small carrots,
     sliced
1 large onion, chopped
½ sweet red pepper, thinly
     sliced

Steamed Mixed Vegetables

It's just as easy to add variety to your steamed vegetables as it is to serve them one at a time.

Combine the vegetables in a metal colander over boiling water in a large kettle. Cover and allow to steam for about 15 minutes, until vegetables are crisp-tender. Serve hot.

Makes six servings
1 head cauliflower
2 tablespoons (30 ml) yogurt
2 tablespoons (30 ml) tomato
     paste
1 teaspoon (5 ml) tamari
⅛ teaspoon (0.5 ml) freshly
     grated nutmeg
2 eggs, separated
2 egg whites

Cauliflower Souffle

Steam cauliflower until soft. Press cauliflower through a sieve with the back of a wooden spoon, then mix with yogurt and tomato paste in a large bowl. Or, place small amounts of cauliflower with some of the yogurt and tomato paste in a blender and process on low speed until smooth, then place in a large bowl.

Stir tamari, nutmeg and two egg yolks into cauliflower mixture. Beat the four egg whites with an eggbeater until they are stiff. Gently fold the egg whites into the cauliflower.

Place the cauliflower mixture in a medium, lightly oiled souffle dish. Bake in a preheated 325° F. (165° C.) oven until firm, about 35 minutes.

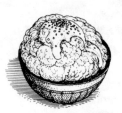

Capitol Dome Cauliflower

Makes eight servings
1 head cauliflower
1 tablespoon (15 ml) corn oil
2 tablespoons (30 ml) whole
    wheat flour
½ cup (125 ml) *Chicken Stock*
½ cup (125 ml) skim milk
    soft whole grain bread
        crumbs

A very impressive-looking dish to put on the table.

Steam cauliflower head until tender. This can be done with a colander set inside a large kettle with an inch (2.5 cm) or so of water for steaming. Cover the kettle and check the cauliflower periodically with a sharp fork. When the inside of the cauliflower yields easily to the fork, the cauliflower is done. Meanwhile, in a medium saucepan, heat the oil and add the flour, stirring to combine. Stir one or two minutes over low heat. Add the *Chicken Stock* and milk slowly, stirring constantly to avoid lumping.

When the cauliflower is done cooking, place whole in an ovenproof serving dish, pour the milk sauce over top, sprinkle with bread crumbs, and place in a 400° F. (200° C.) oven until the topping begins to brown. Serve hot.

Variation: Substitute sieved, cooked chestnuts or ground almonds for bread crumbs.

Broccoli Mousse

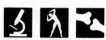

Makes six servings
1 large bunch broccoli
2 tablespoons (30 ml)
    safflower oil
2 tablespoons (30 ml) whole
    wheat flour
1 teaspoon (5 ml) basil
1½ cups (375 ml) skim milk
2 teaspoons (10 ml) tamari
1 tablespoon (15 ml) minced
    fresh parsley
½ teaspoon (2 ml) finely grated
    lemon rind
    dash freshly grated nutmeg
2 eggs, well beaten

Steam broccoli until tender. Rub broccoli with the back of a wooden spoon through a sieve, or blend in small amounts until smooth.

In a saucepan, heat the oil and stir in flour and basil. Stir over low heat two to three minutes. Add milk gradually, stirring between each addition to prevent lumping. Add tamari. Simmer until sauce has thickened. Remove from heat. Stir in parsley, lemon rind and nutmeg.

To beat eggs, have eggs at room temperature. Place the eggs in a warm bowl, or in a bowl set over, not in, hot water. Beat for three to four minutes with an electric mixer until the eggs are quite thick and creamy.

When the milk sauce has cooled a bit, stir in the broccoli and fold in the eggs. Pour into a large, lightly oiled souffle dish.

To bake, place the souffle dish in a larger pan filled with boiling water an inch (2.5 cm) deep. Bake in a preheated 400° F. (200° C.) oven one hour. Serve immediately.

Oven-Braised Brussels Sprouts

Makes four servings
2 cups (500 ml) brussels sprouts
2 teaspoons (10 ml) olive oil
1 tablespoon (15 ml) grated
    Parmesan cheese

Rinse brussels sprouts and trim bottoms. Cut a deep cross in the bottom of each sprout with a paring knife. Steam the sprouts just until slightly tender.

Preheat oven to 350° F. (175° C.). Place brussels sprouts in a casserole or baking dish large enough to hold them all in one or two layers. Drizzle olive oil over sprouts and sprinkle with Parmesan cheese. Place a lightly oiled piece of waxed paper over the sprouts, and place in the oven. Bake for about 20 minutes, until sprouts are tender. Serve hot.

Brussels Sprouts with *Lemon White Sauce*

Makes four servings
2 cups (500 ml) brussels sprouts

Sauce:
1 tablespoon (15 ml) corn oil
2 tablespoons (30 ml) whole
    wheat flour
½ cup (125 ml) skim milk
1 tablespoon (15 ml) lemon
    juice
1 teaspoon (5 ml) finely grated
    lemon rind
    dash freshly grated nutmeg

Pull any wilted outer leaves from the sprouts and cut crosswise slashes in the stem ends. Steam the sprouts just until tender. (Overcooked brussels sprouts develop a very strong taste.) Drain the sprouts in a colander.

In a heavy-bottom skillet, heat the oil and add the flour. Stir the flour and oil over low heat until the flour is "toasted" and begins to turn a slightly deeper brown. This should take about three to four minutes. Add the milk gradually, stirring constantly to avoid lumping. Stir in lemon juice and lemon rind, and add brussels sprouts. Add a few grains of nutmeg. Stir over low heat until the brussels sprouts are coated with sauce and the mixture is hot.

Note: Lemon White Sauce is also tasty on cooked broccoli or over poached fish.

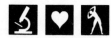

Hi-Pro Sprouts

Makes two servings
¾ cup (175 ml) *V-7 Juice*
½ teaspoon (2 ml) tamari
1 clove garlic, crushed
½ cup (125 ml) sprouted
    sunflower seeds
½ cup (125 ml) sprouted
    soybeans
dash cumin powder
dash cayenne pepper

Place enough *V-7 Juice* in a pan or wok to cover the bottom. Add tamari and garlic and heat until steaming. Add sprouts and steam for five minutes, stirring occasionally. Makes a crunchy kind of vegetable dish that can be eaten plain, used as a taco filler or ingredient in other dishes calling for beans.

MISCELLANEOUS

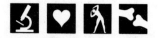

Cauliflower White Sauce I

Makes 2½ cups (625 ml)
1½ cups (375 ml) skim milk
2 cups (500 ml) cauliflower
    florets
freshly grated nutmeg

A tasty and healthful substitute for butter-based white sauces.

Heat milk to a simmer and add florets. Cook until cauliflower is quite tender. Place cauliflower and milk in a blender, add a sprinkling of freshly grated nutmeg, and process on medium speed until smooth. Add more skim milk if a thinner sauce is desired.

Cauliflower White Sauce I can be poured over leftover grains and vegetable combinations for a tasty and attractive casserole. Sprinkle with whole grain bread crumbs and bake until heated through.

Cauliflower White Sauce II

Makes 1½ cups (375 ml)
½ cup (125 ml) *Garlic Broth*
2 cups (500 ml) cauliflower
    florets
¼ cup (60 ml) yogurt

This sauce is especially appropriate for healthier circulation, with its low fat, garlic and yogurt.

Place *Garlic Broth* and cauliflower in a medium saucepan and cook over low heat until cauliflower is very tender and liquid is absorbed. Add a little water, if necessary, to prevent scorching. Place cauliflower in blender and process on medium speed with yogurt until mixture is smooth.

Cauliflower White Sauce II can be served over stuffed fish or fish fillets. To serve fish "au gratin," cover with sauce, sprinkle with a little grated Parmesan cheese or some whole grain bread crumbs and run the dish under the broiler just until topping begins to brown.

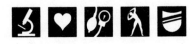

Makes five cups (1.25 l)
4 cups (1 l) tomato juice
2 tablespoons (30 ml) lemon
  juice
2 stalks celery with leaves,
  chopped
1 teaspoon (5 ml) minced fresh
  parsley
1 tablespoon (15 ml) finely
  chopped onions
2 tablespoons (30 ml) diced
  green peppers
¼ teaspoon (1 ml) celery seeds

V-7 Juice

You don't need an expensive or high-powered juice machine for this "vitamin cocktail" which will rival a Bloody Mary at lunch or at "happy hour."

Combine one cup (250 ml) of tomato juice and remaining ingredients in blender. Blend at high speed until smooth. Add remaining juice, continuing to blend until thoroughly mixed. Chill well before serving.

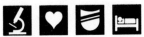

Makes eight servings
3 cups (750 ml) mashed sweet
  potatoes
1 cup (250 ml) applesauce
¼ cup (60 ml) bran
½ cup (125 ml) yogurt
¼ cup (60 ml) honey
2 eggs, beaten
2 teaspoons (10 ml) cinnamon
¼ teaspoon (1 ml) ginger
¼ teaspoon (1 ml) coriander
  dash nutmeg, allspice and
  cloves
9-inch (23-cm) unbaked
  No-Roll Pie Crust

DESSERT

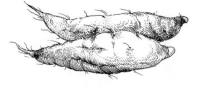

Sweet Potato Pie

Combine ingredients in a large bowl and pour into pie crust. Bake 25 minutes, until browned, in a preheated 350° F. (175° C.) oven. Can be served warm or chilled.

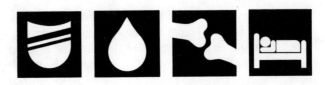

Chapter 7

Getting Stronger Every Day

INCREASING YOUR RESISTANCE

"Resistance" is probably what your parents called it. The "immune function" is more likely to come from the lips of a scientist. But whatever word you use for it, what we are talking about is the reason why the same germs that make one person ill can kill another and do absolutely nothing to a third person.

It's not *one* reason, of course. We know now that the human body has all sorts of weapons at its disposal to fight off invading germs. Some of them go by exotic-sounding names like macrophages and leukocytes, cells to which the body's intelligence agency has given a license to kill. Others go by such mundane-sounding names as sneezes (which kick germs out the front door) and the runs (which kick them out the back door before they can do more damage than they've done already). There are many factors affecting how well these various weapons function, including previous exposure to similar germs, heredity, stress, emotions and nutrition.

All these factors and more are involved in the ever-changing profile of disease resistance. Yet, nutrition stands out as a very special factor indeed, for one simple reason: it is the one factor that lies almost totally under the control of the individual.

Think about that. Sure, heredity is important, but there's not a great deal that we can do to change it. Sure, avoiding piles of germs helps too, but how do you prevent that cute two-year-old from depositing a million germs on the tip of your nose when he suddenly sneezes in your face? Yet even on a strictly limited budget, it's possible to enjoy a wide variety of foods containing high amounts of those elements known to boost the responsiveness of the immune system. While better nutrition may not do everything you hope it will, at least it is a positive step in the right direction, a practical approach that can only do good and cannot harm.

Don't let yourself be discouraged or misled by the ever-present example of the person with terrible health habits who never seems to become ill. He may be blessed with a fantastic array of antibodies, leukocytes, macrophages and all the other forces of immunity. For the time being, at least, they're keeping him out of trouble. Your soldiers of resistance, however, thanks to one or more of those factors we mentioned above, might only be able to function well with a steady supply of good food, fresh air and plenty of rest. In practical terms then, immunity is just like anything else: you have to make the best of what you are given to work with. And that, in a nutshell, is what this section is all about. Let's see how it's done.

STRONG RESISTANCE REQUIRES VITAMIN A

How would you like to have a chemical in your body which—when bacteria or viruses get close enough to even *think* about slipping inside for some fun—comes pouring out like boiling oil from the parapet of a besieged fortress, and literally skins the germs alive? You say it sounds gross . . . but you'll take it all the same? Okay, you've got it. It's called lysozyme, an enzyme contained in tears, saliva, sweat, mucus and other outposts of body defense. It's not 100 percent perfect, but it works against at least *some* bacteria and viruses, dissolving their "skins." And here's where good nutrition comes in: "Lysozyme secretion," writes Samuel Dreizen, D.D.S., M.D., "is markedly diminished or completely abolished in persons with a vitamin A deficiency" (*International Journal of Vitamin and Nutrition Research,* vol. 49, no. 2, 1979).

Vitamin A is of special importance to our whole system of first-line defenses. When vitamin A is in short supply—which it frequently is, according to nutrition surveys —the delicate epithelial linings, or mucous membranes that protect the lungs, urinary tract, eyes, glands and even the hair follicles, become dry, rough and weak. Special cells which, under conditions of good nutrition, would produce those lysozymes, as well as mucus and other factors that fight incoming germs, are replaced by cells that sit down and twiddle their thumbs.

It's not surprising, then, that infections associated with vitamin A deficiency chiefly involve the eyes, skin, lungs and other areas normally protected by moist membranes. A specific example has been provided by Leopoldo F. Montes, M.D., professor of dermatology at the University of Alabama Medical Center. According to Dr. Montes, a fungus infection that goes by the name of thrush when it affects the mouth but is also liable to infect the skin, respiratory tract or vagina, seems more likely to attack people who are deficient in vitamin A. Dr. Montes tested the blood levels of vitamin A in 12 people with the infection and found 7 had lower than normal amounts. In the other 5 people, vitamin A levels were in the lower half of the normal range (*Skin and Allergy News,* September, 1973).

Some of the germs and foreign objects swarming around our skins, mouths, lungs and other portals manage to get by our front-line defenses. Industrial chemicals can easily enter our bodies hidden in the food we eat or the water we drink. One of the most widely occurring chemicals is the industrial pollutant polychlorinated biphenyl or PCB, believed to cause cancer. Researchers from the National Institute of Nutrition, in Tokyo, Japan, found that test animals fed a diet deficient in vitamin A—and laced with PCB— fared worse than animals given a normal diet with PCB. But more interesting was the discovery that those animals given *extra* vitamin A fared best of all. "It is apparent that animals fed a PCB diet require more vitamin A than usual. This indicates that vitamin A may play a role in detoxification of PCB. It is well known that toxic chemicals such as . . . sodium benzoate, nitrite, aflatoxin, DDT, and dieldrin influence vitamin A metabolism in animals. These results strongly suggest that vitamin A is implicated in detoxification mechanisms of toxic chemicals" (*Journal of Nutritional Science and Vitaminology,* October, 1974). The correctness of that assertion was comfirmed subsequently in Europe, where researchers discovered that one of the toxic chemicals that vitamin A protects against is cigarette smoke, a finding we discuss in greater detail in the chapter The Anti-Cancer Diet.

Bacteria and viruses, as well as chemicals, can break through the outermost defense barriers—as we all know too well. But vitamin A helps here too, remarkably increasing our resistance to a wide variety of infectious germs. Benjamin E. Cohen, M.D., and Ronald J. Elin, M.D., Ph.D., from the Massachusetts General Hospital, and the National Institute of Health Clinical Center in Bethesda, Maryland, respectively, challenged two groups of laboratory animals with three different types of infectious organisms. One group also received four consecutive daily injections of 3,000 international units of vitamin A. The vitamin A-treated mice which were infected with what was apparently the most vicious organism were *completely protected.* After 24 hours, *all* the untreated animals were dead from the infection. But the blood of the animals treated with vitamin A was virtually free of infection. Vitamin A-treated animals infected with the other organisms fared decidedly better than untreated animals, too (*Journal of Infectious Diseases,* May, 1974).

Remember, we said that vitamin A increases *resistance* to germs—it doesn't kill them directly. In fact, we don't know of any nutrient that acts directly against germs. They all seem to do their work by feeding, strengthening and somehow encouraging all the natural immune mechanisms in our body to do the dirty work for them.

One scientist who is especially knowledgeable—and enthusiastic—about vitamin A's ability to strengthen resistance is Eli Seifter, Ph.D., associate professor of biochemistry and surgery at Albert Einstein College of Medicine. Back in September of 1975, Dr. Seifter reported in *Infectious Diseases* that vitamin A increases the body's immune response to pox viruses, a group that includes smallpox. In experiments with mice, animals given extra vitamin A in amounts of 5 to 10 times the Recommended Dietary Allowance were less affected by injections of viruses. And in those animals that did get reactions, few "pox" developed. Vitamin A also extended the disease's incubation period, shortened the duration of illness and reduced fever.

Dr. Seifter is particularly fascinated by the *why* and *how* of vitamin A's protection. After a number of experiments, Dr. Seifter told us that many clues point to the importance of vitamin A's effect on two critical glands—the adrenal and the thymus. When the body is subjected to any severe stress—particularly the stress of a serious infection, Dr. Seifter explained—there is a tendency for the adrenal glands to become enlarged and swollen with fat. If the stress is prolonged and severe enough, bleeding and even tissue death of the adrenals can result. That's bad enough, but the adrenal crisis somehow apparently causes the thymus gland to begin shrinking—a process called thymic involution. The thymus, located high in the chest, is a lymphatic organ that plays an essential role in the development of the immune system. It helps govern the production of special surveillance cells which can recognize invading tumor cells and other infectious agents and trigger their destruction before they gain a foothold. When the thymus shrinks, the ranks of those very skillful cells begin to diminish rapidly and the body's resistance weakens.

But when extra vitamin A is on the scene, that whole chain of events never closes one link. The adrenals don't swell, the thymus doesn't shrink, resistance doesn't go down. "For years," Dr. Seifter mentioned to us, "we've been talking about vitamin A's defensive mechanism. But we weren't sure of the mechanism. Now we're a lot closer to it."

In November of 1979, the medical world moved closer yet to that understanding, when an international group of surgeons and scientists published "Reversal of Postoperative Immunosuppression in Man by Vitamin A" in *Surgery, Gynecology and Obstetrics.* The term "postoperative immunosuppression" refers to that well-known state of vulnerability that people experience immediately following surgery—any kind of surgery. As Dr. Benjamin Cohen and colleagues explain it, "It is not clear whether the anesthesia or the operation, or both, are responsible for the observed immunodepression," but the effect is quite clear, "immediate in onset, and lasts for several weeks." Now, when you're in a germ-haunted hospital recovering from surgery, a weakened resistance to infection is about the last thing you want. But another, more sinister dimension may be involved here. There is a "clinical impression" among surgeons that following surgery in which an inoperable tumor is found, it frequently happens that the cancer seems to advance with a vengeance while the patient deteriorates rapidly. Now, you might think such a downhill course could be psychological in cause, because of the patient finding out that his case is inoperable. However, when animals with tumors are operated on, the same thing happens. It's very likely, then, that the trouble is a direct result of surgery crippling the immune system for several weeks.

We now know, thanks to Dr. Cohen's group, that there is a way to prevent the immune system from falling asleep while you're lying in a hospital bed. Extra vitamin A will do the trick. It takes a hefty dose—but it works, "blocking the depression of the immune function associated with an operation and acting as an immunostimulant in man." What isn't yet known is whether giving people extra vitamin A before surgery is actually going to help prevent hospital infections or the spread of cancer, but such knowledge should be forthcoming before too long.

Now, in many of these studies we've been discussing, the doses of vitamin A used were larger than one would normally receive, even with a good diet. Luckily, it's really rather easy to increase your vitamin A intake to higher levels, particularly over a relatively short period of time, like a few weeks. If, for example, you managed to eat six ounces of beef liver, one sweet potato, and two carrots in one day, you'd be getting at least 120,000 international units of vitamin A. That's about 24 times the Recommended Dietary Allowance, yet quite safe for an adult. When you get tired of eating liver, you can have at least one large salad a day made from green leafy vegetables, carrots, and maybe some broccoli buds. When you get tired of the sweet potatoes, try a winter squash like butternut, which is really quite delicious when served hot with a sprinkling of cinnamon and nutmeg. For dessert, turn to dried apricots or pumpkin pie.

VITAMIN C, ANOTHER POWERFUL RESISTANCE BOOSTER

The same month late in 1979 that saw publication of Dr. Cohen's fascinating study on vitamin A also brought us an important insight into how vitamin C protects us against disease. Writing in the *Journal of Immunology* (November, 1979), John P. Manzella, M.D., and Norbert J. Roberts, Jr., M.D., suggested that vitamin C might help us recover faster from viruses such as the flu by somehow instilling renewed vigor into leukocytes, or white blood cells, an important part of the body's immune defenses. The influenza virus itself, interestingly, actually depresses the activity of leukocytes, making it easier for itself to multiply. Vitamin C simply prevents that from happening. Significantly, the researchers also found that higher temperatures, such as those found in a fever, have much the same protective effect.

What this experiment seems to be telling us is rather than taking aspirin when the flu hits, we might be better off taking vitamin C and allowing fever to help combat the germs (unless, of course, the fever gets out of hand). The researchers aren't ready to make that interpretation themselves, being properly cautious. But, whether or not you think it's appropriate to hold off on the aspirin when an infection is raking you over the coals, there are plenty of good reasons you should at least be saturating your system with dietary vitamin C.

An experiment conducted at the University of Witwatersrand, South Africa, suggests that, for one thing, vitamin C can increase the amount of antibodies available to fight disease. Researchers gave a group of healthy students vitamin C supplements— 1,000 milligrams daily for 77 days. They compared levels of immunoglobulins (that part of the blood that contains antibodies) in these students to those in a control group who had not received extra vitamin C. "Our results showed that ascorbic acid [vitamin C] supplementation caused a statistically significant increase" in the antibody-bearing part of the blood, they reported (*International Journal of Vitamin Nutrition Research,* vol.

47, no. 3, 1977). The amount, 1,000 milligrams (one gram) may sound a little steep. By no means, however, is that amount out of reach if you set your mind to it. You could hit it, for example if, during the course of one day, you ate three large navel oranges and two large sweet red peppers.

Recently, researchers have been putting a lot of energy into investigating another natural chemical that the body uses to fight its enemies. Called interferon, it not only destroys viruses, but there are indications it may also promote the destruction of cancer cells. And, according to experiments conducted by Benjamin V. Siegel, Ph.D., professor of pathology at the University of Oregon Health Sciences Center, vitamin C may actually stimulate the body to produce *more* interferon. After giving large doses of vitamin C to a group of mice for several months, Dr. Siegel infected them with a virus that causes leukemia. He also infected a control group that had not received vitamin C. Blood tests showed the mice that had received the vitamin megadose produced twice as much interferon as those that had not. And their leukemia was considerably less severe.

According to other experiments, vitamin C also strengthens the white blood cells that seek out and destroy germs. In one, T-lymphocytes, which have an important role in fighting viruses and fungi, were significantly more energetic in lab animals that had been given extra vitamin C. In another, vitamin C whetted the appetites of white blood cells called phagocytes (from the Greek *phagein:* to eat), which swallow bacteria and other enemy organisms.

A pharmaceutical company not long ago developed a strain of bacteria that can produce enough interferon to be used as a drug. But while it has been used in many experimental trials so far, the results have been confusing, and somewhat disappointing. Apparently, artificially produced interferon may not have the spunk of the real thing. But it's good to know we can increase our own supply of *real* interferon with *real* food. Not that drug companies or even the medical profession are that anxious to get the word out to the public. (*"Don't want to give any false hopes,"* we can hear them saying.)

We could go on for pages detailing the evidence that vitamin C helps the body defend itself against all sorts of enemies, including hepatitis, a large variety of industrial pollutants and more. But by now, we all get the idea. Before leaving vitamin C, let's emphasize one point, though. The person who stands to derive the greatest benefits from a higher intake of vitamin C is not the person who is already in excellent health and wants to become absolutely invulnerable, but the person whose resistance is below par. The person, in other words, who gets five or six colds a year and would be happy to have only one or two, rather than the person who never wants to sneeze again as long as he or she lives. Which means that when we're talking about healing a weak or run-down resistance, vitamin C is just what the doctor ordered.

ZINC, ANOTHER NUTRITIONAL ESSENTIAL FOR STRONG RESISTANCE

If you haven't been following the field of nutrition in the last 10 years or so, you're probably surprised to see that word "zinc" pop up in a book like this. Is it really that important? Or is it one of those strange trace minerals like vanadium that are supposedly essential to health but the kind of thing most of us needn't worry about?

Well, let's put it this way. If your resistance is everything you want it to be, if your skin is in good shape and any injuries you get heal right on schedule, zinc deficiency is probably not one of the major problems in your life. But if you're reading this section with more than academic interest in the importance of nutrition to the body's immune system, zinc is a mineral you need to know about.

Remember the disease-fighting T-lymphocytes we mentioned before? Besides needing vitamin C, scientists have discovered, they also need zinc to keep them at work. When people with low zinc levels and poor immunity were given supplements of the mineral, their T-lymphocytes grew strong, divided, and cleared up some persistent infections they'd been suffering from (*Federation of American Societies for Experimental Biology Abstracts,* April, 1979). A spokesperson for a Sloan-Kettering Cancer Center group that has been studying the importance of zinc to immunity told us that "zinc seems to be necessary for the T-cells to perform their immunological functions correctly." Doctors should be particularly on the alert for zinc deficiency because "it can make sick people sicker." Those who are especially at risk include "patients with liver problems, poor appetites, absorption problems or poor dietary habits, for example," said the Sloan-Kettering spokesperson. (That last category, by the way—poor dietary habits—could include just about anyone in the hospital. A government survey found the average daily intake of zinc on a hospital diet is less than two-thirds the Recommended Dietary Allowance [*Journal of the American Medical Association,* May 4, 1979].)

Other research performed at Sloan-Kettering suggests that zinc also strengthens those lymphocytes that produce antibodies. B-lymphocytes from normal blood were cultured and exposed to sheep red blood cells (which normally stimulates them to secrete antibodies). Zinc, it was found, increased their response to stimulation—it turned up the immune reaction. And the more zinc added to the cell culture (within a certain range), the better the response. "This is a test-tube study, a special study," the Sloan-Kettering spokesperson said. "But it does suggest that zinc may be able to stimulate B cells to make antibodies."

Zinc support of lymphocyte activity in antibody production may explain, at least in part, the long-observed connection between low zinc levels and susceptibility to infections. One study found, for example, that men with prostate infections had on the average only one-tenth as much zinc in their prostatic fluid as healthy men. Similarly, a British physician reported low zinc levels in 15 of his patients who were afflicted with boils, recurrent infections that had plagued them for three years or more. When 8 of these patients were given zinc supplements, their boils disappeared and did not come back.

It's relatively easy, as we saw, to increase your intake of vitamin A and C quite dramatically. With zinc, it isn't. On the other hand, it probably is not necessary or even advisable to consume 10 or more times the Recommended Dietary Allowance of zinc, as it is with vitamin C and vitamin A, when you're fighting off an infection. For zinc, the Recommended Dietary Allowance happens to be 15. Now, if you are low on zinc, a doctor might tell you to take about 50 milligrams a day for a month or so and then go down to a maintenance dose of somewhere between 10 and 30 milligrams a day. Relying on natural food rather than supplements, you can't do that. But you could take a moderate amount of zinc in tablets and then get as much zinc from your diet as possible. To do that, concentrate on liver, lamb, dark meat of turkey, and wheat germ. Beef is also a very good source of zinc but we don't like it because of the excessive fat content. Oysters from the Atlantic Ocean are far and away the best source of zinc, with three ounces supplying about 74 milligrams of zinc. To understand just how high that is, consider that the same amount of beef or liver, both excellent sources, supplies only about 5 milligrams! The problem is, it's difficult to recommend oysters as a regular source of zinc because they tend to accumulate relatively large amounts of potentially harmful minerals such as cadmium, from industrial pollution. There is also a risk of disease if the oysters come from dirty water. The high price is something else again. So for practical purposes over the long haul, the foods we mentioned before are your best bet. If you can manage to eat about six ounces of liver or lamb for dinner, and six tablespoons of wheat germ for breakfast, you've got about 16 milligrams of zinc right there, which is a substantial amount.

OTHER NUTRITIONAL FACTORS THAT HELP KEEP US WELL

Although vitamin A, vitamin C and zinc seem to deserve the most attention in the nutritional approach to increasing our resistance, many other vitamins and minerals are necessary to keep our complex immune systems working at full strength. A review of nutrition and the immune response by Dr. Samuel Dreizen, mentioned earlier, identifies the following nutrients as playing recognized roles in the immune response: vitamin A, niacin, riboflavin, folic acid, vitamin B_{12}, pyridoxine or vitamin B_6, vitamin C, iron, zinc, pantothenic acid, thiamine, biotin, protein and even calories. Although in our society the last two factors are usually not critical, they are of great importance in societies where food is scarce, and among the elderly, debilitated, or long-term hospitalized in any society, including ours. Likewise, a person on a crash diet in any culture may suffer the effects of a shortage of protein, calories, and any or all of the other nutrients we mentioned. So, depending on your individual dietary habits, life-style, health history, or biochemical individuality (such as an absorption difficulty), your resistance could conceivably be hurting for just about any nutrient, because there are precious few that don't come into play at some point.

Vitamin E, for instance, is not usually thought of as being particularly important in building resistance, but some scientists would regard that as a serious oversight. Denham Harman, M.D., Ph.D., believes that vitamin E might help us resist the decrease in our ability to produce lymphocytes and antibodies that usually accompanies aging. The decline in immunity, he theorizes, might be largely due to free radical reactions that impair the cells and chemicals involved in immunity. By inhibiting these free radical reactions, he suggests, vitamin E could preserve the strength in the immune system. When Dr. Harman gave vitamin E to a group of mice, he found that the loss of immune response that normally accompanies aging proceeded more slowly. Their ability to manufacture antibodies and their loss of lymphocyte activity did not decline as steeply as that of untreated animals (*Journal of the American Geriatrics Society,* September, 1977). More recently, experiments using sheep revealed that extra vitamin E could literally be a lifesaver in the face of acute infection. Your best sources of vitamin E from food are wheat germ, sunflower seeds, almonds and peanuts.

Protein, which the body uses as a basic building material for everything from hipbones to antibodies, was in 1979 reported to be necessary for the functioning of what is probably the body's most misunderstood defense mechanism: *fever.*

On extreme occasions, when fever gets out of hand, it may cause bodily damage itself, but it is now generally agreed that fever evolved as a defense mechanism against microorganisms that cannot multiply well when things get hot. So, along with many of the other "annoying" symptoms of infection, such as chills, a runny nose and coughing, fever is actually on *our* side. But when there isn't enough protein available, your body lacks the spark it needs to get a decent fever going. In the words of investigators at the University of Michigan, "an attenuated febrile response during protein malnutrition might result in an impairment of the host's ability to combat infection" (*American Journal of Clinical Nutrition,* July, 1979). Weak fever, weak defense.

The lack of protein decreases production of a natural chemical called endogenous pyrogen, a protein itself, which seems to be the spark for the fever response. And besides weakening immunity, the diagnostic value of a fever is also lost. But there could be a further problem, which involves yet another nutrient.

The Michigan researchers suggest that besides being involved in fever, endogenous pyrogen is somehow involved in a very slick trick the body likes to pull on invading bacteria: as soon as it senses their presence in the body, it rounds up much of the iron circulating in the blood serum and hides it in the liver for the duration. A smart move because bacteria can't breed without access to iron! But when there's not enough protein around to make the endogenous pyrogen, which in turn hides the iron in the closet, the bacteria are free to multiply.

Are there any dietary factors which, when present in large amounts, have a *negative* effect on the immune system the way, for instance, cholesterol does on the circulation? Yes, there are. And, as a matter of fact, one of them happens to be cholesterol—as well as fats in general. In 1978, scientists at the Medical College of Virginia reported that animals fed a cholesterol-rich diet were noticeably more susceptible to a virus challenge (*Atherosclerosis,* November, 1978). Then, in 1979, a broader series of experiments carried out by another team at the same college found that a high-cholesterol diet in animals is "associated with an impairment in the host immune response and increased susceptibility to viral, bacterial, and tumor cell challenge" (*Infection and Immunity,* November, 1979). Besides the obvious implications, the researchers point out that the fact that cholesterol lowers resistance to viruses may be linked to theories that viruses are somehow involved in both heart disease and diabetes. Cholesterol in the blood and arteries, they suggest, could open the door to a group of malevolent microorganisms called group B coxsackieviruses.

Sugar, which in the average American diet provides something on the order of 25 percent of all calories (that's not including the natural sugar in fruit), is suspected of distracting the body in its vigil against infection. It may not be that sugar is directly injurious to the immune system, but that it indirectly weakens it by replacing natural foods, which would supply it with the vitamins, minerals and protein it needs. A fascinating study suggesting this was published in the *Journal of Nutrition* (April, 1972) by B. N. Nalder and colleagues. That research, conducted at Utah State University, showed that "as the nutritional quality of the diet is reduced by progressively diluting the diet with sucrose in 10 percent increments, the production of antibodies was decreased proportionately." The scientists were using mice in these experiments, but experience tells us it's highly likely that similar if not identical effects would occur in human beings. In another experiment, the researchers found that "as the level of iron in a diet is progressively decreased in 10 percent increments, the production of antibodies also is decreased proportionately." To the extent, in other words, that we cut back on such iron-rich foods as liver, fish, beans, potatoes, whole grains and green leafies, we bid adieu to whole regiments of antibodies. And to the extent we replace those iron-rich foods with the likes of cake and ice cream, the damage may be compounded. Add cholesterol and other fats in excessive amounts to your diet and your immune system is hampered even more.

Looking at it the positive way—which is the purpose of this book—we see that shrinking those dietary negatives and emphasizing the positives like C-rich fruits, A-rich vegetables, and the protein-zinc sources like liver and turkey, is going to tell your immune system that you appreciate the beautiful job it's doing to keep you healthy. It's saying you're glad to return the favor by giving it the good food it needs to do that job. Psychology is a major part of the resistance story, and we feel that when you consciously change your diet to encourage stronger resistance, that very decision sends psychosomatic ripples of high morale to every outpost in the body's immune system. Good food, good karma.

SOUPS

Sweet Potato Bisque

Makes four servings
3 medium sweet potatoes
¼ cup (60 ml) *Yogurt Cream Cheese*
1½ cups (375 ml) *Chicken Stock*

Cube sweet potatoes, which have been washed but not peeled, and boil in water to cover until tender. Drain and mash the potatoes, combining with *Yogurt Cream Cheese* and stirring in stock. This can also be made by placing the cooked potatoes and remaining ingredients in a blender and processing on medium speed until smooth. Makes about 3½ cups (875 ml).

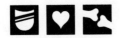

Chili-Pumpkin Soup

Makes eight servings
2 tablespoons (30 ml) corn oil
2 tablespoons (30 ml) whole wheat flour
1 tablespoon (15 ml) brewer's yeast
3 cups (750 ml) skim milk
2 cups (500 ml) cooked pumpkin, mashed
1 cup (250 ml) cooked soybeans or chick-peas
2 teaspoons (10 ml) chili powder
½ teaspoon (2 ml) cumin powder
1 teaspoon (5 ml) blackstrap molasses
1 teaspoon (5 ml) tamari
1 tablespoon (15 ml) tomato paste
dash cayenne pepper

In a heavy saucepan over medium heat, warm oil and stir in flour and brewer's yeast. Lower heat slightly and stir ingredients for two to three minutes. Add the milk slowly, stirring until smooth. Stir in remaining ingredients, and simmer on low heat for 15 minutes. Serve hot. Makes about six cups (1.5 l).

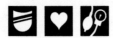

Cream of Carrot Soup

Makes four servings
4–5 carrots (about ½ pound
      [225 g]), shredded
  1 large onion, chopped
  1 tablespoon (15 ml) corn oil
  2 tablespoons (30 ml) whole
      wheat flour
  ¼ teaspoon (1 ml) paprika
  2 cups (500 ml) skim milk
  2 teaspoons (10 ml) tomato
      paste
    dash cayenne pepper

Try it hot or chilled, garnished with a dollop of yogurt or sprigs of parsley.

Place carrots and onion in a skillet with the oil. Saute just until soft. Sprinkle with flour and paprika and stir to combine over medium heat for one or two minutes. Add milk and simmer for five minutes, stirring. Remove from heat and place carrot mixture in a blender with tomato paste and cayenne. Blend on low speed until smooth. Makes 3½ cups (875 ml) of soup.

Chilled Peach Soup

Makes two servings
3 large, very ripe peaches,
    chilled

Here's a perfect use for peaches that are slightly past their prime, but still sweet and delicious.

Wash peaches. Cut off any brown spots, pit, and process in a blender on low speed until smooth. Leave the skins on, as these will give color and texture to the creamy soup. The peaches should be served immediately after blending or the soup will lose its attractive color.

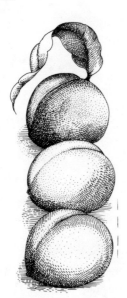

SALADS

Spinach-Mushroom Salad

A classic, this salad features a touch of sesame.

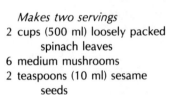

Makes two servings
2 cups (500 ml) loosely packed
    spinach leaves
6 medium mushrooms
2 teaspoons (10 ml) sesame
    seeds
Creamy Garlic Dressing

Thoroughly wash the spinach leaves. Brush off the mushrooms with a wet paper towel, trim stem ends, and slice. Place the sesame seeds in a small, heavy skillet and stir over medium heat until they begin to turn golden. In a serving bowl toss the seeds with the spinach and mushrooms, adding enough dressing to moisten.

Variation: Eliminate the sesame seeds, and arrange the sliced mushrooms over the spinach in individual salad bowls. Garnish with large red onion rings, and spoon on a little of the dressing.

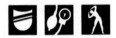

Orange and Grape Salad

Makes two servings
2 oranges
1 cup (250 ml) large grapes,
    halved
½ teaspoon (2 ml) finely grated
    lemon rind
1 teaspoon (5 ml) honey
2 teaspoons (10 ml) lemon
    juice

Section oranges and remove membranes. Place grapes with orange sections and lemon rind in a medium serving bowl. Mix honey and lemon juice together and toss with fruit. Serve chilled.

Variation: Substitute tangerines or a pink grapefruit for oranges. Garnish with mint.

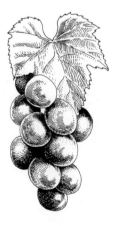

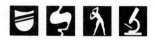

Four Star Cabbage 'n' Fruit Salad

Makes four servings
2 cups (500 ml) finely shredded
    cabbage
1 tablespoon (15 ml) sunflower
    oil
1 orange or tangerine
1 pink grapefruit
1 cup (250 ml) red grapes,
    halved
1 unpeeled apple, chopped
1 tablespoon (15 ml) *Tarragon
    Vinegar*

This salad is bursting with good flavor and is packed with vitamin C.

Place the cabbage in a salad bowl, and toss with the oil until well coated. Section and remove the membranes from the orange and grapefruit and add to the cabbage. Add grapes and apple to the cabbage.

Sprinkle with *Tarragon Vinegar* and toss to combine. Serve chilled. In summer, garnish with chopped fresh mint.

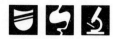

Zingy Spring Salad

Makes two servings
2 cups (500 ml) shredded
    cabbage
½ cup (125 ml) chopped
    dandelion greens
1 clove garlic, minced
    Vinaigrette Dressing

Success here depends upon picking the earliest of spring dandelion greens, before the plants are in flower.

Toss the cabbage, dandelion greens and garlic in enough dressing to moisten. Serve chilled.

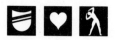

Ruby Tofu Dressing

*Makes about 1¼ cups
    (300 ml)*
2 tablespoons (30 ml) lemon
    juice
1 tablespoon (15 ml) sunflower
    oil
2 teaspoons (10 ml) tamari
2 cloves garlic
½ pound (225 g) tofu, chopped
1 sweet red pepper, chopped

Place lemon juice, oil, tamari and garlic in a blender and process until smooth. Add half of the tofu and blend on low speed until smooth. Add remaining tofu and pepper. Process on low speed until smooth, stopping the blender to scrape down the sides of the container, as necessary.

Serve dressing on tossed green salads, or tuna or chicken salad.

Creamy Vegetable Salad Dressing

A hearty dressing—one of our favorites. Try it!

Makes two cups (500 ml)
1 cup (250 ml) sliced carrots
½ cup (125 ml) chopped red
    onions
¼ cup (60 ml) sesame seeds
½ cup (125 ml) water
2 tablespoons (30 ml) soy oil
2 tablespoons (30 ml) lemon
    juice
1 tablespoon (15 ml) tamari
½ cup (125 ml) chopped sweet
    red peppers (optional)

Combine the ingredients in a blender and process on low speed until dressing is smooth. This will take two to three minutes.

Try the dressing with the red pepper and without to see which flavor you prefer.

Variation: Add ½ cup (125 ml) cubed daikon (white) radishes. Substitute ½ cup (125 ml) chopped scallions for red onions.

BREAD

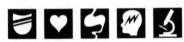

Carrot Bread

Makes one loaf
1½ cups (375 ml) whole wheat
    pastry flour
1½ cups (375 ml) wheat germ
1 tablespoon (15 ml)
    cinnamon
½ cup (125 ml) walnuts,
    chopped
½ teaspoon (2 ml) grated
    orange rind
1 tablespoon (15 ml) *Baking
    Powder*
2 eggs, beaten
¼ cup (60 ml) corn oil
¼ cup (60 ml) honey
½ cup (125 ml) orange juice
1½ cups (375 ml) shredded
    carrots

Combine dry ingredients in a large mixing bowl. In another bowl, beat the eggs with the remaining ingredients. Stir the egg mixture into the dry ingredients and place batter in a lightly oiled 8½ × 4½-inch (22 × 11-cm) bread pan. Bake bread in a 350° F. (175° C.) preheated oven for 50 to 60 minutes, or until a cake tester or toothpick inserted into the bread comes out clean.

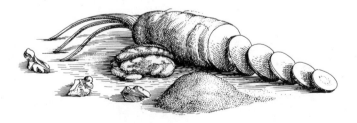

MAIN DISHES

Liver Dressed for Dinner

Liver takes on a new personality with a combination of spices and ingredients guaranteed to please and surprise.

Makes two servings

¾ pound (340 g) calf liver
1 tablespoon (15 ml) soy or
   corn oil
½ sweet red pepper, chopped
4–5 scallions, chopped
3 tablespoons (45 ml) raisins
1 teaspoon (5 ml) chili
   powder
1 teaspoon (5 ml) cinnamon
¼ cup (60 ml) water
1 teaspoon (5 ml) tamari

Rinse the liver, trim away any membranes, and cut into thin pieces. In a skillet, place the oil and add the pepper and scallions. Stir for five minutes, or until the vegetables begin to become tender. Add the raisins and spices, stir, then add the liver, the water and tamari. Put on a lid, and steam for just a few minutes, until the liver is lightly cooked. It should be slightly pink inside; do not overcook. Serve immediately.

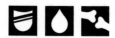

Kale Quiche

Makes six servings

Crust:

1 cup (250 ml) whole wheat
   flour
¼ cup (60 ml) safflower oil
2 tablespoons (30 ml)
   buttermilk

Filling:

4 cups (1 l) packed kale
1 cup (250 ml) cottage cheese
2 tablespoons (30 ml)
   buttermilk
6 scallions
1 egg yolk
2 egg whites
   dash freshly grated nutmeg

Measure the ingredients for the crust directly into a 9-inch (23-cm) pie plate. Toss with a fork until combined, then press against bottom and sides of dish to form the pie shell.

Steam kale five minutes. Coarsely chop. Place in the pie crust.

In a blender, combine the cottage cheese, buttermilk, scallions and the egg yolk. Process on low speed until smooth. Beat the egg whites with an eggbeater or electric mixer set on medium speed. When the whites are stiff, fold into the cottage cheese mixture, along with some nutmeg.

Pour the cheese mixture over the kale in the unbaked pie shell. Place in a preheated 375° F. (190° C.) oven and bake for 35 to 40 minutes, until firm.

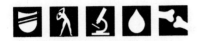

Makes four servings
1 pound spinach (450 g)
1 green or sweet red pepper,
    chopped
1 large onion, chopped
5 stalks celery, chopped
¼ cup (60 ml) raisins
½ teaspoon (2 ml) cinnamon
¼ teaspoon (1 ml) dill seed
    dash cayenne pepper
1 large tomato, chopped
1 cup (250 ml) cottage cheese
¾ cup (175 ml) shredded sharp
    cheese

Mexican Vegetable Casserole

Thoroughly wash spinach. Steam about five minutes, until limp. Set aside to cool.

Combine pepper, onion, and celery in a heavy skillet with the raisins, cinnamon, dill seed and cayenne. Steam-stir, adding a few spoonfuls of water as necessary, until vegetables are tender. Place tomato in a blender and process on medium speed until smooth. Pour over vegetables, stir, and simmer two to three minutes. Remove from heat.

In a medium, lightly oiled casserole, place half of the spinach. Top with half of the vegetable mixture. Spread with the cottage cheese. Spoon over the remaining vegetables, and top with a layer of spinach. Sprinkle with the shredded cheese.

To bake, place the casserole in a preheated 375° F. (190° C.) oven for 30 to 35 minutes. Serve hot.

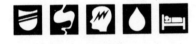

Makes two servings
2 carrots
1 large potato
1 sweet potato
1 yellow onion
1 whole chicken breast, skinned
    and split
½ cup (125 ml) water

Oven-Baked Chicken and Vegetables

Scrub, but do not peel carrots. Cut into large pieces. Wash potatoes and cut them, unpeeled, into thick slices. Peel onion and slice it thin.

In a casserole dish, place the carrots and potato slices, arranging chicken breasts on top. Cover with onion slices. Pour the water over ingredients; cover casserole.

Place in a preheated 350° F. (175° C.) oven for 1½ hours or until chicken and vegetables are tender.

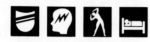

Fettucini with Spinach and Mushrooms

Makes four servings

¾ pound (340 g) whole wheat
   fettucini noodles
1 tablespoon (15 ml) olive oil
½ medium onion, chopped
1 clove garlic, minced
2 tablespoons (30 ml) minced
   fresh parsley
8 medium mushrooms, sliced
1 lemon slice
4 cups (1 l) loosely packed
   spinach, coarsely
   chopped
2–3 tablespoons (30–45 ml)
   grated Parmesan or
   Romano cheese
½ cup (125 ml) ricotta cheese
½ cup (125 ml) yogurt

In a large kettle, bring about three quarts (3 l) of water to a boil. Add noodles and cook until tender but still firm.

While the noodles are cooking, prepare the vegetables. Place a few tablespoons (50 ml) of water—just enough to keep the vegetables from sticking—along with the oil in a large skillet. Over medium heat, steam-stir the onion until transparent. Add the garlic, parsley and mushrooms. Sprinkle with juice squeezed from the lemon slice. Stir often, adding a little more water if necessary. After about three minutes, add the spinach, cover the skillet with a lid, and continue to steam until the spinach is wilted and limp but not soggy.

By this time the noodles should be done. Drain thoroughly, place in a large serving bowl, and immediately sprinkle evenly with cheese. Quickly stir in the ricotta and yogurt, and finally the vegetables. Serve hot.

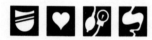

Sweet Potato-Bean Pie

Makes six servings

1 yellow onion, chopped
3 cups (750 ml) shredded
   sweet potatoes (about 2
   pounds [1 kg])
1 teaspoon corn oil
1 cup (250 ml) cooked navy
   beans
1 egg, beaten
¼ teaspoon (1 ml) freshly grated
   nutmeg
¼ teaspoon (1 ml) coriander
9-inch (23-cm) unbaked
   No-Roll Pie Crust

Saute onion and sweet potatoes in the oil in a large skillet until the onions are transparent and the sweet potatoes are limp. Add a few drops of water if necessary to prevent scorching. Place the beans in a blender with a third of the sweet potato mixture. Process on low speed until smooth.

Stir the blended bean mixture with the remaining sweet potatoes and the egg. Season with spices and pour into pie crust. Bake in a preheated 350° F. (175° C.) oven 40 minutes.

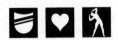

Stuffed Butternut Squash

Makes two servings
1 butternut squash
½ teaspoon (2 ml) corn oil
½ cup (125 ml) cooked lentils
½ cup (125 ml) corn
2 tablespoons (30 ml) sunflower
   seeds, toasted
½ teaspoon (2 ml) tamari
2 tablespoons (30 ml) shredded
   Swiss cheese
1 teaspoon (5 ml) wheat germ

Winter squash like the butternut are especially high in vitamin A. This recipe looks "different" but tastes terrific!

Cut the squash in half and scoop out seeds and stringy pulp from cavity. Rub each cut surface with ¼ teaspoon (1 ml) oil. In a medium bowl, combine the lentils, corn, sunflower seeds and tamari. Divide into two parts, and stuff squash cavities. Sprinkle cheese and wheat germ over stuffing.

Cover the squash with aluminum foil and place in a baking dish with ½ inch (1 cm) of water. To keep the squash level, you may have to place a folded piece of aluminum foil under the neck ends.

Bake in a preheated 350° F. (175° C.) oven for 1½ hours, adding water, if necessary, to the baking dish.

Serve hot.

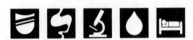

Peanut Butter Tacos

Makes two servings
4 taco shells
6 tablespoons (90 ml) peanut
   butter
½ cup (125 ml) shredded
   lettuce leaves
½ cup (125 ml) shredded
   zucchini
½ cup (125 ml) shredded
   carrots
½ cup (125 ml) alfalfa sprouts
1 tablespoon (15 ml) raisins
   yogurt

Heat taco shells in a moderate oven for four to five minutes. Spread inside of each with peanut butter and fill with lettuce and other vegetables. Add raisins, and top each with a dollop of yogurt.

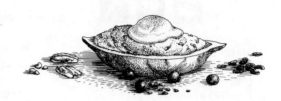

SIDE DISHES

 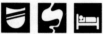

Cranberry-Stuffed Sweet Potatoes

Makes three servings
3 medium sweet potatoes
½ cup (125 ml) cranberries, finely chopped
¼ cup (60 ml) raisins, finely chopped
¼ cup (60 ml) walnuts, finely chopped
1 teaspoon (5 ml) medium unsulfured molasses
¼ teaspoon (1 ml) cinnamon
yogurt (garnish)
dash cinnamon (garnish)

Why wait for the holidays for this special treat?

Leave the sweet potatoes in their jackets and cut them in half lengthwise. Wrap potatoes in aluminum foil and place in a preheated 350° F. (175° C.) oven. Bake for one hour.

Remove potatoes from oven, unwrap and scoop centers from shells, leaving enough to retain shape, and mash the pulp in a medium bowl.

Mix cranberries, raisins, and walnuts with mashed sweet potatoes and add molasses and cinnamon. Place sweet potato mixture into scooped-out shells, place in a shallow baking pan, cover with foil and heat through in oven, about 10 to 15 minutes.

To serve, garnish each half with a dollop of yogurt and sprinkle with a dash of cinnamon. Serve hot.

Sweet Potato-Applesauce Souffle

Makes six to eight servings
3 cups (750 ml) mashed sweet potatoes (about 4–5 potatoes)
2 unpeeled tart apples
½ teaspoon (2 ml) finely grated lemon rind
dash freshly grated nutmeg
2 egg yolks
4 egg whites

Place sweet potatoes in a medium mixing bowl. Run the apples through a blender or food mill to make ½ to ¾ cup (125 to 175 ml) applesauce. Stir applesauce, lemon rind, nutmeg and egg yolks into sweet potatoes. Whip egg whites until stiff with an eggbeater and fold gently into the sweet potato mixture. Prepare a souffle dish by lightly oiling and dusting with a coating of wheat germ or whole wheat flour. Turn souffle mixture into dish and place in preheated 350° F. (175° C.) oven. Bake about 35 minutes. Serve immediately.

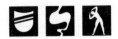

Baked Sweet Potato and Pear

Makes two servings
1 medium sweet potato
1 medium pear
½ cup (125 ml) apple cider
   dash freshly grated nutmeg

A great combination dish to perk up a winter table.

Slice the sweet potato, which has been scrubbed but not peeled, and place the slices around the perimeter of a shallow pie pan. Leave one slice in the center.

Wash, seed, but do not peel pear. Cut pear into thin lengthwise slices and arrange in circular fashion atop sweet potato.

Pour apple cider over pear and sweet potato and dust with nutmeg. Cover with foil.

Bake casserole in a preheated 350° F. (175° C.) oven for 45 minutes, or until tender. Serve hot.

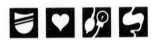

Boiled Sweet Potatoes

Makes two servings
2 medium sweet potatoes
   boiling water to cover

Wash and remove spots from sweet potatoes, but do not peel. Drop them into the boiling water and cook covered about 25 minutes, until tender. Potatoes can be peeled before serving or eaten as is.

To shorten the cooking time, cube potatoes before boiling. Reserve the water for soups.

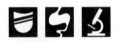

The Ugly Ducklings

Makes four servings
4 medium carrots
4 medium parsnips
2 small pears

The ingredients may look mundane and unpromising, but steamed together they make an astonishingly beautiful medley.

Wash carrots and parsnips thoroughly; trim ends. Cut in two-inch (5 cm) sections, slicing thicker sections in half. Core pears but do not peel. Cut pears in strips of similar size to carrots and parsnips.

In a colander over boiling water, steam vegetables and pears about 8 to 10 minutes, just until tender. Serve hot.

Oven-Baked Carrots

Makes six servings
1 teaspoon (5 ml) sesame oil
¼ cup (60 ml) minced
    shallots
½ clove garlic, crushed
1 tablespoon (15 ml) minced
    parsley
8–10 carrots, cut in strips (about
    1 pound [450 g])
2 tablespoons (30 ml) orange
    juice
¼ cup (60 ml) *Yogurt Cream
    Cheese*
1 teaspoon (5 ml) sesame
    tahini

Oven-baked carrots had been one of our favorite "company's-coming" recipes. Unfortunately, the recipe called for plenty of butter and heavy cream. Working with that recipe, we discovered a dish with much less fat and, surprise!—it tastes even better.

In a large skillet, heat the oil and saute the shallots until slightly tender. Add the garlic, parsley and carrots, and stir until combined. Cook over medium heat, stirring, for about 5 to 8 minutes. In a small bowl, combine orange juice, *Yogurt Cream Cheese* and tahini. Stir into carrots. Place the carrot mixture in a lightly oiled casserole dish and bake, covered, in a preheated 350° F. (175° C.) oven for about 30 to 35 minutes. The carrots should still be a little firm and keep their shape.

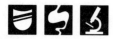

Spicy Ginger Carrots

Makes four servings
5 medium carrots
    fresh ginger root
½ cup (125 ml) apple cider
    dash freshly grated nutmeg

Carrots do so many good things for us we should try to return the favor as often as possible.

Scrub and lightly scrape carrots. Cut in two-inch (5 cm) strips about ¼ inch (6 mm) wide.

Cut a piece of fresh ginger root about the size of a quarter, and mince. In a medium ovenproof dish, toss the carrots with the fresh ginger and apple cider. Top with freshly grated nutmeg.

Cover and bake in a 375° F. (190° C.) oven one hour. When done, the carrots should be crisp-tender, not soft. Serve hot.

Variation: Carrots can also be boiled until just tender with ginger, then drained and sprinkled with nutmeg. Omit apple cider.

Makes six servings

8–10 carrots (about 1 pound
       [450 g])
  1 cup (250 ml) chopped
       scallions
  1 clove garlic, minced
  ½ teaspoon (2 ml) tamari
  ¼ teaspoon (1 ml) paprika
  2 tablespoons (30 ml)
       chopped fresh
       dillweed
  ¼ cup (60 ml) yogurt
     parsley sprigs (garnish)

Dilly Herbed Carrots

Wash, but do not peel carrots, and slice them into long, thin strips. In a skillet, steam-stir scallions and garlic in a small amount of water until nearly tender. Stir in the carrots, tamari, paprika and dill-weed and toss together over medium heat. When ingredients are combined, transfer carrot mixture to a lightly oiled casserole dish and pour yogurt over all. Cover, and bake in a preheated 350° F. (175° C.) oven 35 to 40 minutes. The carrots will retain some crispness. Transfer to a serving dish and garnish with parsley sprigs.

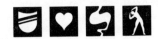

Makes six servings

  1 cup (250 ml) brown rice
2¼ cups (550 ml) water
  2 cups (500 ml) finely
       shredded cabbage
  1 cup (250 ml) thinly sliced
       carrots
  1 cup (250 ml) thinly sliced
       celery
  ½ cup (125 ml) chopped
       onions
  2 teaspoons (10 ml) corn oil
  2 medium pears (10 ml),
       chopped
  2 tablespoons (30 ml)
       chopped fresh parsley
  1 tablespoon (15 ml) chopped
       fresh dillweed
  ½ teaspoon (2 ml) cinnamon
  ¼ teaspoon (1 ml) dry mustard

Rice with Pears

A "nice change," said one enthusiast; "good and different."

Place rice in a medium saucepan with the water. Bring to a boil, reduce heat and simmer, covered, for about 30 to 40 minutes, until the water is absorbed. Meanwhile, in a large heavy-bottom saucepan, saute cabbage, carrots, celery and onions in the oil until crisp-tender, about 3 minutes. Add a few spoonfuls of water, if necessary, to prevent scorching. Stir in pears, parsley, dillweed, cinnamon and mustard. Add cooked rice to the pear mixture.

Cover pan and heat over very low flame about five minutes. Serve hot.

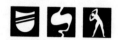

Squash Medley

Makes four servings
3 cups (750 ml) peeled, cubed
    butternut squash
1 cup (250 ml) diced carrots
1 cup (250 ml) cubed pears
½ cup (125 ml) apple cider
½ teaspoon (2 ml) cinnamon

Combine ingredients and place in an 8 × 8-inch (20 × 20-cm) casserole dish. Bake, uncovered, in a preheated 350° F. (175° C.) oven for one hour, or until ingredients are tender.

MISCELLANEOUS

Pimiento

2 sweet red peppers

Place whole, washed peppers over an open flame on a gas stove or under a hot broiler. As the skins begin to blacken, turn the pimientos to darken all sides.

When the peppers are charred, remove from the stove and wrap in a wet kitchen towel for 10 minutes. Cut the peppers in half and remove seeds.

Hold the pepper halves under a slow stream of water from the faucet to remove all traces of skins. Store in corn oil, covered, in the refrigerator. To use, wipe or rinse oil from the peppers.

Dried Apricot "Jam"

Makes ⅓ cup (80 ml)
¼ cup (60 ml) dried apricots,
    soaked
2 tablespoons (30 ml) orange
    juice
1 tablespoon (15 ml) walnuts

Soak apricots until soft. Place in a blender with the juice and nuts. Process on medium speed until smooth.

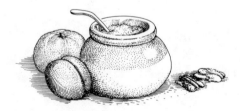

Strawberry-Nut Spread

Makes ⅔ cup (150 ml)
½ cup (125 ml) strawberries
2 tablespoons (30 ml) walnuts
1 tablespoon (15 ml) honey
1 teaspoon (5 ml) wheat germ

Tastes better than jam because the fruit is fresh.

Process the ingredients on medium speed in a blender until smooth. Chill.

Strawberry Topping

Makes ¾ cup (175 ml)
¾ cup (175 ml) strawberries
1 tablespoon (15 ml) orange
    juice

Crush ripe strawberries with a fork and add orange juice, mixing thoroughly. Ingredients can also be combined in a blender until liquified. Serve over desserts, whole grain pancakes or melon.

BEVERAGES

Icy Melon Delight

Makes two servings
½ cup (125 ml) chopped
    cantaloupe
½ cup (125 ml) chopped
    pineapple
2 tablespoons (30 ml) yogurt or
    buttermilk
3 ice cubes
¼ teaspoon (1 ml) *Vanilla
    Extract*
    dash freshly grated nutmeg
    mint sprigs (garnish)

An outstanding summer beverage: delicious, vitamin-packed and ready in minutes.

Place ingredients in a blender and process on high speed until smooth. Serve over ice in a tall, chilled glass. Garnish with mint.

Pineapple Punch

Makes one serving
¼ cup (60 ml) pineapple juice
¼ cup (60 ml) orange juice
¼ cup (60 ml) grapefruit juice
1 teaspoon (5 ml) lemon juice
¼ cup (60 ml) sparkling mineral
    water (optional)

Combine juices and serve over ice. Add sparkling mineral water if desired.

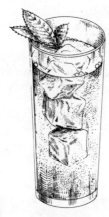

Lemon Tea

Makes one serving
½ lemon
1½ cups (375 ml) water
¼ teaspoon (1 ml) dried mint
    leaves
1 teaspoon (5 ml) honey

This is a Turkish variation on an old cold remedy.

Cut up the lemon coarsely and boil it in the water for about 10 minutes. Just before removing from heat, stir in the mint. Remove the pieces of lemon, pressing them to extract all juice. Stir in honey and drink hot.

DESERTS

Carrot Yogurt Cake

Imagine a carrot cake that's not only delicious, but highly nourishing and positively healing. But why just imagine it when you can eat it?

Place the carrots, yogurt, orange juice, molasses, raisins, sunflower seeds, oil, eggs and vanilla in a large mixing bowl. Beat these ingredients together until well combined.

In a medium bowl, thoroughly combine the flour, wheat germ, bran, baking soda, cinnamon and nutmeg. Fold the dry ingredients gradually into the carrot mixture until blended.

Place the batter in a lightly oiled 8 × 8-inch (20 × 20-cm) baking pan. Bake in a preheated 325° F. (165° C.) oven for about one hour.

Makes 16 servings
1 cup (250 ml) grated carrots
1 cup (250 ml) yogurt
½ cup (125 ml) orange juice
½ cup (125 ml) medium
    unsulfured molasses
½ cup (125 ml) raisins
½ cup (125 ml) sunflower
    seeds
¼ cup (60 ml) sunflower oil
2 eggs, beaten
½ teaspoon (2 ml) *Vanilla
    Extract*
2 cups (500 ml) whole wheat
    pastry flour
½ cup (125 ml) wheat germ
½ cup (125 ml) bran
1½ teaspoons (7 ml) baking
    soda
2 teaspoons (10 ml) cinnamon
¼ teaspoon (1 ml) nutmeg

Pumpkin Pie

In a large mixing bowl, combine the pumpkin, eggs and spices. Place the tofu and honey in a blender and process on low speed until smooth. Stir this into the pumpkin mixture until thoroughly combined.

Pour the pumpkin mixture into the pie crust and place in a preheated 425° F. (220° C.) oven to bake for 15 minutes. Turn heat down to 350° F. (175° C.) and continue to bake 45 minutes longer, until a knife inserted into the filling comes out clean.

Makes six servings
2 cups (500 ml) cooked
    pumpkin
2 eggs, beaten
1 teaspoon (5 ml) cinnamon
½ teaspoon (2 ml) ginger
¼ teaspoon (1 ml) cloves
¼ teaspoon (1 ml) nutmeg
⅛ teaspoon (0.5 ml) allspice
6 ounces (170 g) tofu
¼ cup (60 ml) honey
9-inch (23-cm) unbaked
    No-Roll Pie Crust

ENERGIZING YOUR BLOOD

Body energy is a very complicated business, affected by such different factors as physical fitness, emotions, time of day, infection, medication, even the weather. And we haven't even mentioned nutrition yet! But as complicated as it may be, the lack of energy often boils down to one thing: iron deficiency. Not *always,* but just often enough so that it should always be given consideration. In fact, recent discoveries suggest we ought to be thinking about iron even if we *aren't* feeling particularly pooped. Because despite what health authorities were teaching a generation ago (and what many are probably still teaching), putting more iron into your diet can increase your level of energy even if you have no symptoms whatsoever of iron deficiency. And even if a blood test shows your iron is "normal." But we're getting ahead of ourselves here. First, you may be wondering why it is that iron deficiency should even exist in areas such as Great Britain or North America, where iron-rich meat is so readily available.

Good question. But there are so many answers, you may be sorry you asked. First of all, a woman who is menstruating needs to replace very significant amounts of iron which she loses in her blood. That's hard enough, but if that woman does not perform a great deal of physical work and have the appetite to match it, it can be very difficult for her to get enough iron in her regular diet. Second, although meat is readily available, many people simply don't like the taste of it, while others can't afford it. Women on diets often avoid meat and subsist largely on the likes of cottage cheese, yogurt, lettuce and fresh fruit, none of which have a useful amount of iron. Children who drink large amounts of milk—a quart or more a day—can become anemic simply because the milk fills them up without delivering any iron.

But aren't some foods "enriched" with iron? Sure they are—technically. In reality, though, they're impoverished. Here's why: When wheat and other grains are refined and the processors add iron to the commercial product, the mineral they add has nowhere near the biological value of the iron that was originally in that grain. In one study, investigators found that 15 of 21 infants eating iron-fortified cereals were actually iron-deficient. Their research showed that the infants were absorbing less than one percent of the cereal's iron (*Pediatrics,* May, 1975). In another study, over 100 iron-deficient elderly people were given iron-fortified grain products to eat for six months or longer. The products did *not* boost their iron levels (*American Journal of Clinical Nutrition,* February, 1977). There *are* other kinds of iron, kinds the body *can* absorb, but these kinds may have undesirable effects on the product, such as turning white bread gray, or interfering with baking. So instead, a form of iron that the body can't absorb is used in many products, and the manufacturers (as well as many dietitians) tell the public there is nothing wrong with refined wheat products because they are "enriched with iron."

Processed foods may also be spiked with EDTA, one of the most commonly used preservatives—and a preservative that reduces iron absorption. Research shows the amount of EDTA found in a typical American diet cuts iron absorption in half (*American Journal of Clinical Nutrition,* June, 1976).

Phosphates—food additives used in soft drinks, ice cream, baked goods, candy, beer and a lot of other foods—also reduce the absorption of iron. So do eggs. So do cadmium and lead, pollutants that are found everywhere in the environment.

As if all that weren't enough, heavy tea drinkers may also become iron-deficient because the tannic acid in tea hinders absorption of the mineral. Some researchers have even suggested that the trend away from the old-fashioned iron skillet may also be contributing to widespread iron deficiency. When acidic foods such as tomato sauce are cooked in these pans, small but important amounts of iron are pulled out of the skillet and introduced into the diet.

But what's the difference? Why is iron all that important to energy anyway? Well, mostly, what iron actually imparts to the body is *oxygen.* That's because the oxygen we breathe can only be carried around our bodies and delivered to our cells by hemoglobin, a substance in red blood cells. But without iron, there wouldn't be any hemoglobin. In a state of iron deficiency, there's a hemoglobin deficiency, followed by an oxygen deficiency at the cell level. And the result of *that?* Well, oxygen is so basic to tissue health, that all sorts of things can go wrong. Fatigue, obviously. Weakness. Headaches. But more, too: heartburn, dizziness, loss of hair. Irritability. Itching. Pale skin. Loss of appetite.

DIAGNOSING ANEMIA: A TRICKY BUSINESS

The fact that there are so many possible symptoms of iron deficiency—and that many of them could easily be caused by other factors—has made some physicians very skeptical about diagnosing iron deficiency. Unless a blood test clearly shows values of iron below the normal range, the doctor, nurse, or nutritionist may say your fatigue or other symptoms must be a result of something else—probably just nerves. And there's no sense taking iron "just to see," they may tell you, because if you don't have out-and-out anemia, iron won't help. Today, although you may still hear those kinds of statements, they can no longer be justified.

For one thing, we know that the presence of iron deficiency is not necessarily a yes-or-no affair, like infection. You don't have to be falling over on your feet to benefit from more iron. "Milder degrees of anemia may affect work output in everyday tasks" is the way one study put it (*Agricultural and Food Chemistry,* March, 1978).

Not many people seem to be aware of a most important study carried out in Sweden. There, scientists studied the effect of iron supplementation on the work capacity of healthy, nonanemic men and women between the ages of 58 and 71. Half were given iron supplements twice daily for a period of three months, and half were given a placebo (a pill containing nothing of value). Their capacity for work was measured throughout the three months using an exercise bicycle, and the performance of the two groups was compared. While the average work performance improved in both groups as a result of regular exercise, the improvement was about *four times greater* in the group taking iron. That, in itself, is extremely important because all these people appeared to be perfectly healthy before taking iron. But there's more. Researcher Per Ericsson reported that "in spite of the fact that there was a significant increase in physical work capacity in the iron-supplemented group, no correlations were found between the increase in physical work capacity and the initial values or changes of other measures of the state of iron nutrition" (*Acta Medica Scandinavica,* November, 1970).

In other words, despite the astonishing improvement in endurance experienced by this group, blood tests failed to show that hemoglobin levels were going up. So what was happening?

A likely answer was offered some years later when American scientists discovered that besides its function of delivering oxygen to tissues, iron may also be working in an enzyme inside muscles. It's possible, then, that the extra iron consumed by those older folks in Sweden didn't show up on blood tests because it wasn't circulating—it was hard at work helping produce energy inside muscles. And it's conceivable that you could be short of iron deep in your muscles but never know it from blood tests.

Another reason why blood tests for anemia are less than perfect is that different people apparently need different amounts of iron. "I know of cases where people suffering from appreciable fatigue responded to iron therapy even though initial blood tests did not show an abnormally low level in their blood," James D. Cook, M.D., professor of medicine and director of hematology at the University of Kansas Medical Center, says. "This is not, of course, to say that some people feign improvement. It's just that what is considered a 'normal' iron level for one person may represent an iron deficiency in another. The key is individualized hemoglobin levels."

Now that we have some idea why iron deficiency exists, and what it can do, it's important to put this whole business of iron deficiency and energy into perspective. First, as we mentioned before, symptoms such as fatigue and tiredness can be caused by many different things. If you are not normally fatigued, but suddenly become so and remain that way for more than a few days, you should receive a thorough medical evaluation. And if you are diagnosed anemic, you should receive careful medical evaluation to rule out internal bleeding or other problems.

The next point we want to make is that even if the problem *is* nutritional in nature, a number of factors other than iron may be involved. Be sure to read our entries on "Fatigue" and "Low Blood Sugar (Hypoglycemia)." While iron deficiency is only one possible aspect of fatigue, we have given it a symbol of its own because in a dietary approach such as this, which emphasizes foods of vegetable origin, it is not as easy to get iron as it is to get some of the other nutrients involved in energy, such as potassium and magnesium.

That brings us right down to the question of iron in the diet. If you look at the table below, you'll immediately notice that meat products in general have very high

Selected Dietary Sources of Iron

Food	Portion Size	Milligrams	Food	Portion Size	Milligrams
Beef liver	3 ounces	7.5	Cod	6 ounces	1.8
Sunflower seeds	½ cup	5.1	Spinach		
Apricots			chopped	1 cup	1.7
dried	½ cup	3.6	Brussels sprouts	1 cup	1.7
Blackstrap molasses	1 tablespoon	3.2	Peanuts	½ cup	1.6
Almonds			Peas	½ cup	1.4
slivered	½ cup	2.7	Brewer's yeast	1 tablespoon	1.4
Cashews	½ cup	2.6	Beet greens		
Soybeans	½ cup	2.5	cooked	½ cup	1.4
Raisins	½ cup	2.5	Turkey		
Lentils	½ cup	2.1	light meat	3 ounces	1
Turkey			Endive or escarole		
dark meat	3 ounces	2	shredded	1 cup	1
Lima beans	½ cup	2	Whole grain bread	1 1-ounce slice	0.8
Haddock	6 ounces	1.8	Wheat germ	1 tablespoon	0.5

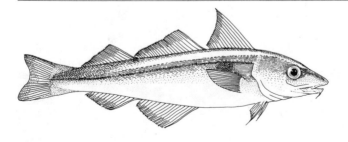

levels of iron, while grains, beans, and potatoes have less, and dairy products practically none. But there's more to it than that. Vegetables not only have less iron than meat products to begin with, but they have *a different kind of iron*. They contain what's known as "nonheme" iron, while meat has "heme" iron. The heme iron in meat is six times more absorbable than nonheme iron. But that doesn't necessarily mean you should wolf down a pound of meat at every meal and skip the potatoes. All the iron in the meal forms a common pool in the stomach, and *the heme iron increases the amount of nonheme iron that can be absorbed.* One study showed that the amount of iron absorbed from corn doubled when it was eaten with fish or beef (*Federation Proceedings,* June, 1977).

Scientists don't understand how meat acts to boost iron absorption. But they have discovered that meat is only one of *two* substances with this ability. The other is vitamin C. In one study, for instance, adding 60 milligrams of vitamin C (the amount in half a cup of orange juice) to a meal of rice more than *tripled* iron absorption. In another study, adding papaya containing 66 milligrams of vitamin C to a meal of corn boosted iron absorption by more than 500 percent (*Federation Proceedings,* June, 1977). In general, says one authority, if you eat some fruits or vegetables high in vitamin C with each meal, you can actually triple the absorption of iron in your diet.

If you have reason to believe that you may be deficient in iron, you will probably want to eat a certain amount of meat. (That is, unless you are vegetarian). Liver, as everyone knows, is probably the best source of iron, not only because it contains a lot of that mineral, but because it is rich in other blood-building factors such as vitamin B_{12} and folate. As an organ meat, however, liver does have a substantial amount of cholesterol, so we don't suggest eating it more than about once a week. Other than the cholesterol, there is nothing at all wrong with liver. We sometimes read that liver contains residues of various toxins because of the way cattle and chickens are raised in the United States. But when we had one of the most respected laboratories in the country analyze six samples of beef liver for us, they reported they could find no residues whatsoever of the hormone DES, no residues of tetracycline, and no residues of 10 different insecticides. Without a doubt, liver is one of the most nutritious foods available. And we think that if you try some of our recipes, you will learn to like it a lot—if you don't already.

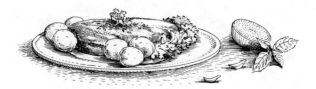

BREAKFAST

Breakfast Spice Cake with Streusel Topping

Makes eight servings

Cake:

2 cups (500 ml) whole wheat
   flour
2 tablespoons (30 ml) bran
2 tablespoons (30 ml) brewer's
   yeast
2 tablespoons (30 ml) lecithin
   granules
2 tablespoons (30 ml) wheat
   germ
1 teaspoon (5 ml) baking soda
1½ teaspoons (7 ml) freshly
   grated nutmeg
1 teaspoon (5 ml) cinnamon
½ teaspoon (2 ml) mace
½ teaspoon (2 ml) cloves
¼ teaspoon (1 ml) cardamom
   (optional)
½ teaspoon (2 ml) allspice
1 egg
¼ cup (60 ml) safflower oil
½ cup (125 ml) buttermilk or
   yogurt
½ cup (125 ml) blackstrap
   molasses
¾ cup (175 ml) raisins

Topping:

1 tablespoon (15 ml) corn oil
1 tablespoon (15 ml) honey
½ cup (125 ml) rolled oats
1 tablespoon (15 ml) wheat
   germ
1 tablespoon (15 ml) bran
1 tablespoon (15 ml) lecithin
   granules
1 teaspoon (5 ml) cinnamon

For the cake, combine dry ingredients in a large mixing bowl. Beat egg in a small bowl and add oil, buttermilk and molasses; beat together. Toss raisins with dry ingredients until they are coated. Add egg mixture to dry ingredients and stir only until ingredients are blended. Some lumps can remain. Pour into a greased 8 × 8-inch (20-cm) baking pan.

For the topping, combine ingredients. Sprinkle over batter. Bake cake at 350° F. (175° C.) for 30 to 35 minutes.

SALADS

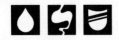

Grapefruit and Prune Salad

Makes two servings
1 pink grapefruit
5–6 soft or soaked pitted prunes,
   chopped
Vinaigrette Dressing
lettuce leaves

You'll enjoy this salad for a change of pace!

Peel grapefruit and section, removing membranes. Toss grapefruit and prunes with *Vinaigrette Dressing*. Serve on a bed of lettuce.

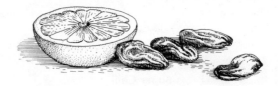

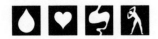

Kidney Bean Salad

Makes eight servings
2 cups (500 ml) dried kidney
   beans
1 cup (250 ml) chopped celery
1 green or sweet red pepper,
   chopped
¼ cup (60 ml) chopped fresh
   parsley
4 scallions, chopped
¼ cup (60 ml) olive oil
6 tablespoons (90 ml) mild
   vinegar
1 tablespoon (15 ml) blackstrap
   molasses
2 teaspoons (10 ml) tamari
lettuce leaves
8 radishes, sliced (garnish)
4 tomatoes, quartered (garnish)

Soak beans overnight. Cook until soft (See *Index* "Cooking Beans").

Combine cooked kidney beans, celery, pepper, parsley and scallions in a large bowl. Combine oil, vinegar, molasses and tamari in a jar; shake with lid on. Pour dressing over bean mixture. Allow to marinate several hours or overnight.

To serve, place salad on lettuce leaves and garnish with sliced radishes and quartered tomatoes.

Unused salad stores well in the refrigerator.

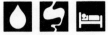

Winter Fruit Salad

Makes two servings
1 unpeeled apple, cubed
1 ripe banana, cubed
5–6 soft or soaked pitted prunes,
    chopped
1 tablespoon (15 ml) walnuts,
    chopped
Lemon Vinaigrette Dressing

Toss all ingredients together with enough dressing to moisten.

MAIN DISHES

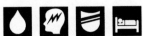

Super Chili

No one will guess that this flavorful chili is made with liver.

Makes eight servings
2 cups (500 ml) dried kidney
    beans
1½ cups (375 ml) reserved
    liquid from cooking
    beans
1 pound (450 g) lean ground
    beef
½ pound (225 g) calf liver
1 large yellow onion,
    quartered
1 green or sweet red pepper,
    chopped
3 cloves garlic, crushed
3–4 tablespoons (45–60 ml) chili
    powder
2 teaspoons (10 ml) cumin
    powder
2 teaspoons (10 ml) oregano
⅔ cup (150 ml) tomato paste
1 cup (250 ml) fresh or frozen
    corn
4 teaspoons (20 ml) tamari
1 tablespoon (15 ml)
    blackstrap molasses
dash cayenne pepper
    (optional)

Soak beans overnight. Cook until soft (see *Index,* "Cooking Beans"). Drain, and reserve liquid.

To make chili, begin browning beef in a large, hot, lightly oiled skillet. Place the liver with ¼ of the onion in a blender and process on low to medium speed until smooth. Stir into the browning meat. When meat is cooked through, chop and add remainder of the onion, the pepper, garlic, chili powder, cumin and oregano. Cook together until the onion becomes transparent.

Stir in tomato paste, cooked kidney beans, reserved bean stock, corn, tamari and molasses. Simmer chili until onions and peppers are tender. Serve hot.

Note: For hotter chili, stir in cayenne pepper or hot red pepper flakes to taste. Freeze leftovers for another meal.

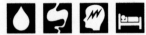

Pate Meatloaf

Makes eight servings

1 pound (450 g) lean ground beef
½ pound (225 g) beef liver
1 tablespoon (15 ml) grated onions
½ green pepper, minced
1 carrot, grated
1 tablespoon (15 ml) minced fresh parsley
1 egg
1 cup (250 ml) soft whole grain bread crumbs
1 cup (250 ml) rolled oats
2 teaspoons (10 ml) tamari
½ teaspoon (2 ml) thyme
½ teaspoon (2 ml) marjoram
¼ teaspoon (1 ml) oregano
¼ teaspoon (1 ml) basil

A perfect balance between meats and vegetables, and quite incredibly delicious to boot.

Place ground beef in a large mixing bowl. In a blender, puree liver and add to beef. Stir in remaining ingredients. Place mixture in an 8½ × 4½-inch (22 × 11-cm) loaf pan. Cover tightly with aluminum foil. Bake in a preheated 350° F. (175° C.) oven one hour, removing foil for last 15 minutes, and glazing, if desired, with *Barbeque Sauce.*

Note: Leftover meatloaf can be sliced, wrapped, and frozen for future use.

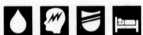

Polynesian Liver

Makes four servings

¼ pineapple (about 1½ cups [375 ml] sliced)
1 large green pepper, thinly sliced
1 cup *Chicken Stock*
1 pound (450 g) calf liver, cut in thin strips

A tropical twist on old-fashioned liver. Great new taste!

Remove skin from pineapple and core. Slice pineapple and cut slices into matchstick-size strips. Steam-stir green pepper slices in a few tablespoons (50 ml) of the stock until it begins to become tender. Add liver strips and cook over medium heat, stirring, until liver is still pink on the inside and juicy, adding more stock as needed to keep mixture from sticking. Add pineapple strips and heat through, with enough of the stock to provide a sauce. Serve over brown rice.

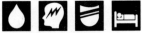

Chicken Livers, Mushrooms and Walnuts

Makes four servings

2½ cups (625 ml) sliced
    mushrooms (about ½
    pound [225 g])
2 gloves garlic, minced
2 tablespoons (30 ml)
    sunflower oil
1 teaspoon (5 ml) tamari
1 pound (450 g) chicken
    livers, cut into small
    pieces
¼ cup (60 ml) walnuts,
    chopped
1 teaspoon (5 ml) basil
1 tablespoon (15 ml) minced
    fresh parsley
½ cup (125 ml) *Chicken Stock*

In a heavy skillet, place mushrooms and garlic with the oil and tamari and stir until water has evaporated from the mushrooms and they are tender. Set aside.

Steam-stir the livers the in the same pan, adding a few table-spoons (50 ml) of water as necessary to prevent sticking. When livers are still pink inside, add mushroom mixture, walnuts and remaining ingredients to the pan and heat through. Serve immediately over cooked whole wheat pasta.

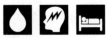

Liver 'n' Onions

Makes two servings

2 large yellow onions, diced
2 cloves garlic, minced
½ teaspoon (2 ml) tamari
½ pound (225 g) beef liver
1 teaspoon (5 ml) basil
½ teaspoon (2 ml) marjoram

Our version of a classic home-cooking dish. The secret is in the herbs and not cooking the liver to the point where it's brown in the middle.

Combine onions with garlic and tamari in a skillet. Steam-stir in a small amount of water until tender and browned slightly. This will take about 20 minutes over medium heat. Add liver and herbs to onion mixture and cook, covered, just until liver is pink inside and has clear juices. Serve hot with steamed new potatoes, or with boiled potatoes garnished with parsley.

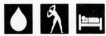

Chicken with Mushrooms

Makes four servings

2 whole chicken breasts,
    skinned and split
¼ cup (60 ml) whole wheat
    flour
2 teaspoons (10 ml) corn oil
2 tablespoons (30 ml) chopped
    shallots
1 clove garlic, minced
3 tablespoons (45 ml) tomato
    paste
2 cups (500 ml) *Chicken Stock*
½ bay leaf
½ teaspoon (2 ml) basil,
    crumbled
⅛ teaspoon (0.5 ml) thyme
⅛ teaspoon (0.5 ml) marjoram
5 cups (1.25 l) sliced
    mushrooms (about 1
    pound [450 g])

Place halves of chicken breasts, which have been coated with the flour, in a large, hot skillet with the oil. Brown the chicken on both sides, adding chopped shallots when the chicken is turned. Add a few drops of water, if needed, to prevent sticking. When chicken is golden and shallots are tender, add the remaining ingredients. Simmer the chicken, covered, one hour, or until tender. Serve over pasta, brown rice, polenta or with boiled potatoes.

Liver Yucatan

Makes four servings

2 onions, sliced in rings
1 green pepper, thinly sliced
2 tomatoes, chopped
1 pound (450 g) beef liver, cut
    in thin strips
1 tablespoon (15 ml) chili
    powder
1 teaspoon (5 ml) cumin
    powder
½ teaspoon (2 ml) tamari

Tasters gave this liver dish an "A-plus" and said they enjoyed seeing liver "dressed up."

Place onion rings and green pepper slices in a large skillet, and steam-stir in enough water to prevent sticking until onion begins to turn transparent. Add tomatoes and stir over medium heat until onion and pepper are tender. Place liver strips over the onion mixture, add spices, and cover. Steam liver just until tender; pink juices should remain in slices. Add tamari, stirring liver and vegetables to combine, and serve with rice or boiled potatoes.

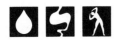

Tortillas Buenas

Makes two servings
2 corn tortillas
1 cup (250 ml) *Lentil Stew,*
    Savory Lentils, or
    Mexican Lentils
1 tablespoon (15 ml) shredded
    cheddar cheese
  lettuce, chopped
  scallions, chopped
  tomatoes, chopped
  alfalfa sprouts

Why not double the recipe and invite some friends to enjoy a mountain of nutritious food, Mexican-style?

Top each corn tortilla with some *Lentil Stew, Savory Lentils* or *Mexican Lentils.* Sprinkle with the cheese and place under a broiler until the cheese melts. Top with a big mound of fresh lettuce, scallions, tomatoes and sprouts. Looks delicious, and it is!

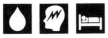

Thick Beef Spaghetti Sauce

Makes two quarts (2 l)
1 onion, chopped
2 tablespoons (30 ml) corn oil
1 pound (450 g) lean beef
    cubes
¼ cup (60 ml) whole wheat
    flour
4 cups (1 l) Italian plum
    tomatoes with juice
½ teaspoon (2 ml) thyme
½ teaspoon (2 ml) marjoram
½ teaspoon (2 ml) basil
½ teaspoon (2 ml) oregano
1 sweet red pepper, chopped
2½ cups (625 ml) sliced
    mushrooms (about ½
    pound [225 g])
1 teaspoon (5 ml) blackstrap
    molasses

Saute onion in one tablespoon (15 ml) of oil until translucent; remove from pan.

Remove all visible fat from the beef cubes and dredge the dry cubes in the flour. The cubes should be bite-size. In a large, heavy-bottom saucepan, brown the beef cubes, a few at a time, over high heat in the remaining oil. Do not have more than one layer of beef cubes on the bottom of the pan while browning.

When all of the beef cubes have been browned, place them along with the sauteed onion, tomatoes, herbs, pepper, mushrooms and molasses in the big saucepan. Simmer over low heat for 1½ to 2 hours, stirring occasionally. If the sauce becomes too thick, add some water or tomato juice.

Serve over cooked whole wheat spaghetti.

This recipe will yield about 10 servings. The excess can be easily frozen for later use.

Note: Using beef cubes rather than ground beef insures that the cook can remove all visible traces of fat.

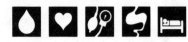

Savory Lentils

Makes about three cups (750 ml)

1 cup (250 ml) dried lentils
2½ cups (625 ml) water
1 medium onion
5 cloves garlic
1 tablespoon (15 ml) chili powder
½ teaspoon (2 ml) cumin powder
½ cup (125 ml) raisins
1 tablespoon (15 ml) blackstrap molasses
5 tablespoons (75 ml) tomato paste

Bring lentils to a boil in the water and simmer 20 to 25 minutes with the onion and garlic. Add remaining ingredients and cook about 20 minutes longer, until the lentils are tender, but not mushy.

Note: These lentils can be used in tacos, tortillas or served with corn bread.

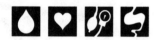

Mexican Lentils

Makes eight servings

1½ cups (375 ml) dried lentils
¼ cup (60 ml) raisins
4 cups (1 l) water
½ green pepper, chopped
4 cloves garlic, minced
½ teaspoon (2 ml) dried hot red pepper flakes
1 tablespoon (15 ml) chili powder
1 teaspoon (5 ml) cumin powder
½ teaspoon (2 ml) basil
⅔ cup (150 ml) tomato paste

A sweet, savory version of a food that's a dietary staple for millions.

Place lentils and raisins in large skillet or saucepan with three cups (750 ml) of the water. Simmer lentils about 10 minutes. Add pepper, garlic, seasonings, tomato paste and remaining cup of water. Simmer mixture 30 to 45 minutes, until lentils are tender, adding water if mixture becomes too thick. Makes about five cups (1.25 l). Lentils can be served over brown rice, whole wheat noodles or corn tortillas.

Note: Refrigerate or freeze unused portion for later use.

Pureed Lentils

Makes about one quart (1 l)
1 cup (250 ml) dried lentils
2 bay leaves
1 medium onion
2 cloves garlic
1 medium carrot
½ stalk celery
1 tablespoon (15 ml) fresh
   parsley
1 tablespoon (15 ml) raisins
3 cups (750 ml) water
1 tablespoon (15 ml) chili
   powder
½ teaspoon (2 ml) cumin
   powder

Can be used as a sandwich spread or served with tacos or tortillas.

Wash lentils and combine ingredients in a 3-quart (3 l) saucepan. Bring to a boil, reduce heat, and simmer for 35 to 45 minutes, or until lentils are tender and water is absorbed. (Add a little boiling water, if necessary, to prevent sticking as the ingredients cook.) When lentils are done, remove bay leaves, place ingredients in a blender and, on medium speed, process until smooth.

Variation: To serve pureed lentils as a dinner vegetable, omit chili and cumin powders, and add ¼ to ½ cup (60 to 125 ml) yogurt, when blending, to thin the puree. Garnish with strips of *Pimiento.*

SIDE DISHES

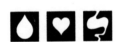

Pennsylvania Dutch Baked Lima Beans

Makes 10 servings
2 cups (500 ml) dried lima
   beans
   water
2 large yellow onions, chopped
2 teaspoons (10 ml) tamari
⅔ cup (150 ml) tomato paste
1 tablespoon (15 ml) sesame
   tahini
¼ cup (60 ml) blackstrap
   molasses
1 orange

Here's a hearty bean dish with lots of flavor which develops a culinary theme popular among Pennsylvania farmers.

Soak beans overnight in six cups (1.5 l) of water; drain. For quick-soak method, bring six cups (1.5 l) of water to a boil, add beans and simmer two minutes. Remove from heat, cover tightly, and set aside one hour or longer. Drain. To cook beans, add water to cover, and boil 30 to 40 minutes, or until tender.

Meanwhile, in a large skillet or Dutch oven, steam-stir onions in just enough water to prevent scorching. When the onions are golden, add tamari, tomato paste, ½ cup (125 ml) of water, tahini and molasses. Slice orange in half. From each half, cut two thin slices of orange. Squeeze juice from remaining orange halves. Add juice to tomato paste mixture, and add beans. Simmer mixture until ingredients are heated through. Place in an 8 × 8-inch (20 × 20-cm) casserole dish and garnish with the orange slices. Bake, covered, for one hour at 350° F. (175° C.). Remove cover and continue baking 30 minutes. Makes about 2 quarts (2 l).

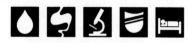

Curried Rice

Makes four servings

½ cup (125 ml) dried apricots, chopped
¼ cup (60 ml) raisins
2 cups (500 ml) cooked brown rice
¼ cup (60 ml) chopped scallions
¼ cup (60 ml) chopped green peppers
1 teaspoon (5 ml) sesame oil
¼ cup (60 ml) walnuts, toasted
½ teaspoon (2 ml) curry
¼ teaspoon (1 ml) coriander
dash freshly grated nutmeg

A piquant example of the wonderful things that can be done with rice and fruit.

Combine apricots, raisins and brown rice in a medium bowl.

In a large skillet, saute scallions and green peppers in oil until crisp-tender. In a small skillet, place walnuts over medium heat and stir until golden. Stir walnuts, seasonings and apricot-rice mixture into scallions and green peppers. Heat through and serve.

Variation: For a protein-rich main course, stir in one cup (250 ml) cooked soybeans or cooked red lentils.

Creamed Spinach

Makes two servings

10 ounces (280 g) spinach
1 clove garlic, minced
½ teaspoon (2 ml) tamari
2 tablespoons (30 ml) yogurt
1 tablespoon (15 ml) grated Parmesan cheese

Wash spinach, remove large stems, and shake excess water from leaves. Reserve stems for making soup stock. Place spinach, along with garlic and tamari, in a large saucepan and steam in the small amount of water that clings to the leaves. When spinach is limp and has turned a deep green, remove from heat. Place spinach, drained if necessary, in a blender with yogurt and cheese. Process on low speed until spinach is pureed. Serve immediately.

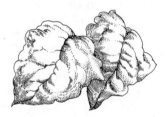

MISCELLANEOUS

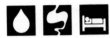

Lentil Pate

Makes three cups (750 ml)
1½ cups (375 ml) dried lentils
1 carrot, shredded
2 cups (500 ml) water
1 bay leaf
1½ teaspoons (7 ml) tamari
¼ cup (60 ml) *Tofu
    Mayonnaise*
½ teaspoon (2 ml) basil
⅛ teaspoon (0.5 ml) mace
⅛ teaspoon (0.5 ml) allspice
dash cayenne pepper

Place lentils, carrot and water in a medium saucepan. Add bay leaf and simmer mixture, covered, until lentils are quite tender and the liquid is absorbed, about 45 to 55 minutes. Add a few tablespoons (50 ml) of water, if necessary, to prevent scorching. Remove from heat. Place lentils in mixing bowl; remove bay leaf. Mash lentils with fork or potato masher, and combine with remaining ingredients. Continue mashing mixture until smooth.

Press into a bread pan; chill thoroughly, then invert and serve as a party pate, or use as a sandwich spread.

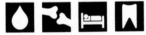

Fig Bars

Makes two dozen
1 cup (250 ml) whole wheat
    flour
2 tablespoons (30 ml) brewer's
    yeast
1 tablespoon (15 ml) bone meal
1 teaspoon (5 ml) kelp powder
1 teaspoon (5 ml) *Baking
    Powder*
2 teaspoons (10 ml) cinnamon
¼ teaspoon (1 ml) coriander
¼ teaspoon (1 ml) allspice
3 eggs
¼ cup (60 ml) honey
1 teaspoon (5 ml) *Vanilla
    Extract*
1 cup (250 ml) chopped figs
½ cup (125 ml) walnuts,
    chopped

Great snacks for kids of any age. We love 'em!

Combine the dry ingredients in a medium mixing bowl. In another bowl, beat eggs, and add honey, *Vanilla Extract* and figs. Stir to combine. Add liquid ingredients to dry ingredients, add nuts, and stir until combined. Lightly oil a 13 × 9-inch (33 × 23-cm) baking pan and spread the mixture across the bottom. Bake in a 350° F. (175° C.) preheated oven 20 to 25 minutes, until browned.

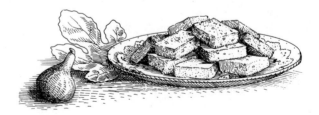

Prune Butter

Makes ½ cup (125 ml)
½ cup (125 ml) soft or soaked
  pitted prunes
1 teaspoon (5 ml) medium
  unsulfured molasses

Replace sugar-packed jams with this tasty alternative.

Combine ingredients in a blender and process on low speed until smooth. Store, covered, in the refrigerator.

DESSERTS

Wet-Bottom Molasses Cake

Makes 8 to 10 servings
2½ cups (625 ml) whole wheat
  flour
1½ teaspoons (7 ml) baking
  soda
½ cup (125 ml) corn oil
½ cup (125 ml) medium
  unsulfured molasses
½ cup (125 ml) hot water
¼ cup (60 ml) blackstrap
  molasses

Combine the flour and baking soda in a large bowl. Stir in the oil and medium molasses. Remove one cup (250 ml) of this mixture and set aside.

In a small bowl, combine the hot water and blackstrap molasses. Add to the flour mixture in the large bowl, and stir until thoroughly combined.

Place the batter in a lightly oiled 8-inch (20-cm) round cake pan. Sprinkle the remaining cup of flour mixture over top of the batter.

Bake in a preheated 375° F. (190° C.) oven for 25 to 30 minutes, until done.

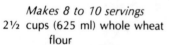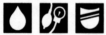

Cantaloupe-Raisin Pie

Makes eight servings
¾ cup (175 ml) raisins
2 cups (500 ml) apple juice
2 heaping tablespoons (40 ml)
  agar-agar flakes
½ teaspoon (2 ml) dried
  spearmint leaves
1½ cups (375 ml) diced
  cantaloupe
9-inch (23-cm) prebaked
  No-Roll Pie Crust

Cook raisins in apple juice in a medium saucepan until they begin to swell. Sprinkle agar-agar and spearmint over mixture and simmer five more minutes. Cool slightly, and stir in cantaloupe. Pour cantaloupe mixture into pie crust and chill until firm.

No-Roll Pie Crust

*Makes one 9-inch (23 cm)
pie crust*
1 cup (250 ml) whole wheat
    pastry flour
¼ cup (60 ml) corn oil
2 tablespoons (30 ml)
    buttermilk

Combine ingredients in a pie plate. Toss with a fork until thoroughly combined, then press on bottom and sides of pie plate. Fill and bake as with a regular crust.

Variation: For sweet pies, two teaspoons (10 ml) of honey can be added to the crust.

BUILDING A STRONGER FOUNDATION

Loss of bone strength is probably the most unseen, unsuspected epidemic disease among adults in our society. Unseen, that is, for what it really is. Because in one form or another, we've all seen the condition doctors call osteoporosis, which means simply a loss of the density and strength of bones.

• A 64-year-old woman who never had backaches in her life suddenly gets them in the low part of her spine. One doctor prescribes aspirin. Another heat treatments. The third, muscle relaxants. Probably arthritis, says another. But what she's really suffering from is bone weakness—osteoporosis.

• The last time you saw Aunt Mae must have been 20 years ago. Now she's 80, and still looks pretty healthy, except that she seems to have actually shrunk a good four or five inches. And developed a noticeable hump in her upper back. "Is that what happens when you get old?" asks one of your children. "No. That's what happens when you have osteoporosis."

• Mrs. Conners was walking her dog one fine day in June, thinking about how nice it was to be out again after a long winter, when she stepped off the curb and wound up sprawled in the street with a fractured hip. "A freak accident," one relative said. "It was just age; Bea was 75, you know," said another. But both were wrong. Bea Conners was knocked off her feet by osteoporosis.

Osteoporosis is the single leading cause of disability among all women over the age of 60. It has more women laid up than stroke, heart disease, cancer or high blood pressure. If that sounds hard to believe, consider that what happened to Bea Conners is believed to happen no less than six million times a year in the United States. And five million of those fractures—which have absolutely no cause except the weakness of the bone—strike down women. It's estimated that more than one woman in four over the age of 60 has osteoporosis severe enough to cause pain, loss of height and spinal deformity.

But why? Is it natural or inevitable that bones should become weak with advancing age? And how could *diet* prevent or heal such a serious epidemic? Surely it's not possible that American diets are so deficient in calcium as to cause such suffering. *Is it?*

Actually, it wasn't too many years ago that researchers and doctors were asking those same questions. Within the last 10 to 20 years, however, we have learned a lot about osteoporosis, and very simply, it boils down to this:

All but one percent of the body's calcium is stored in the bones and teeth. But as important as our bones and teeth are to our health, that little bit that's left over, the one percent, is even *more* important. That's the calcium that circulates along with the blood throughout the body, and makes it possible for the nervous system to function. Were the concentration of calcium to drop below a certain minimal level, the result would be convulsions. It's no surprise, then, that the body has a very powerful built-in calcium-regulating system to keep that from happening. That system is so efficient that even a person with very poor eating habits usually has a "normal" level of calcium in his blood.

The system operates on the principle of robbing Peter to pay Paul. Whenever our nerves need more calcium, the body simply withdraws it from the bones and puts it to work circulating around the body. Now, that might be a little hard to imagine, because most of us picture the bones as being more or less like inert pillars of marble. But in fact, there is almost always a lively interchange of calcium between the bones and the blood, with some of the mineral being withdrawn and some being replaced every day. During youth, when bones are actively growing, there is more calcium being deposited than withdrawn. During early adulthood, the balance is usually even. But as we head into maturity, what usually happens is that we begin withdrawing more than we're depositing.

We said before that four out of every five osteoporotic fractures victimize women. Usually, older women. The major reason seems to be that the calcium metabolism of women is largely dependent upon estrogen. After menopause, when levels of that hormone diminish dramatically, the bones lose some of their ability to hold on to calcium. But trouble can begin long before menopause: in one medical survey, some women as young as 25 were found to have bone density levels from 10 to 25 percent below average.

Meanwhile, at the same point in life where estrogen levels have dipped low, the ability to *absorb* calcium through the intestinal wall may also be faltering. So the mature woman has at least two challenges. But maybe more.

Sex and aging aside, scientists recently discovered that eating a high-protein diet (as many people in the Western countries do) tends to wash substantial amounts of calcium right out of the body. Ingesting that high amount of protein is likely only if you are eating generous portions of meat or fish at least twice a day. Eating meat only occasionally, and getting protein from vegetable sources (as we do in this book) prevents that calcium washout from occurring. The fact that only people in Western countries can *afford* to eat such large amounts of meat is the apparent explanation for the fact that Westerners have just as much osteoporosis as people in the other countries who consume far less calcium. Vegetable eaters can get by with much less calcium than people regularly consuming fish, poultry and meat.

But if you don't eat a particularly high-protein diet, is it still necessary to go out of your way to get extra calcium into your diet? That depends. Do you smoke? If so, your lungs aren't the only organs suffering from your habit. Smoking tends to demineralize the bones.

Do you get but a smidgen of exercise each day? Exercise is very important in keeping a positive balance of calcium. Just a few weeks of bed rest can cause significant bone weakness. But so can years of sedentary habits. If you don't do a lot of long, hard walking, you may need extra calcium to make up for it.

Do you spend most of your time indoors? When the sun strikes the skin, it causes vitamin D to be synthesized, and vitamin D is necessary for calcium to be absorbed and transported to the bones. People who live in northern climates are at a real disadvantage here, because even when the sun does shine during the winter, it's so weak as to be almost useless as far as vitamin D is concerned. And while you can store up on vitamin D during the summer, it tends to disappear by early spring. And so does calcium. English researchers found that bone density actually varies from season to season, with the lowest density occurring from April to June, when stores of vitamin D from the previous summer are exhausted. That explains, perhaps, why our friend Bea had her fracture in June.

WHY CALCIUM SUPPLEMENTS ARE NATURAL

Menopause. Absorption problems that come with age. A high-protein diet. Smoking. Lack of exercise. Lack of sunshine. All of them can cause a calcium shortage. Does that mean taking extra calcium is a kind of unnatural thing we have to do in order to live in our unnatural environment? Not at all. Primitive peoples all over the world routinely and normally make calcium supplements a part of their diet. They may not buy them at a health food store, but they do eat special foods that are rich in calcium. Most often, perhaps, the calcium comes in the form of bone. The Eskimos eat small birds, when they can catch them, bones and all. In Ecuador, the Vilcabamba people, who are fabled for their strength and strong bones, cook beef bones all day with a few vegetables to make a soup that is very high in calcium (vinegar or acidic vegetables such as tomatoes help get the calcium out of the bones). Asian Indians also eat small bones in their curry dishes, although they are said to avoid doing this when having Westerners as guests, for fear of offending them. Mexican peasants add limestone, which is basically calcium carbonate, to the cornmeal they use to make their tortillas. In the American Southwest, the Papago and Hopi Indians eat cholla cactus buds—half an ounce of which contains about 400 milligrams of calcium (four times more than the same amount of cheddar cheese!).

Maybe it would be more helpful if, instead of saying that people all over the world take calcium supplements, we said that such apparently unusual foods as bone or mineral powders aren't really supplements at all, but foods. Special foods, yes, but natural, nonetheless. We therefore regard bone meal and dolomite (a natural mineral powder containing mostly calcium and magnesium) as perfectly natural foods.

We apologize if this discussion of our need for calcium seems long-winded, but remember, we're talking about *the* most common cause of disability in older women, and we want to make sure that everyone understands why it's important to protect against it with appropriate dietary measures. And to understand that you *can* fight it off. Stop it. Even turn it around.

Anthony A. Albanese, Ph.D., one of the leading figures in osteoporosis research, has been administering calcium supplements in doses ranging from 750 to 1,000 milligrams a day to over 500 women in a rehabilitation setting. Over and over again, he has seen what it does. In one series of tests, women who were given 750 milligrams of calcium a day along with 375 units of vitamin D for a period of three years actually *increased* the density of their bones, even though their average age was 82. Meanwhile, another group of women, the same age, who hadn't received extra calcium, experienced a decrease of bone density. When you can turn back physical deterioration at the age of 82, you must be doing something right.

At least two other studies, both published in major medical journals, likewise show that osteoporosis can be stopped with a calcium intake of between 1,200 and 1,400 milligrams a day. Still another study, which used a combination of calcium, phosphorus, vitamin D and two ounces of cheese a day, showed that after six months, the density of the finger bones in elderly women, all with a history of osteoporosis, actually increased by 25 percent.

While some old-fashioned doctors are still telling their patients that adults have no particular need for calcium, the word is now getting out to most of the profession, so the idea of taking extra calcium can no longer be considered especially controversial.

"Bone loss and fracture risk may be minimized or reversed by a daily intake of approximately 1 gram [1,000 milligrams] of calcium derived from the diet or through supplements," readers of the *American Family Physician* in October of 1978 were told.

Another article making a very strong argument for the use of calcium in osteoporosis appeared in the *American Journal of Medicine* in December, 1978. In August of 1976, an orthopedic specialist from the Mayo Clinic, Jenifer Jowsey, Ph.D., recommended that "calcium supplements should probably be given from age 25, when bone loss starts. This may seem to be an extraordinary recommendation, but if calcium supplementation is initiated at this early age, by the time the individual is 70, he or she may retain the bone mass, and therefore the bone strength, of a 40-year-old" *(Postgraduate Medicine)*. Even the readers of the conservative *Journal of the American Medical Association* were informed in the issue of October 20, 1978, that middle-aged or older persons with histories of low calcium intake and signs of osteoporosis should "probably" be receiving 1,000 milligrams of supplemental calcium a day. They were even told that absorption is better when calcium is taken in several small portions and that supplemental vitamin D may also help.

Some people may be thinking, why not wait until I *know* I need the calcium, or when the doctor tells me I have early osteoporosis? The problem with trying to be very precise about meeting your calcium needs is that osteoporosis doesn't show up on x-rays until about one-third of the bone mass is already gone. Too often, the first sign of osteoporosis is a major bone fracture.

Now, what about getting calcium from your food? Some people make it sound easy—all you have to do is drink a quart of milk a day. That's easy for *them* to say. But how many adults do you know who drink even half that much milk? Many adults don't drink *any* milk. Where are they to get their calcium from, then?

You can't leave it to chance, that's for sure. A quick glance at the following table, "Common Foods Low in Calcium," should prove that. Remember, you're aiming for at least 1,000 milligrams a day of calcium. Yet, you can see that these very common foods—all of them wholesome and nourishing—are uniformly low in this mineral. In fact, if you ate double portions of all the foods listed, you'd only get a total of a little over 400 milligrams of calcium (but nearly 3,000 calories!). Further, that list includes grain products, fruits, vegetables, meat, fish and eggs, so even if you eat a variety of foods, you can still be grossly deficient in calcium.

In the next table, "Selected Good Sources of Calcium," you'll notice there really aren't that many commonly eaten foods that deliver a great deal of calcium. You'll also notice the list doesn't include certain dark, green leafy vegetables that are high in calcium. That's because most of them are also high in oxalate, which renders the calcium largely or entirely unabsorbable.

At this point, we can begin to better understand why so many cultures have developed special sources of dietary calcium, such as limestone. And why people in our own culture often turn to bone meal or dolomite.

Our last table details the calcium and other food values in cheese. Although cheese is generally high in fat and often contains substantial amounts of cholesterol, we think that an ounce of hard cheese a day is not excessive, because of the valuable calcium it contains. Larger amounts of ricotta can be eaten because of the greater moisture content. Of all the hard or firm cheeses, your best bet is probably Swiss, which is not only very rich in calcium, but exceptionally low in sodium. Ricotta is the best soft cheese, while cream cheese, which contains more fat than any other kind of cheese, but is extremely low in calcium, is the worst.

Common Foods Low in Calcium

Food	Portion Size	Calcium (milligrams)	Calories
Apple	1 medium	10	80
Brown rice	1 cup	23	232
Chicken			
light meat	1 breast	6	83
Cod	4 ounces	36	192
Corn	1 ear	2	70
Egg	1 large	27	82
Hamburger	4 ounces	14	202
Orange juice	1 cup	27	112
Potato	1 large	14	145
Spaghetti			
enriched	1 cup	14	192
Tomato			
raw	1 large	16	27
Whole wheat bread	1 slice	25	61

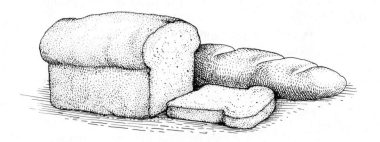

Selected Good Sources of Calcium

Food	Portion Size	Milligrams	Calories
Bone meal powder	1 teaspoon	1,000	—
Dolomite powder	1 teaspoon	981	—
Salmon			
with bones	3 ounces	275	388
Sardines	4 ounces	496	232
Yogurt			
skim-milk	1 cup	294	123
Bone meal tablets	1 tablet	166	—
Dolomite tablets	1 tablet	158	—
Chick-peas	½ cup	150	360
Buttermilk	½ cup	148	44
Milk			
skim	½ cup	148	44
Tofu (soybean curd)	4 ounces	145	1
Milk			
whole	½ cup	144	80
Blackstrap molasses	1 tablespoon	137	43
Turnip greens			
cooked	½ cup	134	15
Collards			
cooked	½ cup	110	21
Kale			
cooked	½ cup	103	22
Cream			
light	½ cup	99	112
Mustard greens			
cooked	½ cup	97	16
Sunflower seeds	½ cup	87	406
Dandelion greens			
cooked	½ cup	74	18
Okra			
cooked	½ cup	74	23
Broccoli			
cooked	½ cup	68	20
Soybeans	½ cup	66	117
Cheese	see table on following page		

Food Values in One Ounce of Cheese

Type	Calcium (milligrams)	Calories	Protein (grams)	Fat (grams)	Cholesterol (milligrams)	Sodium (milligrams)
Blue	150	100	6	8	21	396
Brick	191	105	7	8	27	159
Brie	52	95	6	8	28	178
Camembert	110	85	6	7	20	239
Cheddar	204	114	7	9	30	176
Colby	194	112	7	9	27	171
Cottage						
Creamed	17	29	4	1	4	114
Unsalted, dry-curd	9	24	5	0.1	2	4
Low-fat (made with						
1% milk fat)	17	21	4	0.25	1	115
Cream	23	99	2	10	31	84
Edam	207	101	7	8	25	274
Feta	140	75	4	6	25	316
Gouda	198	101	7	8	32	232
Limburger	141	93	6	8	26	227
Mozzarella	147	90	6	7	16	118
Mozzarella, part skim	183	72	7	5	16	132
Muenster	203	104	7	9	27	178
Parmesan, grated	390	129	12	9	22	528
Process American						
Cheese Food	163	93	6	7	18	337
Cheese Spread	159	82	5	6	16	381
Ricotta	63	54	4	4	16	26
Swiss or Jarlsburg	272	107	8	8	26	74

BREAKFASTS

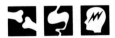

Brown Rice Pancakes

Makes two servings
½ cup (125 ml) cooked brown
    rice
1 cup (250 ml) skim milk
1 tablespoon (15 ml) medium
    unsulfured molasses
½ cup (125 ml) whole wheat
    flour
1 teaspoon (5 ml) *Baking
    Powder*
1 egg, beaten

Place rice, milk and molasses in a saucepan and bring to a boil over medium heat. Lower heat and simmer five minutes. Set aside to cool.

Combine flour and *Baking Powder* in a large bowl. When rice mixture is lukewarm, stir into flour along with egg. Cook in a hot, lightly oiled skillet, turning once, and serve with *One-Minute Cinnamon Applesauce* or fresh fruit.

Broiled Cinnamon Pancake

Makes two servings
¼ cup (60 ml) cottage or
    ricotta cheese
½ cup (125 ml) yogurt
1½ cups (375 ml) soft whole
    grain bread cubes
½ medium unpeeled apple,
    chopped
1 teaspoon (5 ml) cinnamon

Place all ingredients in a blender and blend on medium speed until smooth. Pour entire batter into a hot, lightly oiled medium skillet and cook until bottom is browned. Do not turn, but place pan under broiler until top is brown and pancake is baked through. Cut in half for serving.

Variation: For *Fruited Cinnamon Pancake,* prepare broiled cinnamon pancake as above. When bottom is brown, add thin apple slices to top before broiling. Press fruit down slightly into surface of pancake, so it does not scorch. Strawberry slices, peach slices or blueberries can also be used.

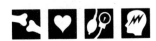

Sweet Sugarless Muesli

Makes one serving
¾ cup (175 ml) yogurt
½ cup (125 ml) *Dutch Muesli*
½ very ripe banana
    dash freshly grated nutmeg
    dash cinnamon

Beat the yogurt with a spoon to thin out the consistency so that it's somewhere between buttermilk and regular yogurt. Mix this with the *Dutch Muesli,* slice in the banana, and sprinkle on the nutmeg and cinnamon.

SOUPS

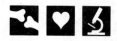

Broccoli Soup

Makes six servings
1 tablespoon (15 ml) corn oil
1 tablespoon (15 ml) whole
    wheat flour
½ teaspoon (2 ml) basil
1 cup (250 ml) skim milk
1½ cups (375 ml) *Chicken
    Stock* or *Vegetable
    Stock*
2 cups (500 ml) broccoli
    florets
2 teaspoons (10 ml) sesame
    tahini
½ cup (125 ml) yogurt
1 teaspoon (5 ml) tamari
    dash freshly grated nutmeg

In a skillet, heat oil and stir in flour and basil. Add milk slowly, stirring constantly to avoid lumps. Add stock and bring to a boil. Add broccoli florets (save stems for another vegetable combination) and simmer five to eight minutes, until slightly tender. Place tahini and yogurt in a blender. Add cooked broccoli mixture, tamari and nutmeg. Process on low, then medium speed until smooth. Serve hot. Makes about one quart. (1 l).

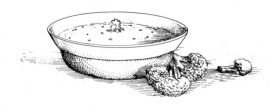

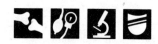

Chilled Apricot Soup

Makes four servings
½ cup (125 ml) dried apricots
    juice of 1 orange
2 cups (500 ml) yogurt
1 teaspoon (5 ml) sesame tahini
1 cup (250 ml) skim milk
    dash freshly grated nutmeg
    mint sprigs or orange slices
        (garnish)

In a saucepan, bring apricots and orange juice to a boil and set aside until apricots are softened. In a blender, combine yogurt, tahini, milk and apricot mixture with a little nutmeg. Process on low speed until smooth. Serve with a sprig of mint or an orange slice.

Blueberry Soup with Yogurt

Makes four servings
2 cups (500 ml) blueberries
¼ cup (60 ml) orange juice
    dash allspice
    dash freshly grated nutmeg
2 cups (500 ml) yogurt
2 thin orange slices, halved

Has a very striking, beautiful appearance and a fresh, sweet taste. Recommended for summertime entertaining.

Mix blueberries, orange juice, allspice and nutmeg in a blender on low speed. Chill in refrigerator. To serve, ladle soup into individual bowls and spoon ½ cup (125 ml) yogurt into the center of each. Garnish with half a slice of fresh orange.

SALADS

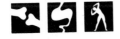

Dairy and Fruit Salad

Makes one serving
¼ cup (60 ml) low-fat cottage
    cheese
¼ cup (60 ml) yogurt
½ banana, sliced
1 large plum, sliced
1 tablespoon (15 ml) wheat
    germ
1 tablespoon (15 ml) bran
    dash cinnamon
    dash freshly grated nutmeg

Try this for breakfast or lunch.

Combine ingredients in a serving bowl. This dish is quite filling, and gives very good protein and calcium values, two nutrients that may be deficient in the diets of people who overdo a reducing regimen.

Variation: An apple, melon or a small peach may be substituted for the plum.

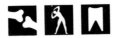

Garden Cottage Cheese Salad

Makes four servings
1 cup (250 ml) cottage cheese
1 stalk celery, finely chopped
1 carrot, grated
1 scallion, finely chopped
2 tablespoons (30 ml) chopped
    walnuts
2 tablespoons (30 ml) minced
    fresh parsley
¼ teaspoon (1 ml) basil
    lettuce leaves

Combine cottage cheese with vegetables and herbs. Serve on a bed of lettuce.

Persian Cucumber Salad

Makes six to eight servings
2 cups (500 ml) yogurt
3–3½ cups (750–875 ml) finely
     chopped cucumbers
1 scallion, finely chopped
1 teaspoon (5 ml) minced
     fresh mint
1 teaspoon (5 ml) minced
     fresh basil
2 tablespoons (30 ml)
     raisins
2 tablespoons (30 ml)
     chopped walnuts

A refreshing salad in summer, and delightful with curried dishes. "Wonderful" was the tasters' verdicts.

Combine ingredients in a large bowl and chill before serving.

Variation: Substitute finely shredded cabbage for the cucumber.

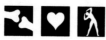

Yogurt-Dill Dressing

Makes 1¼ cups (300 ml)
1 cup (250 ml) yogurt
2 tablespoons (30 ml) fresh
     dillweed
1 tablespoon (15 ml) lemon
     juice
½ small yellow onion or 1
     scallion

A favorite at Fitness House, the health food dining room for Rodale Press employees.

Process ingredients in a blender on medium speed until smooth. Use fresh dillweed and fresh lemon juice for the best flavor. Chill and serve over cooked vegetables or fish.

Rosy Sesame Dressing

Makes ¾ cup (175 ml)
1 tablespoon (15 ml) sesame
     tahini
¾ cup (175 ml) yogurt
1 teaspoon (5 ml) tamari
1 tablespoon (15 ml) tomato
     paste

Beat together the ingredients in a small bowl until well blended. Serve over lightly steamed, chilled vegetables, raw vegetables or on salad. Try it, too, with cold, sliced chicken breast.

Sesame-Tofu Dressing

Makes 1¼ cups (300 ml)
6 ounces (170 g) tofu
2 tablespoons (30 ml) mild
      vinegar
½ teaspoon (2 ml) Dijon-style
      mustard
1 tablespoon (30 ml) sesame
      tahini
1 teaspoon (5 ml) honey

This is a fine dressing for chicken salad or raw vegetable salad.

Place ingredients in a blender and process on medium speed until smooth.

BREADS

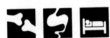

Apricot-Corn Bread

Makes eight servings
¾ cup (175 ml) dried apricots
2 cups (500 ml) whole grain
      cornmeal
1 tablespoon (15 ml) brewer's
      yeast
1 tablespoon (15 ml) lecithin
      granules
1 teaspoon (5 ml) baking soda
1 tablespoon (15 ml) corn oil
1 cup (250 ml) buttermilk
1 cup (250 ml) yogurt
2 eggs, separated

Soak, drain and chop the apricots finely. In a large mixing bowl, combine cornmeal, brewer's yeast, lecithin and baking soda; toss apricots with the dry ingredients. In a separate bowl, combine oil, buttermilk, yogurt and egg yolks. Beat the egg whites until stiff. Add the liquid ingredients to the cornmeal mixture and combine until smooth. Fold in stiffly beaten egg whites. Pour batter into an oiled 8 × 8-inch (20 × 20-cm) baking pan and place in a preheated 350° F. (175° C.) oven for about 25 minutes. Serve hot, or reheat by splitting and toasting corn bread in a broiler.

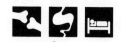

Quick Date Bread

Makes two loaves
5½ cups (1.4 l) whole wheat
     flour
 4 teaspoons (20 ml) baking
     soda
½ cup (125 ml) chopped pitted
     dates
 4 cups (1 l) yogurt or
     buttermilk
¾ cup (175 ml) medium
     unsulfured molasses

A tasty bread that's a good choice for take-along food.

Combine flour and baking soda in a large bowl. Stir in dates. Mix yogurt and molasses together in a separate bowl; then stir into flour mixture.

Place batter in two lightly oiled 8½ × 4½-inch (22 × 11-cm) bread pans. Bake in a preheated 350° F. (175° C.) oven about one hour, or until browned and baked through.

MAIN DISHES

Fish Fillets Florentine

Makes four servings
1 pound (450 g) spinach
2 tablespoons (30 ml) soy oil
4 scallions or 1 small onion,
     chopped
2 tablespoons (30 ml) whole
     wheat flour
½ teaspoon (2 ml) paprika
     dash cayenne pepper
1½ cups (375 ml) skim milk
2 teaspoons (10 ml) tamari
½ cup (125 ml) shredded
     cheddar cheese
1½ pounds (675 g) fish fillets
     (cod, flounder or
     haddock)
½ cup (125 ml) soft whole
     grain bread crumbs

Colorful and appealing, this dressed-up fish entree is also a nutritional star.

Steam spinach until wilted, chop and set aside. In a large skillet, warm the oil, then place the scallions in the pan. Reduce heat and stir until tender.

Add the flour, paprika and cayenne and stir until the onions are coated. Add the milk slowly, stirring, and heat over low flame until thick. Stir in spinach mixture, tamari and cheese, and when cheese is melted, remove from heat.

Arrange fish fillets in the bottom of an 8 × 8-inch (20 × 20-cm) baking dish. Pour spinach sauce over top. Place in a preheated 350° F. (175° C.) oven for 25 to 30 minutes, until the fish is done. Sprinkle with bread crumbs in the final 10 to 15 minutes of baking.

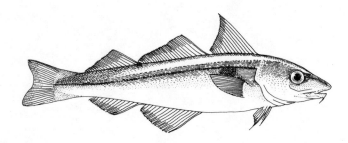

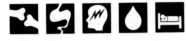

Whole Wheat Crepes with Spinach-Ricotta Filling

Makes 10 crepes

A beautiful balance of flavors, textures and healing nutrients.

Crepes:

2 eggs
2 egg whites
1 tablespoon (15 ml) sunflower oil
1 cup (250 ml) skim milk
⅔ cup (150 ml) whole wheat pastry flour

Filling:

2 cups (500 ml) ricotta cheese (1 pound [450 g])
1 egg, beaten
10 ounces (280 g) spinach, cooked and chopped
¼ cup (60 ml) grated Parmesan cheese
2 tablespoons (30 ml) chopped fresh parsley
¼ cup (60 ml) finely chopped scallions
¼ teaspoon (1 ml) freshly grated nutmeg

Mix the ingredients together with an electric mixer or on medium speed in a blender, processing the batter until completely smooth. Cover, and allow the batter to chill for about two hours before making crepes. Stir again before using.

To make crepes, heat a small, 6-inch (15-cm) skillet and oil lightly. Pour in two to three tablespoons (30 to 45 ml) of batter, and swirl the pan in a circle, gently, to distribute the batter in a thin layer across the bottom of the pan. Cook for about one minute, or until the surface of the crepe appears dry. Remove from the pan and place on a kitchen towel draped over cooling racks.

For the filling, beat ricotta with egg in a medium bowl until light. Add remaining ingredients and beat again until thoroughly combined.

Fill each crepe with about ¼ cup (60 ml) of filling, with uncooked side of the crepe to the outside. Roll like a jelly roll and place seam-side down in a shallow baking dish which has been lightly oiled.

Top, if desired, with a tomato sauce (see *Index* for several suggestions). Bake at 300° F. (150° C.) for 15 minutes, or until heated through. Sauce can also be added at the table.

Better-Than-Lox-and-Cream-Cheese Sandwich

Makes two servings

6 tablespoons (90 ml) *Yogurt Cream Cheese*
4 slices rye bread
7 ounces (198 g) salmon with bones
3 tablespoons (45 ml) *Tofu Mayonnaise*
1 stalk celery, chopped
¼ cup (60 ml) chopped onions
½ tomato, sliced
½ cup (125 ml) alfalfa sprouts

Besides not having nitrites and an overload of salt and fat, this combination gives you calcium from the salmon, the Tofu Mayonnaise, *and the* Yogurt Cream Cheese.

Spread *Yogurt Cream Cheese* on all four pieces of bread. Mix together the salmon, *Tofu Mayonnaise,* celery and onions and spread on two pieces of bread. Place tomato slices on the other two pieces and top with sprouts. Serve open-faced—just because the sandwich is so attractive—but close before eating.

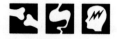

Fancy Stuffed Macaroni Shells

Makes four servings

16 jumbo whole wheat
        macaroni shells
½ cup (125 ml) finely chopped
        celery
 2 tablespoons (30 ml) finely
        chopped onions
 2 cups (500 ml) ricotta cheese
¾ pound (340 g) spinach
 1 clove garlic, minced
 1 egg, beaten
⅛ teaspoon (0.5 ml) oregano,
        crumbled
⅛ teaspoon (0.5 ml) freshly
        grated nutmeg
 1 tablespoon (15 ml) corn oil
 1 tablespoon (15 ml) finely
        chopped shallots
 2 tablespoons (30 ml) whole
        wheat flour
 2 cups (500 ml) *Chicken
        Stock,* milk or
        combination
 2 tablespoons (30 ml) grated
        Parmesan cheese

Cook macaroni shells in a large pot of water until slightly tender, but still firm (al dente). Rinse in cold water, separate and set aside. Steam-stir celery and onion in a few drops of water until translucent. Add ricotta cheese. Steam spinach in water that clings to the leaves after washing, adding garlic to the pot. Chop cooked spinach finely. Stir spinach, egg, oregano and nutmeg into ricotta mixture.

For sauce, place oil in a heated skillet, and saute shallots for one or two minutes. Add flour and stir to coat shallots. Gradually add *Chicken Stock* or milk, stirring after each addition, to make a paste. When all the liquid is incorporated, simmer until thickened.

In an 8 × 8-inch (20 × 20-cm) casserole dish, pour half the sauce. Stuff shells with the ricotta mixture, and arrange in casserole. Pour remaining sauce over shells. Sprinkle with grated Parmesan; cover casserole. Bake in a preheated 375° F. (190° C.) oven for 20 minutes. Remove cover and continue to bake an additional 15 minutes.

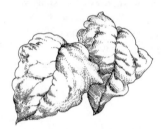

Welsh Leek Tart

Makes six servings

Crust:

- ¾ cup (175 ml) buttermilk
- ¼ cup (60 ml) corn oil
- 1 tablespoon (15 ml) active dry yeast
- 1 teaspoon (5 ml) honey
- 2 tablespoons (30 ml) lukewarm water
- 2 cups (500 ml) whole wheat pastry flour

Filling:

- 6 leeks, chopped
- 2 teaspoons (10 ml) soy or corn oil
- 1½ cups (375 ml) cottage cheese
- 1 egg, beaten
- ¼ cup (60 ml) yogurt
- ¼ cup (60 ml) wheat germ
- ¼ cup (60 ml) minced fresh basil or dillweed
- 1 egg white, lightly beaten

Place buttermilk and oil in a small saucepan and scald. Set aside to cool. In a large bowl, combine yeast with honey and lukewarm water until dissolved. After the milk has cooled to lukewarm, add to yeast mixture. Add to yeast mixture one cup (250 ml) of the flour and stir briskly with a wooden spoon until smooth. Add remaining flour, stirring with the spoon. Place dough in a lightly oiled bowl and set aside in a warm place to rise.

Meanwhile, to make filling, saute leeks in oil until they are slightly tender. Combine sauteed leeks in a large bowl with cottage cheese, egg, yogurt, wheat germ and herbs.

Punch down dough and divide in two. Dust pastry board with flour and roll dough to fit a 9-inch (23-cm) pie plate. Lift carefully into pie plate and press into place. The dough is a little tricky to handle, but is very tender after baking, so just handle gently.

Brush pie shell with beaten egg white. Allow to dry. Fill pie shell with leek mixture. Roll out remaining dough and place over leek filling. Trim edges and crimp to seal. Make several slashes in top crust to allow steam to escape. Bake leek tart in a preheated 350° F. (175° C.) oven for 35 minutes. Serve at room temperature.

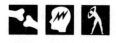

MISCELLANEOUS

Yogurt Cream Cheese

Makes 1½ to 2 cups (375 to 500 ml)
1 quart (1 l) yogurt

Do you adore the taste of cream cheese, but feel queasy about its overwhelming fat content? Here's the answer—surprisingly simple, too. Your taste buds will hardly believe what you're eating has just one-quarter of the calories, one-fifteenth of the saturated fat, but double the calcium of regular cream cheese (when made with low-fat yogurt).

Line a colander with a double layer of cheesecloth or with a linen kitchen towel. Material must be clean and damp. Gently pour the yogurt into the fabric-lined colander. Gather the ends of the fabric together to create a "bag" for the draining yogurt. This can be hung with string from the kitchen faucet or from another spot where it can be left for six to eight hours or overnight. Hang the draining curd over a container, so whey can be saved for use in baking breads or boiling rice.

Note: If using homemade yogurt, chill before making *Yogurt Cream Cheese.* This seems to make the curd more stable, allowing a higher yield.

Garlic-Yogurt Spread

Makes one cup (250 ml)
1 cup (250 ml) *Yogurt Cream Cheese*
2 cloves garlic

A zesty and versatile way to get more calcium.

Place *Yogurt Cream Cheese* in small mixing bowl. Crush garlic in garlic press or with heavy knife handle between two layers of waxed paper. Stir to combine garlic with *Yogurt Cream Cheese.*
Garlic-Yogurt Spread can be used on whole grain crackers, vegetable sticks, or spread on whole wheat bread and placed under the broiler until it begins to brown. Try a tablespoonful (15 ml) tossed with steamed vegetables, or stir some into soups when they are about to be served.

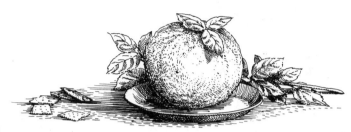

Herbed Cheese Ball

Makes one cup (250 ml)
1 cup (250 ml) ricotta cheese
¼ cup (60 ml) minced fresh
    basil
1 teaspoon (5 ml) dried basil
2 cloves garlic, crushed
1 tablespoon (15 ml) grated
    Parmesan cheese
1 teaspoon (5 ml) kelp powder
3 tablespoons (45 ml) minced
    fresh parsley

Serve with whole wheat crackers for healthful, delicious made-from-scratch party fare!

Combine the ricotta with the basil, garlic, Parmesan cheese and kelp powder. Form into a ball and roll in minced parsley. Delicious with *Sesame Crackers.*

Garlic Dip

Makes one cup (250 ml)
1 cup (250 ml) cottage cheese
2 tablespoons (30 ml) yogurt
1 tablespoon (15 ml) minced
    fresh parsley
1 clove garlic, minced

People really dive for this dip!

Place cottage cheese in a blender with the yogurt and process on medium speed until smooth, or press cottage cheese through a sieve and stir together with yogurt. Combine with remaining ingredients and chill. Serve with raw vegetables such as cauliflower, carrots, celery, broccoli, mushrooms, scallions or Jerusalem artichokes.

Whole Wheat White Sauce

Makes 1¼ cups (300 ml)
2 tablespoons (30 ml) corn oil
3 tablespoons (45 ml) whole
    wheat flour
½ teaspoon (2 ml) brewer's
    yeast
1¼ cups (300 ml) skim milk

Place oil in a medium saucepan over medium heat. Add flour and brewer's yeast and stir together over the heat for two to three minutes. Add the milk slowly, stirring after each addition until mixture is smooth. When the sauce begins to thicken, remove from heat.

Can be used over vegetables or casseroles.

Creamy Tofu Sauce

Makes two cups (500 ml)
2 tablespoons (30 ml) corn oil
2 tablespoons (30 ml) whole
    wheat flour
1 cup (250 ml) *Vegetable Stock*
4 ounces (115 g) tofu

A nondairy alternative to white sauce.

Place oil in a saucepan over medium heat. Add flour and stir over heat for two to three minutes. Add stock slowly, stirring after each addition until mixture is a smooth paste. Simmer two to three minutes. Remove from heat. Break up tofu into blender. Pour hot sauce over tofu and process on low, then medium speed until smooth.

Variation: Add 6½ ounces (184 g) water-packed tuna, drained, and serve over rice or noodles. Add one cup (250 ml) cooked, drained broccoli and one teaspoon (5 ml) basil and serve over fettucini.

Zesty Lemon Sauce

Makes 1¼ cups (300 ml)
½ cup (125 ml) tofu
¾ cup (175 ml) buttermilk
3 tablespoons (45 ml) lemon
    juice
½ teaspoon (2 ml) finely grated
    lemon rind
1 tablespoon (15 ml) sesame
    tahini
½ teaspoon (2 ml) tamari
½ teaspoon (2 ml) Dijon-style
    mustard

A delicious accompaniment to fish cakes or broiled fish. It's flavorful, too, with a baked potato or steamed broccoli.

Combine tofu and buttermilk in a blender and process on low speed until smooth. Add remaining ingredients and blend just until combined.

Onion Sauce

Makes 3½ cups (875 ml)
1 large Spanish onion, chopped
    (about 2 cups [500 ml])
2 teaspoons (10 ml) corn oil
1 tablespoon (15 ml) whole
    wheat flour
1 cup (250 ml) skim milk
1 cup (250 ml) *Chicken Stock*
1 tablespoon (15 ml) sesame
    tahini
½ cup (125 ml) yogurt
    dash freshly grated nutmeg

Adds a special touch to vegetables or chicken.

Saute onion in oil in a large skillet until slightly tender and translucent. Do not brown. Stir in flour and add milk slowly. Stir in *Chicken Stock* and boil 10 minutes. Place tahini, yogurt and nutmeg in blender. Add onion mixture and process on medium speed until smooth.

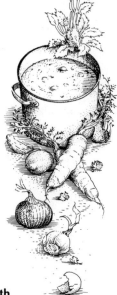

Turkey Broth

Makes two quarts (2 l)
1 carcass from cooked turkey
    breast
3 carrots, chopped
2 stalks celery, chopped
1 yellow onion, chopped
3–4 eggshells, washed
½ cup (125 ml) fresh parsley
3 cloves garlic
1 teaspoon (5 ml) lemon juice
8 cups (2 l) water

This high-calcium broth can be used in soups, stews and sauces or as liquid to cook rice.

Place ingredients in a large stockpot, and cover with the water. Bring to a boil, then lower heat to a gentle simmer. Simmer for about 2 hours.

Strain and cool broth. Refrigerate.

Note: Broths made without salt are subject to more rapid spoilage than those containing salt. Therefore, unless the stock will be used in a day or two, it is best frozen.

BEVERAGES

Banana Curd Shake

Makes one serving
1 very ripe banana, chilled
1 cup (250 ml) yogurt

This is an ever-popular "thick shake" among travelers in Nepal. A thinner mixture results from using a blender, so everyone asks for the beverage to be made by hand, which leaves it so thick it is then eaten with a spoon. Try it for breakfast or a snack!

In a small bowl, mash the banana witha fork. Stir in the yogurt. Place in a glass and serve with a spoon.

Hot Milk Unwinder

Makes one serving
1 cup (250 ml) skim milk
1 teaspoon (5 ml) honey
1 teaspoon (5 ml) wheat germ
½ teaspoon (2 ml) brewer's
    yeast

Place ingredients in a saucepan and heat to just below boiling. Serve in a warmed mug with a spoon.

Frosted Banana Whip

Makes two servings
1 banana, sliced
1 cup (250 ml) buttermilk
1 tablespoon (15 ml) peanut
    butter
1 tablespoon (15 ml) brewer's
    yeast
1 tablespoon (15 ml) wheat
    germ
½ teaspoon (2 ml) *Vanilla
    Extract*
¼ teaspoon (1 ml) cinnamon
2 ice cubes

Looking for potassium, magnesium, calcium, protein and B vitamins? Drink up!

Place ingredients in a blender and process on medium speed until smooth. Serve in chilled glasses.

DESSERT

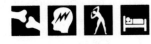

Makes 12 servings

Filling:

  2 cups (500 ml) cottage
      cheese
  1 cup (250 ml) *Yogurt Cream
      Cheese*
  ¼ cup (60 ml) honey
  3 eggs, beaten

Crust:

  ½ cup (125 ml) wheat germ
  2 tablespoons (30 ml) bran
  3 tablespoons (45 ml) corn oil

Topping:

1½ cups (375 ml) *Yogurt
      Cream Cheese*
  ¼ cup (60 ml) honey

Body-Shaper Cheesecake

The high-calcium and low-fat-and-sugar content means a piece of this cake builds up your hipbones instead of your hips.

Combine cottage cheese with *Yogurt Cream Cheese* and honey in a blender; process on low speed until smooth. In a large bowl, fold together the cheese mixture with the eggs. The cottage cheese can also be pressed through a sieve, and combined with the *Yogurt Cream Cheese,* honey and egg. Preheat the oven to 350° F. (175° C.).

For the crust, combine the wheat germ, bran and oil in the bottom of a 9-inch (23-cm) springform pan. Press into bottom and halfway up sides of the pan. Pour cheese mixture into the crust and bake 30 minutes at 350° F. (175° C.). Remove from the oven and be sure to cool for 45 minutes.

Meanwhile, in a medium bowl, stir together the *Yogurt Cream Cheese* and honey for the topping. When the cheesecake has cooled, spread the topping over the surface and return to the 350° F. (175° C.) oven for 30 minutes.

Turn off the oven and let the cheesecake remain inside with door ajar for 30 minutes. Remove from the oven and cool to room temperature. Refrigerate for eight hours before serving.

RECUPERATING FASTER

The injured body has a miraculous power to heal itself but sometimes it seems as though it has forgotten how the miracle works. Bones that should mend, don't. Incisions that should melt into smooth skin remain incisions. Fatigue that should be swept away by sleep refuses to budge. And recuperation that should take a few weeks becomes a major ordeal.

The problem, though, may not be with the miracle so much as the raw materials. Healing is the kind of process that can be brought to a complete halt by a shortage of just *one* of the many components needed to do the job. And supplying all those components is not always the easiest thing in the world. Poor appetite or poor digestion may be a problem. Pain, for instance, can produce stress, which not only burns up extra nutrients but ruins the appetite needed to replace them. Infection can have the same effect. Medication may be making the problem worse yet. The result is that the patient who needs excellent nutritional support the most is usually the same patient who is eating the least. And the result? Well, many of us have seen it in an older relative who has gone through surgery or some other medical treatment, only to grow weaker and weaker instead of stronger and stronger.

Until recently, doctors—by their own admission—paid scant attention to the nutritional situation of their patients. Somehow, they were so engrossed with the more technological side of medical care that they were literally blind to cases of gross malnutrition occurring right under their noses—and in some of the biggest and best hospitals around! Even today, as an increasing number of doctors claim to be more sensitive to nutrition, the responsiblity of providing the raw materials of healing is exclusively yours —especially once you've been discharged from the hospital. Drugs may kill germs that are infecting an incision and preventing healing, but there is no drug yet invented that participates in the actual healing process. The substances involved in healing go by names like vitamin A, vitamin C, protein, zinc—all of them nutrients, all of them found in food.

The recipes we give here are suitable for most cases where very specific instructions have not been given by a physician. Our plan is that food at this time should be considerably higher than usual in protein, iron, zinc, calcium, a wide range of vitamins and—if necessary—calories. Since your appetite during this period is probably something less than boundless, if you want to get substantial amounts of these nutrients, you have to go to foods that contain them in high concentration. Often, that means animal-source foods such as liver, meat, poultry, fish and cheese. It's not that you want a diet full of fat: only that you are *temporarily* willing to exchange a moderate increase in fat content for an increase in nutrients needed *right now* to do an emergency job.

There is another reason for giving more attention than usual to animal-source foods at this time. While certain high-fiber foods, like whole wheat products, may contain goodly amounts of minerals such as iron or zinc, the minerals in these plant foods are not ordinarily absorbed by the body as effectively as minerals from animal sources. You can increase the amount of iron you absorb from vegetable-source foods by making sure to eat a lot of vitamin C foods at the same time, but at present there is no way to insure high absorption of other minerals, such as zinc.

There's no question about it—animal products are important. But what you *don't* want to do is go on a diet consisting almost exclusively of milk and meat. Your elimination function is probably not what it should be at this point either, and if you cut fiber out of your diet completely, you are only going to make matters worse and wind up with a good case of constipation. If you don't have the appetite to eat potatoes, carrots, soybeans, oats, beans and other high-fiber foods, now is the time to make good use of bran. Somewhere between one and three tablespoons a day of this concentrated fiber source, eaten along with plentiful fluids, should take care of any elimination problems.

Many nutrients, as we said, are vital ingredients of the healing process. Here's a quick look at the key components—those that are not only important, but whose shortage in the diet is a real possibility.

Vitamin C. Vitamin C is the chief healing vitamin because it is essential to the manufacture of collagen—a tough, fibrous substance which gives strength to new tissue by cementing cells together. Without collagen, a wound remains just that—a wound. Vitamin C also heals indirectly by encouraging capillaries to renew themselves in the wound area, which brings in more red blood cells, nutrients, and antibodies that fight infectious bacteria. The body's stores of vitamin C are rapidly depleted by disease, injury, stress, fever and infection. The more severe the stress, the faster the rate of depletion. A therapeutic dose of vitamin C is usually considered to be about 500 milligrams, although it could go higher than that in cases of severe injury such as major burns.

Vitamin A. Vitamin A's major role in healing is the maintenance and repair of the epithelium, the very thin tissue that lines organs and covers the body. Vitamin A also influences the rate at which collagen is laid down between cells. Vitamin A deficiency is one of the most common nutritional shortfalls—not only in America but around the world—so it's no wonder that boosting the amount of vitamin A has been shown to speed wound healing.

B Vitamins. The family of B vitamins are involved in many jobs that relate to healing, but the one that needs the most looking after is probably folate. A Danish study showed that of 46 long-term surgical patients in one hospital ward, most were eating very inadequate levels of folate, and only borderline amounts of vitamin B_{12}. Both folate and vitamin B_{12} help maintain the red blood cells which deliver vital nutrients to all parts of the body, including those involved in wound healing. And don't think that the poor intake of folate of those Danish patients was solely a result of the fact that they were eating hospital food. A recent survey of nutritional status of medical patients in one American hospital showed that 69 percent *entered* the hospital with low blood folate levels. But, after two weeks there, even those who were admitted with normal levels left with folate levels almost 50 percent lower. The physicians involved in this study mentioned that multivitamin supplements aren't always the answer either since folate is usually missing from the formula (*American Journal of Clinical Nutrition,* February, 1979). B vitamin tables are included in the chapter Take a Load Off Your Nerves.

Zinc. Until about two years ago, you didn't hear very much about the importance of zinc. One thing that helped bring it to the forefront was the increased use of artificial feeding formulas for patients unable to eat normal food. Over long periods of time, many of these patients developed skin problems and very slow healing of wounds which, we didn't realize till later, were linked to a lack of zinc in this dietary formula.

(continued on page 318)

Selected Good Sources of Vitamin C

Recommended Dietary Allowance (milligrams)		Therapeutic Requirement (milligrams)
60		500–3,000 or more

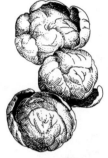

Food	Portion Size	Milligrams
Broccoli raw*	1 small stalk	128
Orange juice	¾ cup	93
Cantaloupe	½ melon	90
Strawberries	½ cup	88
Brussels sprouts cooked	4 sprouts	73
Green peppers raw*	½ cup	64
Cauliflower raw*	½ cup	33
Potato baked	1 large	31
Tomato juice	¾ cup	29
Tomato raw*	1 medium	21
Mung bean sprouts	½ cup	10

*Vitamin C is heat-sensitive and water-soluble; therefore, values for equal amounts of cooked vegetables will be lower than they are for raw vegetables.

Selected Good Sources of Vitamin A

Recommended Dietary Allowance (international units)		*Therapeutic Requirement (international units)*
5,000 (men) *4,000 (women)*		*10,000 (adults)*

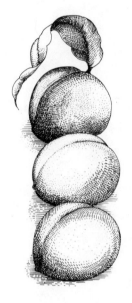

Food	*Portion Size*	*International Units*
Beef liver	3 ounces	45,390
Sweet potato cooked	½ cup	10,075
Cantaloupe	½ melon	9,240
Dandelion greens cooked	½ cup	6,145
Swiss chard cooked	½ cup	4,725
Squash, winter	½ cup	4,305
Beet greens cooked	½ cup	3,700
Broccoli raw	1 small stalk	2,835
Peach	1 medium	2,030
Endive chopped	1 cup	1,650
Tomato juice	¾ cup	1,460
Scallions raw, tops only	¼ cup	1,000

Selected Good Sources of Zinc

Recommended Dietary Allowance (milligrams)		Therapeutic Requirement (milligrams)
15		30

Food	Portion Size	Milligrams
Beef liver	3 ounces	4
Turkey dark meat, without skin	3 ounces	4
Brazil nuts	½ cup	2.4
Turkey light meat, without skin	3 ounces	2
Fish white varieties	6 ounces	2
Wheat germ	1 tablespoon	1
Chick-peas	½ cup	1
Black-eyed peas cooked	½ cup	1

NOTE: Adapted from "Provisional Tables on Zinc Content of Foods," Journal of the American Dietetic Association, April, 1975.

Zinc, we now understand, is one of the most important minerals in the body. It is vital to the whole process by which new cells are produced and protein metabolized for repair of body tissues. In addition, zinc seems to spark the release of vitamin A from the liver and enhances that vitamin's role in healing. A shortage of zinc can also retard the development of the sex organs in young people and diminish the sexual potency of adults.

Iron. Many women, as we saw earlier in this chapter, are deficient in iron. That situation arises from iron losses in menstruation, compounded by a poor intake of iron to begin with. But anyone, of any age, can develop an iron deficiency as a result of losing blood from an injury or surgery. A person with a hearty appetite, particularly a man, might be able to eat his way out of that confrontation with anemia without much trouble. For someone with a lesser appetite, or who has a history of being anemic, however, it's time to get serious about iron. For a table detailing the iron content of foods, see the section on "Energizing Your Blood." In our recipes for people on the mend, we lean heavily on liver because it is far out in front of all other foods as a source of easily absorbed iron.

Calcium. Repeated studies have shown that when people are laid up in bed for a length of time, anything more than a few days, really—they begin to lose calcium in their bones at an astonishing rate. It's difficult to say why this should be so. All we can do is guess that the body is going into a kind of frenzy of negative adaptation. If you aren't going to use your bones to support yourself and move around, it seems to be telling us they'll be recycled. Actually, this tendency is so strong that although you might be able to slow it down by taking in a lot of calcium, you probably can't stop it—at least while you're still laid up. If you are able to move around, do as much walking as you can. Get plenty of calcium from skim milk, skim milk yogurt, tofu, and recipes that incorporate bone meal. For a detailed look at the calcium content of foods, see our earlier section on "Building a Stronger Foundation" in this chapter.

Protein. When the body undergoes an injury, even if that injury is surgery, it temporarily goes into a state called negative nitrogen balance—which is simply another way of saying that it loses protein and no one knows exactly why. When the injury has been stabilized and recuperation begins, the body seems willing to begin putting back the protein it lost. Our job is to make sure it gets the raw materials. Once again, we have a situation where the healthy person with a hearty appetite is going to have no problem getting enough protein, while the person who needs protein the most may have a very poor appetite, or be the kind of person who lives on noodles, tea and dessert.

When you think about protein, don't automatically think steak. Steak, like such other traditional protein sources as whole milk and eggs, contains more fat than you need —even if you're recuperating. You can get plenty of protein from fish and poultry. Ordinarily you can also get plenty of protein from plant-source foods, but if your appetite isn't up to snuff, and you have lost considerable weight during your illness or surgery, you may want to eat one serving a day of a very high-protein food such as chicken, turkey or fish.

It's a good idea to check with your physician to see if he or she has any special instructions or cautions for you about diet during your recuperation. A patient recovering from a serious burn injury, for instance, requires an exceptionally high intake of virtually all nutrients—including calories. But that approach might well be far too high in calories

(continued on page 322)

Selected Dietary Sources of Protein, Listed According to Fat Content

Food	Portion Size	Protein (grams)	Calories	Fat (grams)	Percentage of Total Calories from Fat
Lentils	½ cup	8	106	trace	less than 1
Buttermilk	¾ cup	7	66	0.2	2
Milk					
skim	¾ cup	7	66	0.2	2
Split peas	½ cup	8	115	0.3	2
Cottage cheese					
dry-curd	½ cup	12	63	0.2	2
Brewer's yeast	1 tablespoon	3	23	0.1	4
Lima beans					
fresh, cooked	½ cup	6.5	95	0.5	4
Navy beans	½ cup	7.5	112	0.5	4
Kidney beans	½ cup	7	109	0.5	4
Shrimp	10 large	14	67	0.6	8
Scallops	6 ounces	35	169	2	11
Turkey					
light meat, without skin	3 ounces	28	150	3	18
Chicken					
light meat, without skin	3 ounces	26	147	3.8	23
Cod	6 ounces	49	288	9	28
Yogurt					
skim-milk	1 cup	8	123	4	29
Sirloin steak					
trimmed of fat	6 ounces	55	352	13	33
Haddock	6 ounces	34	282	11	35
Flounder	6 ounces	51	342	14	36
Turkey					
dark meat, without skin	3 ounces	26	173	7	36
Tuna					
packed in oil, drained	½ cup	23	158	6.5	37
Halibut	6 ounces	43	288	12	38
Soybeans	½ cup	10	117	5	38
Ham					
lean, trimmed of fat	3 ounces	25	184	8.5	41

Selected Dietary Sources of Protein, Listed According to Fat Content (continued)

Food	Portion Size	Protein (grams)	Calories	Fat (grams)	Percentage of Total Calories from Fat
Beef liver	3 ounces	22	195	9	42
Chicken dark meat, without skin	3 ounces	23	174	8.3	43
Ground beef lean	3 ounces	23	186	10	45
Yogurt whole-milk	1 cup	7	152	8	47
Milk whole	6 ounces	6	119	6	48
Salmon sockeye	3 ounces	23	188	10	48
Sardines	4	12	96	5	49
Prime rib of beef trimmed of fat	3 ounces	24	205	11.4	50
Pork chops	3 ounces	26	229	13.1	51
Tofu (soybean curd)	4 ounces	9.5	86	5	52
Mackerel	6 ounces	37	402	27	60
Ground beef regular	2.9 ounces	20	235	17	65
Egg hard-cooked	1 large	6.5	82	6	66
Cheddar cheese	1 ounce	7	113	9	72
Sirloin steak not trimmed of fat	6 ounces	39	658	54	74
Corned beef	3 ounces	21	337	28	75
Salami	3 1-ounce slices	15	264	22	75
Bologna	3 1-ounce slices	10	258	23	80
Prime rib of beef, not trimmed of fat	6 ounces	34	748	67	81
Sausages	3 1-ounce links	7	186	17	82
Hot dogs	2	14	352	32	82

or fat for someone on the mend after gallbladder surgery (an overly rich diet probably contributed to the gallbladder troubles in the first place). And the person whose broken hip kept him in bed for several weeks should be consuming a lot more calcium than the person with a broken arm, because bed rest causes calcium to be lost from the body—in this case, just when it's needed most!

BREAKFASTS

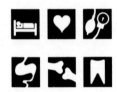

Makes about five cups
(1.25 l)
¾ cup (175 ml) sunflower seeds
½ cup (125 ml) slivered
   Blanched Almonds
¼ cup (60 ml) pumpkin seeds
2 cups (500 ml) rolled oats
1 cup (250 ml) wheat germ
1 tablespoon (15 ml) bone
   meal
½ cup (125 ml) bran
8 medium dried figs
16 small dried apricots
3 tablespoons (45 ml) brewer's
   yeast flakes

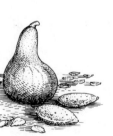

Royal Elizabethan Breakfast

We made this for our friend Liz when she was recuperating and needed something special to perk up her appetite, rev up her sluggish digestion and get the healing process rolling.

Ordinarily we avoid toasting the ingredients in our muesli-type granola mixtures, but this is a special case, designed to be tasty enough to be eaten even by someone not particularly interested in food (but in serious need of fiber and good nutrition). Of course, you don't have to be recuperating to enjoy this breakfast, which is rich in vitamins A, B complex, vitamin E, iron, magnesium, phosphorus, potassium, zinc, polyunsaturated oils, protein and fiber. The oil-rich seeds and nuts pack a considerable caloric punch as well, but when this breakfast is eaten with low-fat milk and fresh fruit, the caloric density is greatly reduced.

The first thing we want to do is toast the sunflower seeds and almonds. Turn your oven on to "broil" and cover a tray with aluminum foil. Distribute the sunflower seeds and almonds over the foil and place on the next-to-the-top rung. Once the broiler is on full blast, the toasting will only take about two or three minutes, but you must watch the tray at all times. Leave the oven door open a generous crack so you can watch. Just before the almonds and sunflower seeds are done, they will turn a golden brown. A wonderful aroma will begin to fill the kitchen (and drift through the whole house as well). Remove the nuts and seeds from the broiler immediately and let cool.

Pumpkin seeds, probably because of their flat shape, seem to toast much faster than sunflower seeds, and will explode with a loud *pop* in less than a minute under a hot broiler, so they can't be toasted at the same time you're browning the seeds and nuts. However, if you wish to give them a light toasting separately, you can, but be prepared to remove them as soon as you hear the first pop or two.

While the almonds and sunflower seeds are cooling, pour the required amounts of oats, wheat germ, bone meal, bran and pumpkin seeds into a large bowl. Put the figs on a cutting board, remove their stems, and slice into small pieces. Slice the apricots, and then add both fruits to the bowl of grains. Mix in the sunflower seeds, almonds and pumpkin seeds and stir well.

We've saved the step of adding the yeast flakes until last, because depending on how the taste strikes you, you may want to use slightly more or less than our recipe calls for. Note that we're using yeast *flakes* here, rather than brewer's yeast powder. Yeast flakes have a much less potent taste. Most people learn to enjoy the taste of yeast flakes quite rapidly, and the taste seems to blend especially well with this breakfast mixture.

When all the ingredients are mixed, store in a container in the refrigerator until ready to use. Serve with milk, or milk plus yogurt, and top with fresh fruit such as sliced apples, bananas or berries.

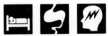

High-Protein Buttermilk Pancakes

Makes two to three servings

1 cup (250 ml) whole wheat flour

2 tablespoons (30 ml) soy flour

2 tablespoons (30 ml) wheat germ

1½ teaspoons (7 ml) *Baking Powder*

1 egg

1 egg white

1¼–1½ cups (300–375 ml) buttermilk

1 tablespoon (15 ml) medium unsulfured molasses

Combine the flours, wheat germ and *Baking Powder* in a large bowl. In a separate bowl, beat egg and additional white together, then add one cup (250 ml) of buttermilk and the molasses. Beat until combined.

Stir egg mixture into the dry ingredients just until combined. If batter is too stiff, add a little additional buttermilk.

On a hot, lightly oiled griddle or skillet, cook the pancakes in any desired size. Turn over when bubbles appear on the uncooked surface.

Serve with fresh fruit or a fruit sauce.

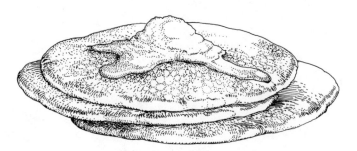

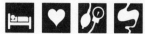

Apricot-Brown Rice Cereal

Makes two servings
1¾ cups (425 ml) water
½ cup (125 ml) brown rice
¼ cup (60 ml) soy flakes
¼ cup (60 ml) chopped dried
    apricots
1 tablespoon (15 ml) sesame
    seeds

Place all ingredients in a saucepan and bring to a boil over medium heat. Stir, reduce heat to low, and simmer with lid on for 25 to 30 minutes, until water is absorbed and rice is tender. Do not stir.

Serve hot, as is, or with some orange juice instead of milk.

SOUPS

T.L.C. Chicken Soup

Makes eight servings
1 chicken, cut up, with skin
    removed
3–4 medium onions, chopped
2 carrots, sliced
8 cloves garlic, minced
8 cups (2 l) water
½ cup (125 ml) brown rice
2 tablespoons (30 ml) minced
    fresh parsley
¼ teaspoon (1 ml) cayenne
    pepper
4 teaspoons (20 ml) tamari

The tender loving care in this soup not only eases a cold but gives you nourishment and healing factors when you're on the mend from just about anything.

Place the chicken pieces, onions, carrots, garlic and water in a large kettle. Bring to a boil, reduce heat, and simmer.

After 50 minutes, add the rice, parsley and cayenne. Simmer an additional 30 to 40 minutes, until the rice is cooked. Stir in the tamari at the end of cooking.

To prepare for serving, allow the soup to cool somewhat, then remove the bones from the chicken, returning the chicken meat to the soup. Reheat soup before serving. Makes about 10 cups (2.5 l), with bones removed.

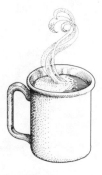

Tuna Chowder

Makes six to eight servings

1½ cups (375 ml) diced celery
3 cups (750 ml) diced potatoes
1 cup (250 ml) diced onions
1 clove garlic, minced
3 cups (750 ml) *Chicken Stock* or *Vegetable Stock*
2 bay leaves
1 tablespoon (15 ml) minced fresh parsley
1 teaspoon (5 ml) basil, crumbled
½ teaspoon (2 ml) paprika
6 ounces (170 g) tofu
6½ ounces (184 g) water-packed tuna, drained

This can be a main course, served with a crisp salad and Whole Wheat Popovers.

In a large skillet or saucepan, steam-stir celery, potatoes, onions and garlic in a small amount of water until onion is translucent. Add stock, bay leaves and seasonings. Bring to a boil, reduce heat, and simmer until potatoes are just tender. Remove bay leaves. Place tofu in a blender, add two cups (500 ml) of soup, and process on low speed until smooth. Return tofu-soup mixture to pan and add drained tuna. Stir until heated through. Serve hot.

BREADS

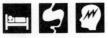

Banana Bread

Makes one loaf

¼ cup (60 ml) medium unsulfured molasses
3 tablespoons (45 ml) corn oil
1 teaspoon (5 ml) baking soda
¼ cup (60 ml) yogurt
2 eggs, beaten
1½ cups mashed bananas
½ teaspoon (2 ml) cinnamon
1 teaspoon (5 ml) brewer's yeast
1¾ cups (425 ml) whole wheat flour
½ cup (125 ml) bran
½ cup (125 ml) walnuts, chopped

Combine molasses and oil in a large mixing bowl. Dissolve the baking soda in the yogurt and add with eggs to molasses mixture. Add remaining ingredients and stir until combined. Place batter in a lightly greased 8½ × 4½-inch (22 × 11-cm) bread pan. Bake in a preheated 350° F. (175° C.) oven one hour. Remove from pan and cool on a rack before slicing.

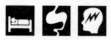

New England Blueberry Muffins

Makes one dozen
1½ cups (375 ml) whole wheat
    pastry flour
2½ teaspoons (12 ml) *Baking*
    Powder
½ cup (125 ml) wheat germ
½ cup (125 ml) bran
2 tablespoons (30 ml) lecithin
    granules
1 cup (250 ml) walnuts, chopped
1 cup (250 ml) blueberries
¾ cup (175 ml) buttermilk or
    yogurt
2 eggs, beaten
⅓ cup (80 ml) maple syrup
1 tablespoon (15 ml) sesame
    tahini

Besides being packed with fiber, these big muffins are bursting with luscious blueberries and crunchy walnuts.

Combine the dry ingredients, including nuts and blueberries. Beat together buttermilk with eggs, syrup and tahini. Stir into dry ingredients just enough to moisten; some lumps can remain. Divide batter between 12 muffin cups. Bake in a preheated 400° F. (200° C.) oven for 20 to 25 minutes, or until golden brown.

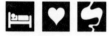

Holiday Fruit 'n' Nut Bread

Makes one loaf
2 cups (500 ml) whole wheat
    flour
2 tablespoons (30 ml) lecithin
    granules
2 teaspoons (10 ml) *Baking*
    Powder
2 teaspoons (10 ml) brewer's
    yeast
2 teaspoons (10 ml) cinnamon
½ teaspoon (2 ml) mace
¼ cup (60 ml) corn oil
¼ cup (60 ml) honey
½ cup (125 ml) yogurt
2 eggs, beaten
1 teaspoon (5 ml) tamari
1 cup (250 ml) chopped pitted
    dates
½ cup (125 ml) walnuts, chopped
2 teaspoons (10 ml) grated
    orange rind

A good Christmas gift idea—a lot healthier than fruitcake.

In a medium mixing bowl, combine the dry ingredients. In a larger bowl, place oil, honey, yogurt, eggs and tamari. Stir to combine. Stir dates, walnuts and orange rind into the liquid ingredients. Add the dry ingredients to the egg mixture slowly, stirring after each addition.

Lightly oil an 8½ × 4½-inch (22 × 11-cm) bread pan. Pour batter into bread pan and bake in a preheated 325° F. (165° C.) oven for about an hour, or until a cake tester comes out clean.

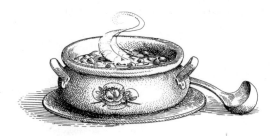

MAIN DISHES

Four-Star Beef Stew

Makes eight servings
1½ pounds (675 g) beef cubes
½ cup (125 ml) whole wheat
    flour
2 tablespoons (30 ml) corn oil
1 yellow onion, chopped
1 clove garlic, crushed
2 cups (500 ml) *Vegetable
    Stock*
4 cups (1 l) Italian plum
    tomatoes with juice
¼ teaspoon (1 ml) rosemary,
    crushed
¼ teaspoon (1 ml) oregano
½ teaspoon (2 ml) thyme
½ teaspoon (2 ml) marjoram
½ teaspoon (2 ml) basil
1 cup (250 ml) mushrooms,
    quartered (about ¼
    pound [115 g])
5 carrots, cut in thick slices
6 white onions, halved
2 sweet red peppers
1 cup (250 ml) broccoli florets
¼ cup (60 ml) minced fresh
    parsley or chives

Here's a truly delicious version of beef stew in which the meat is both taste-complemented and health-balanced by onions, garlic, carrots, peppers and even broccoli.

Trim all visible fat from the meat, dry, and dredge in the flour. In a large, heavy-bottom saucepan, brown the beef cubes in the oil over high heat. Do not have more than one layer on the bottom of the pan while browning the meat.

When all the meat has been browned, place it in the large pot with the chopped onion and saute briefly until the onion begins to grow translucent. Then add the garlic, *Vegetable Stock,* tomatoes and seasonings, except for parsley. Bring to a boil. Reduce heat, cover, and simmer slowly for one hour, stirring occasionally.

Add the mushrooms, carrots and the white onions. Simmer an additional 45 minutes.

Seed and slice the red peppers lengthwise into thin pieces. If the pepper slices are too long to be easily managed for eating, cut them in half. Add the red peppers to the stew after 1½ hours of cooking. Fifteen minutes after adding the red peppers, stir in the separated broccoli florets.

Cook stew an additional 10 to 15 minutes, just until the broccoli is tender but still bright green.

Remove from heat, stir in minced fresh parsley or chives, and serve. A crisp salad and bread or popovers hot from the oven make excellent accompaniments.

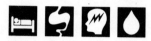

Vegetable Meatloaf

Economical and healthfully robust—a good family dish.

Makes six servings

1 small onion, finely chopped
2 cups (500 ml) shredded
    carrots
1 cup (250 ml) chopped
    mushrooms (about ¼
    pound [115 g])
2 stalks celery, finely chopped
1 pound (450 g) lean ground
    beef
1 egg
1 cup (250 ml) soft whole grain
    bread cubes
1 cup (250 ml) rolled oats
¼ cup (60 ml) skim milk
3 tablespoons (45 ml) tomato
    paste
2 teaspoons (10 ml) tamari
2 teaspoons (10 ml) oregano
2 teaspoons (10 ml) basil
1 teaspoon (5 ml) marjoram
½ teaspoon (2 ml) thyme

Place the onion, carrots, mushrooms, and celery in a heavy skillet; add a few tablespoons (50 ml) of water, and steam-stir until the vegetables are soft and the water has evaporated. Set aside.

In a large mixing bowl, combine the ground beef, egg, bread cubes, oats, milk, two tablespoons (30 ml) of the tomato paste, and the herbs. Add the vegetables and stir together.

Place the mixture in a two-quart (2 l) oven casserole, and glaze the surface with the remaining tomato paste. Bake in a 350° F. (175° C.) oven for one hour.

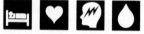

Baked Chicken Breasts with Raisin Stuffing

Makes four servings

2 cups (500 ml) soft whole
    grain bread cubes
2 stalks celery, finely chopped
1 scallion, minced
¼ cup (60 ml) raisins
2 tablespoons (30 ml) walnuts,
    chopped
1 egg, beaten
⅓ cup (80 ml) skim milk
½ teaspoon (2 ml) basil
¼ teaspoon (1 ml) thyme
2 whole chicken breasts,
    skinned

In a medium bowl, combine bread cubes with celery, scallion, raisins and walnuts. Stir together egg with skim milk in a separate bowl. Combine with bread cube mixture and season with basil and thyme.

Divide stuffing between chicken breasts, holding in place with aluminum foil over opening. Place chicken breasts in a lightly oiled shallow baking dish and cover loosely with aluminum foil to keep meat moist. Bake in a preheated 350° F. (175° C.) oven about one hour, until chicken is tender.

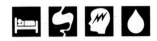

Roasted Turkey Breast with Apple and Prune Stuffing

Makes four servings

1 whole turkey breast (about 4
  pounds [1.8 kg])
3 cups (750 ml) soft whole
  grain bread cubes
1 cup (250 ml) chopped
  unpeeled apple
1 stalk celery, chopped
½ cup (125 ml) chopped,
  cooked prunes
¼ cup (60 ml) walnuts, chopped
1 egg, beaten
¼ cup (60 ml) skim milk
½ teaspoon (2 ml) finely grated
  orange rind
¼ teaspoon (1 ml) thyme
¾ cup (175 ml) *Chicken Stock*
  or *Vegetable Stock*

Clean turkey breast and remove skin.

Combine bread cubes, apple, celery, prunes, walnuts, egg, milk, orange rind and thyme. Mix thoroughly. Stuff into breast cavity, and place aluminum foil over the stuffing and halfway up the sides of the breast.

Place breast right side up in a shallow baking dish and baste lightly with stock. Place in a preheated 350° F. (175° C.) oven. Bake about 30 minutes per pound (450 g) including stuffing, or until meat is tender. Baste occasionally with stock. To serve, slice meat from turkey breast and place on a warmed serving platter with the stuffing. There will probably be leftover turkey meat.

Try with *Cranberry-Stuffed Sweet Potatoes.*

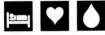

Apple-Chicken Casserole

Makes two servings

3 unpeeled tart apples, cubed
½ cup (125 ml) yogurt
1 chicken breast, skinned and
  split
1 orange

Place apples in the bottom of a lightly oiled casserole dish, pour yogurt over them and stir lightly to combine. Place chicken breast halves over apple-yogurt mixture. Cut unpeeled orange into thin slices, and place these over the chicken breasts to keep chicken from drying out. Bake in a preheated 350° F. (175° C.) oven for 1¼ hours. Remove orange slices before serving.

Savory Chicken Curry

Makes four servings
2 whole chicken breasts,
   skinned and split
¼ cup (60 ml) whole wheat
   flour
2 teaspoons (10 ml) corn oil
1 finely chopped shallot
   (optional)
¼ cup (60 ml) finely chopped
   onions
½ cup (125 ml) finely chopped
   green peppers
1 clove garlic, minced
2–4 teaspoons (10–20 ml) curry
½ teaspoon (2 ml) thyme
1 teaspoon (5 ml) kelp
   powder
2 cups (500 ml) cooked
   tomatoes
3 tablespoons (45 ml) currants

If you've never had curry, here's a good introduction. Go easy on it the first time out.

Dredge chicken breast halves in flour and place in the oil in a hot skillet. Brown chicken, turning several times. If desired, you may add the shallot toward the end of the browning period to give the chicken additional flavor. Remove the chicken from the skillet and place in a casserole dish. In the skillet, simmer the onions and green peppers in the remaining oil, adding a few drops of water if necessary to prevent scorching. When onion is translucent, add garlic and seasonings, stirring until all are combined. Add tomatoes and simmer two to three minutes, stirring constantly. Pour the sauce over the chicken in the casserole dish. Bake in a preheated 350° F. (175° C.) oven about 45 minutes, until the chicken is tender. Add the currants during the last 5 to 10 minutes of cooking. Serve over boiled brown rice.

Herbed Fish Stuffing

Makes 1½ cups (375 ml)
2 tablespoons (30 ml) chopped
   shallots
1 teaspoon (5 ml) corn oil
1 egg
½ cup (125 ml) chopped celery
   with leaves
½ cup (125 ml) fresh parsley
¼ cup (60 ml) watercress leaves
¼ teaspoon (1 ml) basil
1 cup (250 ml) soft whole grain
   bread crumbs
2 tablespoons (30 ml) walnuts,
   crushed

Tasty, yet subtle enough so that it will not overpower the delicate flavor of fish.

Saute the shallots in the oil, adding a few drops of water if necessary to prevent scorching. When the shallots are transparent, remove them from the heat and cool slightly. Place the shallots in a blender with the remaining ingredients, reserving ½ cup (125 ml) of bread crumbs and the walnuts. Process on medium speed until smooth. With a fork, stir in the remaining bread crumbs and nuts.

Makes four servings
1 pound (450 g) haddock
 fillets
1½ cups (375 ml) *Herbed Fish
 Stuffing*
2 cups (500 ml) *Cauliflower
 White Sauce II*
2 tablespoons (30 ml) grated
 Parmesan cheese

Stuffed Haddock Fillets au Gratin

Separate haddock fillets into four servings. Place some of the *Herbed Fish Stuffing* on half of each serving and either roll or fold the fillets, with stuffing in center. Place the stuffed fillets into a casserole dish and cover with *Cauliflower White Sauce II.* Cover loosely with aluminum foil. Place casserole dish in a preheated 350° F. (175° C.) oven and bake 30 to 40 minutes, just until fish is flaky and opaque. Remove foil. Sprinkle with grated Parmesan and broil until the top begins to brown.

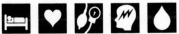

Makes three servings
1 pound (450 g) fish fillets
 (cod, flounder or
 haddock)
1 tablespoon (15 ml) cider
 vinegar
1 tablespoon (15 ml) honey
2 tablespoons (30 ml) tomato
 paste
2 tablespoons (30 ml) finely
 chopped onions
¼ cup (60 ml) water

Saucy Fish Fillets

No one will ever accuse you of serving bland fish if you give them this dish.

Place the fish fillets in a single layer in the bottom of a shallow, 8 × 8-inch (20 × 20-cm) ovenproof dish. Combine the remaining ingredients in a small saucepan, and bring to a boil over medium heat. Pour the sauce over the fish, and place casserole in a preheated 350° F. (175° C.) oven for about 25 minutes, or just until the fish is opaque and cooked through.

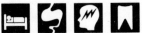

Makes three servings
½ pound (225 g) whole wheat
 pasta
¼ cup (60 ml) olive oil
2½ cups (625 ml) coarsely
 chopped mushrooms
 (about ½ pound
 [225 g])
½ cup (125 ml) walnuts,
 chopped

Mushroom-Walnut Sauce with Whole Wheat Pasta

Place the pasta in a large kettle half-filled with boiling water. Bring the pasta to a boil, stir, reduce heat, and simmer until the pasta is tender, yet still a bit chewy.

Meanwhile, heat oil in a heavy skillet, and add the mushrooms. Saute until the mushrooms have released their juices and the juices have nearly evaporated. Stir in walnuts briefly and remove from heat.

When pasta is done, drain and toss with the sauce.

SIDE DISHES

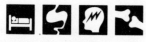

Rice Waffles

Makes four servings
1 cup (250 ml) whole wheat
    flour
2 teaspoons (10 ml) baking
    soda
½ cup (125 ml) cooked brown
    rice
1 egg, beaten
1¼ cups (300 ml) buttermilk
2 tablespoons (30 ml) corn oil
1 tablespoon (15 ml) medium
    unsulfured molasses

Combine the flour and baking soda in a medium bowl, and add remaining ingredients. Heat a waffle iron and pour batter.

These waffles can be served for breakfast, topped with applesauce or fresh fruit. They are also delicious as a light luncheon meal topped with *Creamed Fish and Pimiento.*

Steamed Stuffed Potatoes

Makes four servings
4 potatoes
2 tablespoons (30 ml) *Yogurt
    Cream Cheese*
1 egg yolk
½ teaspoon (2 ml) fresh
    dillweed or fennel, or
    pinch of basil
1 teaspoon (5 ml) grated
    Parmesan cheese

Steam potatoes until tender. Cut in half and remove center, leaving enough potato next to skin to allow the jacket to keep its shape. Press the potato that was removed from the skins through a sieve, then mash with *Yogurt Cream Cheese* and egg yolk. Add herb seasoning.

Place the filling in the potato jackets and sprinkle with grated Parmesan. Bake in a moderate oven, about 350° F. (175° C.), until the tops begin to brown. Serve hot.

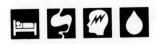

MISCELLANEOUS

Fabulous Date Bars

Makes 1½ dozen
⅓ cup (80 ml) soy oil
1 egg, beaten
2 tablespoons (30 ml) honey
1 tablespoon (15 ml)
    blackstrap molasses
1 teaspoon (5 ml) finely grated
    lemon and/or orange
    rind
1 teaspoon (5 ml) *Vanilla*
    Extract
1 cup (250 ml) pitted dates,
    chopped
1 cup (250 ml) rolled oats
½ cup (125 ml) whole wheat
    flour
½ cup (125 ml) wheat germ
2 tablespoons (30 ml)
    brewer's yeast
1 teaspoon (5 ml) cinnamon
¼ teaspoon (1 ml) cardamom
¼ teaspoon (1 ml) ginger
⅛ teaspoon (0.5 ml) allspice
⅛ teaspoon (0.5 ml) freshly
    grated nutmeg
⅔ cup (150 ml) buttermilk
1½ teaspoons (7 ml) baking
    soda
½ cup (125 ml) walnuts,
    chopped
¼ cup (60 ml) sunflower seeds

These make super high-energy, high-nutrition snacks at home or on the road. Just make sure you don't eat them all 15 minutes after you leave home!

In a large mixing bowl, combine the oil with the egg, honey and molasses. Stir in the grated rind, *Vanilla Extract* and dates.

In a medium bowl, combine the oats, flour, wheat germ, brewer's yeast and spices. Measure out buttermilk into a small bowl and add baking soda, stirring until the soda is dissolved.

Add the dry ingredients to the oil and egg mixture, alternating with the addition of the buttermilk. Beat while adding ingredients until they are blended. Spread the batter in a lightly oiled 15 × 10-inch (38 × 25-cm) baking pan. Sprinkle with the walnuts and raw sunflower seeds, pressing these down a bit into the batter.

Bake in a preheated 325° F. (165° C.) oven for 25 minutes, or until done. Cut into bars.

Peanut Sauce

Makes two servings
1 cup (250 ml) *Vegetable Stock*
4 tablespoons (60 ml) peanut
    butter
½ teaspoon (2 ml) tamari
1 clove garlic, crushed
¼ cup (60 ml) finely chopped
    green peppers

Combine ingredients in a saucepan and simmer over medium heat until pepper is tender, about 10 to 15 minutes.

Serve over vegetables or combination rice and vegetable dishes.

Stuffed Prunes

Makes four servings
¼ cup (60 ml) cottage cheese
1 tablespoon (15 ml) walnuts,
    chopped
dash cinnamon
12 soft or soaked pitted prunes
lemon slices (garnish)
mint sprigs (garnish)

Stuff prunes and serve as a tempting appetizer, dessert or luncheon snack.

Combine cottage cheese and walnuts, add a dash of cinnamon, and stuff prunes. Place on a serving dish and garnish with lemon slices and mint sprigs.

Tofu-Banana-Peanut Spread

Makes one cup (250 ml)
6 ounces (170 g) tofu
2 tablespoons (30 ml) peanut
    butter
½ banana
1 teaspoon (5 ml) lemon juice
dash cinnamon

Try this unique version for your next peanut butter sandwich.

Combine ingredients in a blender and process on low speed until smooth.

Banana-Date-Nut Spread

Makes ¾ cup (175 ml)
1 small or ½ large banana
¼ cup (60 ml) pitted dates
¼ cup (60 ml) walnuts

Place ingredients in a blender and process on low speed until smooth. Store unused portion in the refrigerator.

Date-Nut-Raisin "Jam"

Makes ¾ cup (175 ml)
¼ cup (60 ml) pitted dates
¼ cup (60 ml) walnuts
¼ cup (60 ml) seedless raisins
2 tablespoons (30 ml) orange
juice

A spread that's packed with nutrition and flavor.

Combine ingredients in a blender, and process on low speed until smooth, stopping the blender to scrape down the sides of the blender jar, as necessary. Store in the refrigerator.

Fresh Applebutter

Makes ¾ cup (175 ml)
1 medium unpeeled apple,
chopped
¼ cup (60 ml) pitted dates
1 tablespoon (15 ml) walnuts
1 tablespoon (15 ml) apple
juice
dash cinnamon

Place ingredients in a blender and process on low speed until smooth, stopping the blender to scrape down the sides of the container, as necessary. Store in the refrigerator.

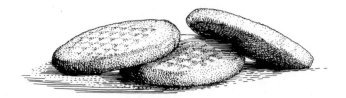

Peanut Butter Cookies

Makes three dozen
1¾ cups (425 ml) whole wheat
pastry flour
2½ teaspoons (12 ml) *Baking
Powder*
½ cup (125 ml) honey
¼ cup (60 ml) sesame tahini
2 tablespoons (30 ml) corn oil
½ cup (125 ml) peanut butter
1 large egg, beaten

Combine flour and *Baking Powder.* Cream together honey, tahini, oil, peanut butter and egg. Add to dry ingredients. Using a tablespoon, take pieces of dough, roll into balls, and place on a lightly oiled baking sheet. Using a fork, press dough flat, leaving a crosshatch design in the cookie. Bake cookies in a preheated 350° F. (175° C.) oven 8 to 10 minutes.

Carob Syrup

Makes 1¾ cups (425 ml)
1 cup (250 ml) water
1 cup (250 ml) carob powder
¼ cup (60 ml) honey or
medium unsulfured
molasses
½ teaspoon (2 ml) *Vanilla Extract*

Coat fresh fruit chunks for a fondue-style dessert.

In a medium saucepan, place the water and stir in carob powder until blended. Add honey and bring to a boil. Simmer about five minutes, or until syrup is smooth. Remove from heat and stir in *Vanilla Extract.*

Carob Syrup can be used to add flavor to milk, either hot or cold. Just stir in two tablespoons (30 ml) per cup (250 ml), or more to taste.

Keep tightly covered in the refrigerator.

Blanched Almonds

Makes one cup (250 ml)
1 cup (250 ml) shelled almonds

Put about two inches (5 cm) of water in a medium pan and bring to a rolling boil. Toss in the almonds and immediately remove from the heat. Two or three minutes later, pour off the hot water, rinse once with cold water and drain.

Freeing the almonds of their skins will now be very easy. Grasp the blunt end of the nut between your thumb and forefinger and squeeze sharply. This will cause the almond to literally jump out of its skin and into your waiting hand. In two or three minutes, all your almonds will be peeled.

Variation: For slivered almonds, choose a knife with a good heavy blade. Divide each almond in half along the split; this can be done by hand. Place each half flat-side down and cut into about five slivers. This is facilitated by putting the point of the knife about five inches (13 cm) in front of the almond and guiding the blade so that the thick, bottom part of the blade does the slicing.

To toast, place the almond slivers on a cookie sheet. Place under the broiler—a good distance away so that the almonds will not scorch—and toast just until lightly golden. This will take only a minute or two, and the almonds must be carefully watched. Or, place cookie sheet in a 350° F. (175° C.) oven and bake, stirring occasionally, just until the almonds are golden.

Sesame Milk

Makes three cups (750 ml)
¼ cup (60 ml) unhulled sesame
    seeds
3 cups (750 ml) water
2 tablespoons (30 ml) honey

A refreshingly different beverage which can be used as a substitute for cow's milk in recipes, beverages or on cereal.

Blend sesame seeds and water in a blender on medium, then high speed for two minutes. Strain the hulls from the milk by pouring through several layers of cheesecloth. Return the milk to the blender and process with honey on medium speed until combined. Refrigerate.

DESSERTS

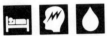

Peanut Butter Pie

Makes 10 servings

Filling:
2 eggs
1 pound (450 g) tofu
¼ cup (60 ml) medium
    unsulfured molasses
¾ cup (175 ml) peanut butter
1 banana

Crust:
1 cup (250 ml) whole wheat
    pastry flour
¼ cup (60 ml) soy oil
2 tablespoons (30 ml)
    buttermilk

Place eggs, tofu and molasses in a blender and process on low speed until smooth. Place in a large bowl. Blend peanut butter and banana on low speed until smooth. Combine thoroughly with tofu mixture.

In a 9-inch (23-cm) pie plate, place the flour, oil and buttermilk. Toss with a fork until combined, then press into the pie plate for crust.

Pour the peanut mixture into the pie crust. Bake in a preheated 350° F. (175° C.) oven for 20 to 25 minutes, until top is slightly browned.

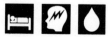

Orange-Almond Cake

Makes 12 servings

2 large oranges, preferably seedless naval variety
¾ cup (175 ml) ground almonds
¼ cup (60 ml) ground sunflower seeds
½ cup (125 ml) whole wheat pastry flour
1½ teaspoons (7 ml) baking soda
3 eggs
2 egg whites
½ cup (125 ml) honey
1 teaspoon (5 ml) *Vanilla Extract*

Orange marmalade-lovers will go nuts over this one!

Place the oranges in a large pot with enough water to cover. Bring to a boil, then reduce heat and simmer 30 minutes.

Meanwhile, in a large bowl, combine the almonds and sunflower seeds with the flour and baking soda. (To grind your own nuts and seeds, place in a blender and process with short bursts at high speed until powdery.)

In a medium bowl, beat the eggs with the additional egg whites, and add the honey and *Vanilla Extract.*

When the oranges are finished cooking, remove from water and chop them, peel and all, removing any seeds. Place the chopped oranges, a little at a time, in a blender and process on low speed just until finely chopped. They should not be too smooth. Stir the orange into the egg mixture, then combine with the dry ingredients in the large bowl.

Place the batter in a lightly oiled 9-inch (23-cm) springform pan, and bake in a preheated 375° F. (190° C.) oven one hour or more, until firm. Turn off the oven, open the door and allow to cool slowly. Remove from oven and remove ring from springform pan. Serve cake at room temperature or chilled. This cake is so rich-tasting that no frosting is needed.

Note: The cake can be decorated with orange slices, if desired.

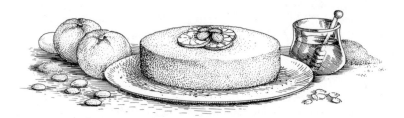

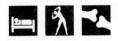

Baked Apple Custard

Makes four servings
1 unpeeled apple, finely
    chopped
3½ cups (875 ml) water
¼ teaspoon (1 ml) cinnamon
1½ cups (375 ml) skim milk
1 egg
1 egg white
2 tablespoons (30 ml) maple
    syrup or honey
½ teaspoon (2 ml) *Vanilla*
    Extract
dash freshly grated nutmeg

Cook the chopped apple about five minutes in ½ cup (125 ml) of water in a small saucepan. Drain and toss with cinnamon in the pan. Divide apple between four custard cups. (Custard can also be baked in a pie plate, placing the cooked apple in the bottom.)

Place milk in saucepan and heat over medium heat. Beat egg and egg white with maple syrup or honey in a medium bowl. When milk is hot, not boiling, stir ½ cup (125 ml) of the milk into the egg mixture, then add remaining milk. Stir in *Vanilla Extract*.

Divide the custard between the four cups. Sprinkle each with a dash of freshly grated nutmeg.

Bring three cups (750 ml) of water to a boil. Place the boiling water in an 11 × 8-inch (28 × 20-cm) baking pan. Place custard cups in the water, which should come halfway up the sides. Place baking pan with custard cups into a preheated 325° F. (165° C.) oven and bake about one hour, or until a knife inserted in the center comes out clean.

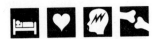

Stovetop Rice Pudding

Makes six servings
2 cups (500 ml) cooked brown
    rice
3 cups (750 ml) skim milk
½ cup (125 ml) raisins
3 tablespoons (45 ml) honey
1 teaspoon (5 ml) *Vanilla*
    Extract
¼ teaspoon (1 ml) cardamom

Mix the ingredients, except *Vanilla Extract,* together in a large saucepan. Bring to a boil, reduce heat and simmer about 30 minutes, stirring often, until pudding has begun to thicken. Remove from heat, add *Vanilla Extract* and cool; chill before serving.

Chapter 8

Healthier Teeth and Gums

If you have problems in your mouth, chances are that it isn't with cavities. No matter how many cavities you had as a youngster, the rate at which you developed new ones probably dropped off dramatically in your early 20s. By 25 or 30, a new cavity is a rare occurrence for most people. Curiously, the reason why this is so remains a mystery.

It's no mystery to dentists, though, that just about the time you stop getting cavities, you become vulnerable to something far more serious—periodontal disease. Gums that were once pink, firm and stippled become whitish, puffy and smooth. They may bleed when you brush, or become inflamed with gingivitis. They may also recede, exposing more and more of the teeth as the years go by—a common happening which gave rise to the colloquial phrase "long in the teeth" as a synonym for advanced age. Finally, the teeth begin to fall out.

Maybe we shouldn't have said "finally," because tooth loss is not the last step. For millions of people, it's only the beginning of more aggravation. Because even if a set of dentures fits beautifully at first, it's likely that it won't after a while. One national health survey found that almost 30 percent of denture wearers thought their appliances either "needed refitting or that they needed new dentures."

The problem is not that the dentures change their shape in time. It's the *wearer* who's changing. "In a great percentage of denture wearers, the jawbone keeps shrinking away," says Kenneth E. Wical, D.D.S., chairman of the removable prostodontics department at Loma Linda University School of Dentistry in California. "Some dentists accept this shrinkage as normal, but it probably isn't normal at all," he told us.

"As the jawbone grows smaller, it becomes more difficult for these people to wear their dentures. Some have gradually lost half of their original jawbone or even more. Eventually they reach the point where they can no longer wear their dentures. There's nothing left for the denture to fit around!"

Rather than being the last straw, though, what we're onto here may well be a clue to preventing, or at least minimizing, the whole nasty process of periodontal disease from the word go.

Long before people even think about the possibility of dentures, some very knowledgeable experts in the field believe, they begin to lose bone from their jaws. In women, you may remember from our earlier discussion of osteoporosis, this loss of bone begins at age 25. For some reason, the crests of the jawbone are hit the hardest by this loss. And the erosion of those crests, the scientists believe, in a sense paves the way for future periodontal disease. Although the teeth are not directly connected to the jawbone, they are anchored in it. When that anchorage begins to drift away, the teeth become loose and wobbly, and damage the surrounding gums in such a way as to invite inflammation.

Lennart Krook, D.V.M., Ph.D., of Cornell University, one of the major authorities in this field, and several of his colleagues, have some interesting experimental data to back up this theory. First, they noticed that of 10 people they examined with periodontal disease, 9 had an estimated daily calcium intake of 400 milligrams or less—far below the Recommended Dietary Allowance of 800 milligrams. When the patients were given 500 milligrams of extra calcium twice a day for six months, remarkable reversals in the disease process were noted. "All patients had gingivitis and bleeding at the start," the scientists said. "After treatment, inflammation was improved in all cases and absent in three. Calculus [mineral deposits] was reduced in half the cases. Pockets along the roots were recorded in 8 patients before the study. Pocket depth was reduced in all cases after treatment. Tooth mobility was likewise recorded in 8 patients. It was reduced in 7 patients, and in 1 there was no mobility after treatment."

Of special interest was the fact that x-rays taken after calcium supplementation showed the appearance of *new bone* in the jaw. Instead of continuing to shrink away from the teeth, the jawbone was actually laying down new growth (*Cornell Veterinarian,* January, 1972).

Your first dietary step to putting a stop to periodontal disease, therefore, is to substantially increase the amount of calcium in your diet. Skim milk, low-fat yogurt and low-fat cheese are excellent calcium sources. Broccoli is an exceptionally fine vegetable source of calcium. (For a list of good food sources of calcium, see the *Index.*)

As we noted earlier in our discussion of osteoporosis, most primitive people throughout the world actually supplement their regular food with calcium in one form or another, such as bones, lime or culinary ash. Therefore, we feel it is not only reasonable, but entirely natural for us to do the same, using tablets of bone meal, dolomite or calcium carbonate. There is very little difference between that and the Navajo Indian custom of eating certain berries which contain a core of practically pure calcium. It's likely that you'll have to use supplements in one form or another, because adding 1,000 milligrams of calcium to your diet, as was done in the study described, may not be all that easy unless you have a big appetite. Of course, you could always bulk up on cheese, but you'd be getting a lot more calories and fat than are good for you.

Vitamin C is also extremely important in controlling periodontal disease and other problems with the mouth. For one thing, it seems to help calcium do its job of halting the loss of bone. Animal studies at the Harvard School of Dental Medicine showed that vitamin C can inhibit bone shrinkage by 50 percent or more. But vitamin C does a lot more for your mouth. Dental scientists have pointed out that the plaque that develops in the gum crevice "constitutes one of the most dense concentrations of bacteria to which man is exposed." Dominick T. DePaola, D.D.S., Ph.D., and Michael C. Alfano, D.M.D., Ph.D., recommend that this bacterial mass be cleaned away in order to prevent or arrest the development of periodontal disease. But beyond that, nutrition is an important factor in protecting against the destructive effects of plaque. They note that the cells lining the gum crevice have one of the highest turnover rates in the body —completely renewing themselves every three to seven days. This thin lining or epithelial tissue is in what they call "a continuous critical period."

"Nutritional stress during this period may impair the renewal of the epithelium and compromise its barrier function," they warn. "Animal studies from our laboratories have indicated that an acute deficiency of vitamin C almost doubles the ease with which bacterial toxins can penetrate the tissues of the mouth. More recently, we have noted similar effects on permeability caused by zinc and protein deficiencies" (*Nutrition Today,* May/June, 1977).

Vitamin C is also essential to construct the protein fibers, called collagen, which actually connect the teeth to the jawbone. When Irish scientists supplemented the diet of patients with 1,000 to 3,000 milligrams of vitamin C a day for five months, they noticed a marked improvement in periodontal health.

The importance of vitamin C and other nutrients for older people is emphasized by Maury Massler, D.D.S., of the College of Dentistry at the University of Illinois, in an article entitled "Oral Aspects of Aging" (*Postgraduate Medicine,* January, 1971). Dr. Massler points out, for instance, that a number of reports indicate that vitamin C—150 to 200 milligrams a day—given before and after oral surgical procedures "promotes healing and seems to reduce the postoperative morbidity." Dr. Massler also feels that a sufficiency of A and B vitamins is important in maintaining the health of oral tissues, especially since the thin epithelial layer covering them progressively thins with advancing age, so that they are very easily scraped, cut and otherwise injured.

Aside from vitamins and minerals, the general health of the gums can be improved tremendously by eating a diet with more crunch. The gums need the massaging effect these harder foods have in order to keep from getting soft, spongy and ready for a bout of gingivitis. But as our diet has come to include more and more processed foods, it has also become softer. Hard crusty bread has been replaced with something that resembles absorbent cotton. Peanut butter steps in for peanuts. Almonds are ground into flour for cakes. Apples are mashed into applesauce or baked into pies and pastries. Carrots are used raw largely as garnishes; as vegetables, most people cook all the crunch out of them while some "health food" people juice them. And in many homes, a good chew on a bone is so passé that even Fido has to be content with a rawhide imitation.

Dr. Massler makes the interesting observation that the shrinking of our jaw-bones as we grow older may be a result not only of insufficient calcium to balance what we lose every day in our bodily functions, but of a lack of *use* as well. That makes a lot of sense, we think. It's well known that exercise in general is an enormous help in enabling the body to retain calcium and keep the bones strong. It's also known that the best kind of exercise for this purpose is that which causes the feet to come into forceful contact with the ground, as in walking. It seems that the actual, physical shock, or perhaps certain very subtle electrical changes that take place in the body as a result of these impacts, encourages bone to stay put. It's a message that the bone is needed, appreciated, and our bodies seem to listen. Lie in bed day after day during a long convalescence and you will lose bone strength at an absolutely frightening rate.

Now, think what happens when the jawbone becomes invalided, so to speak, by not being able to crunch against nuts, seeds, hard raw vegetables and bones. Maybe that's part of the story behind the fact that the jawbone loses its mass faster than any other part of the body.

A vicious cycle effect is operating here, too. When the gums are tender, and bleed easily, or when ill-fitting dentures are worn, those hard crunchy foods disappear from the diet. The result is that the gums become even weaker.

How do you break out of this cycle? Simple—you've got to go ahead and bite the bullet or, at least, the apple. It's the same thing that happens when you take your periodontal disease to the dentist. Before they get better, your gums will get a little worse, or at least feel that way. When your teeth are cleaned and flossed, your gums will probably bleed if you have gingivitis. And when you are taught the proper way to brush your teeth, that may also cause them to bleed. But only for a few days. As we mentioned before, the outer cells covering the gums are replaced by new generations every few days, and those new generations get the message to shape up very quickly indeed.

The foods you want to be eating now include fresh crisp apples, carrots, celery, radishes, artichokes, water chestnuts, green peppers and nuts. Don't eat all of them the first day, of course. Begin gradually with a raw apple or two every day and a few radishes, cucumber slices, bean sprouts and brown rice. Soon you'll be in good enough shape to tackle raw celery, and even something *really* crunchy like raw broccoli and cauliflower.

If you have been on a severely restricted reducing diet, or if you are convalesc-ing you may also want to pay attention to getting plenty of protein and zinc into your diet as well. They are crucial for healing *any* part of the body. Lots of good recipes for these elements are given in the chapter Getting Stronger Every Day, under the section on "Recuperating Faster."

THE NATURAL WAY TO PREVENT CAVITIES

So far we haven't said anything much about cavities except that most people stop getting them when they're around 25 or so. But maybe you still get more than you want to. Or your children do. In any case, you might be surprised by what we're going to say about them.

Most of us have been led to believe by an unceasing barrage of propaganda that the way to prevent tooth decay is through dental hygiene. And we understand that old-fashioned, rather moralistic phrase to mean brushing and flossing our teeth with religious fervor, drinking fluoridated water and making regular visits to a dentist who will scrape, drill and generally clank around in our mouths until our jaws ache. He'll probably shoot a few x-rays while he's at it, just to make sure we don't have cancer of the teeth. If that sounds a little disrespectful, it's because we believe the whole idea to be false and misleading.

That's right, we're saying people don't have to go through all that rigmarole to prevent tooth decay any more than they need a travel agent to get to work in the morning.

Does that sound hard to believe? Well, look at it this way: if that were *not* the case, then people in relatively remote parts of the world, who have no toothbrushes, no toothpaste, no fluoridated water, no dentists and no x-ray machines ought to have an enormous number of cavities. People in England, Canada, the United States and other countries, who *do* have all those things, ought to have remarkably few cavities. But in fact, *the exact opposite happens to be the case.*

About half a century ago, an energetic and idealistic dentist by the name of Weston A. Price, D.D.S., spent an incredible amount of time traveling around to remote and not-so-remote corners of the world looking into people's mouths, noting the presence of dental pathology, and studying the local eating habits. He studied the inhabitants of the South Pacific, Eskimos, African tribesmen, Swiss villagers and many others. He even examined teeth in the skeletons of American Indians. He recorded his findings in a massive tome with the awesome title of *Nutrition and Physical Degeneration* (new edition by Price-Pottenger Foundation, 1970). Reading that book is like plowing through a year's worth of *National Geographics,* with every article in every issue devoted to teeth. But what the dedicated Dr. Price found, in a nutshell, is that societies that do not consume sugar, candy, cake, jam, canned food and other typically Western staples have an extremely low rate of tooth decay. A tremendous number of individuals Price examined had no signs of decay whatsoever. In many cases, whole tribes had an average number of decayed teeth amounting to less than one per person. He also discovered, conversely, that those societies in a transitional period of being Westernized had a higher rate of tooth decay, while those who regularly ate food and snacks imported from the more industrialized countries had an extremely high rate of tooth decay.

Further, it didn't seem to matter much what these various peoples ate in the way of staples. Whether their diet was based on rice, corn, millet, fish, vegetables, or dairy products and meat, they still had excellent dental health as long as their food was natural, whole, fresh and relatively unprocessed.

Today, although people with such unspoiled diets are becoming increasingly harder to locate, the same rule holds true. People who don't eat junk food don't get cavities. They may not have *beautiful* teeth, because they may be worn down by years of chewing very coarse grains or using their teeth as tools. Occasionally they break a tooth. And yes, they often have food debris in their mouths, but it rarely seems to lead to tooth decay. There are exceptions, of course, but that is the general rule recognized by dental scientists—even though your friendly neighborhood dentist may be more interested in caps, crowns and canals than the international epidemiology of tooth decay.

Let's admit though, that very few of us escaped our share of Tootsie Rolls and Mars Bars while we were growing up, and few of us are going to completely avoid occasional dietary lapses in the future. As far as our children are concerned, we all know that no matter how careful we are with them at home, there's no way we can prevent them from getting their share of junk food when they're away from the house. So to be realistic, we are firmly in favor of proper brushing and flossing and dental checkups, although we draw the line at mandatory water fluoridation and routine x-rays. The point we wish to make is that the most logical and important single step to prevent or reduce tooth decay is eating a proper diet. All the rest is strictly *secondary* prevention, something that's done *after* disease-causing foodstuffs have been permitted to enter the mouth.

Yes, disease is an appropriate word for cavities, or caries as dentists prefer to call them. These products of decay and rot are no more natural or minor than erosions of other parts of the body, such as bedsores or ulcers. They represent the invasive destruction of an important part of the body, which can be disfiguring and disabling. Tooth decay and periodontal disease together, in fact, are the most common disease in the world, even though most people don't think of it that way. And its cause, overwhelmingly, is poor diet.

While the clearest revelations come from comparisons of our own society with those which eat no processed foods at all, there are a number of studies showing that consumption of certain kinds of foods is associated with a greater number of cavities. In an article entitled "Snack Food Intake of Adolescence and Caries Development" appearing in the *Journal of Dental Research* (June, 1977), it's mentioned that foods linked to tooth decay when eaten in large amounts include such items as candy (chocolate candy in particular), cakes, buns and chewing gum. Foods linked with a *low* incidence of cavities when eaten in relatively large amounts include apples, vegetables, berries, fish, bread and cereal.

Let's not forget that the teeth of these young people we are talking about are still developing, and adequate calcium is essential to the development of strong teeth. So are other nutrients, notably magnesium and protein. A young person who avoids milk and won't eat yogurt or cheese should probably be getting some bone meal on a daily basis, as it may be difficult to fulfill calcium requirements with fruits and vegetables. Various nuts and beans are good sources of both magnesium and protein.

Some Japanese dental scientists believe that soybeans, in addition to all the other good things they do for us, also help prevent tooth decay. In an experiment conducted at Tokyo Medical and Dental University, laboratory animals developed fewer cavities when the soybean content of their diet was increased. When researchers studied dental decay in two Japanese villages—one noted for its large consumption of tofu (made from soybeans) and another known for its seaweed consumption—they found that over a four-year period, the villagers eating tofu had much less tooth decay, even though they were very lax about dental hygiene. The scientists attribute the decay-preventing power of the soybean to its content of the amino acid glycine (*Vigor/Sokai,* July, 1979).

Another factor frequently implicated in tooth decay is between-meal snacks. When sweet, mushy food is not rubbed away from the teeth and gums by other foods, or washed out of the mouth with beverages, it begins to ferment and produce the right conditions for cavity development. That only seems to apply, though, to foods that aren't all that good in the first place. Many of the people studied by Dr. Price nibbled on food all day long, yet had no cavities.

The great majority of recipes in this book are perfectly appropriate for most people with periodontal or decay problems. Go light on any dishes that are mushy, sticky, or lack some good honest crunch. Crispy salads with plenty of peppers and carrots, high in vitamins C and A, will do wonders for your gums. The recipes containing bone meal—including those given in the section on osteoporosis (see *Index*) and those which follow—will supply goodly amounts of extra calcium. Lightly cooked or sprouted soybeans deliver protein, the glycine valued by the Japanese scientists, magnesium, B vitamins and good firm texture. A handful of unsalted peanuts would make an excellent snack. If your teeth seem weak or brittle, however, go easy on nuts and seeds. You don't want to take a chance on breaking a tooth. Instead, fresh green peppers, apples, lightly steamed carrots and breakfast cereals made with moistened flakes of oats, wheat and soy, along with fresh fruit, will give your gums plenty of vitalizing massage.

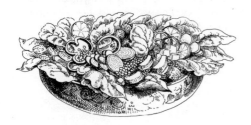

BREAKFASTS

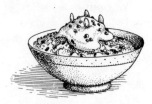

Mat's Himalayan Muesli

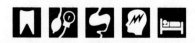

Makes one serving
1 unpeeled apple
1 banana
2 tablespoons (30 ml) raisins
½ cup (125 ml) rolled oats
2 tablespoons (30 ml) wheat
  germ
1 teaspoon (5 ml) bran
½ cup (125 ml) yogurt
1 tablespoon (15 ml) walnuts,
  chopped
4 almonds

Trekking in the Himalayas, Sharon's husband was served a muesli made with apples, papayas and bananas, topped with yogurt and sprinkled with peanuts. Once home, he began experimenting and produced the following formula for a mountainous breakfast with about 600 calories.

Cube apple and banana into a large cereal bowl. Sprinkle with raisins, oats, wheat germ and bran. Spoon yogurt over top and sprinkle with the walnuts. Decorate with the almonds, standing them on end in the yogurt.

Hawaiian Brunch

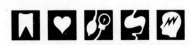

Makes six servings
2 cups (500 ml) rolled oats
½ cup (125 ml) wheat germ
¼ cup (60 ml) sunflower seeds
¼ cup (60 ml) pumpkin seeds
¼ cup (60 ml) walnuts, chopped
  skim milk
  yogurt
  chopped pineapple

Crunchy, creamy and juicy all at the same time, and packed with zinc, fiber and other goodies.

Combine dry ingredients in a bottle, shake well to distribute, and keep in refrigerator until ready to use. (Or keep on shelf if you don't add the wheat germ until serving time.) When serving, add a small amount of milk, just enough to moisten the mix, then top with yogurt in center of bowl. Ring the yogurt with the pineapple, and let stand a minute or two before eating, to let some pineapple juice soak into the oats.

SALADS

Tossed Green Salad with Toasted Sesame Seeds

Makes four servings
4 cups (1 l) loosely packed
    spinach leaves
2 cups (500 ml) loosely packed
    lettuce leaves
½ cup (125 ml) sliced unpeeled
    Jerusalem artichokes or
    zucchini
½ cup (125 ml) thinly sliced
    unpeeled carrots
¼ cup (60 ml) mung bean
    sprouts
1 tablespoon (15 ml) sesame
    seeds
Vinaigrette Dressing

Thoroughly wash the spinach, and rinse and separate lettuce leaves. Tear both into large pieces.

Combine the spinach, lettuce, artichokes, carrots and sprouts. In a small, heavy skillet, toast the sesame seeds briefly over medium heat, until they begin to turn golden. Sprinkle over the salad, then add dressing to taste and toss.

Stuffed Pears with Pineapple

Makes four servings
2 ripe pears
½ cup (125 ml) low-fat cottage
    cheese
2 tablespoons (30 ml) finely
    chopped pineapple
2 tablespoons (30 ml) walnuts,
    chopped
    lettuce leaves
    mint sprigs or walnut halves
    (garnish)

Cut pears in half lengthwise, and remove seeds, leaving a generous cavity for stuffing.

In a small bowl, combine the cottage cheese with the pineapple and walnuts. Divide the cheese mixture between the four pear halves, filling the cavities and spreading over the cut surfaces of the pears.

Serve on a bed of lettuce leaves, garnished with mint or walnut halves. If necessary, remove a slice from the rounded side of the pear halves so that they rest securely on the salad plates.

Cheese-Stuffed Pears

Makes four servings
2 ripe pears
½ cup (125 ml) cottage cheese
1 tablespoon (15 ml) shredded
    Swiss cheese
2 tablespoons (30 ml) walnuts,
    chopped
lettuce leaves

Cut pears in half lengthwise, and remove seeds, leaving a generous cavity for the stuffing.

Combine the cottage cheese with the Swiss cheese and walnuts. Divide the cheese mixture between the four pear halves, filling the cavities and spreading over the cut surfaces of the pears.

Serve on a bed of lettuce leaves. If necessary, remove a slice from the rounded side of the pear halves so that they rest securely on the salad plates.

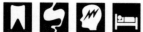

Cottage Cheese Salad with Apple and Raisins

Makes four servings
1 cup (250 ml) cottage cheese
1 carrot, shredded
1 unpeeled apple, chopped
2 tablespoons (30 ml) raisins
2 tablespoons (30 ml) walnuts,
    chopped
lettuce leaves

Combine the cottage cheese with the carrot, apple, raisins and walnuts. Serve on a bed of lettuce leaves.

Carrot-Raisin Salad

Makes four servings
3 medium carrots
¼ cup (60 ml) raisins
¼ cup (60 ml) sunflower seeds
1 tablespoon (15 ml) lemon
    juice
3 tablespoons (45 ml) *Tofu
    Mayonnaise*
lettuce or spinach leaves

Scrub, but do not peel carrots. Grate and combine in a large bowl with raisins and sunflower seeds. Toss with lemon juice, add *Tofu Mayonnaise,* and toss again to combine. Serve chilled on lettuce or spinach leaves.

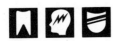

Creamy Fruit Salad

Makes four servings

¼ cup (60 ml) sunflower seeds
2 oranges, chopped
1 pear, cubed
1 unpeeled apple, cubed
2 pitted dates, chopped
¼ cup (60 ml) walnuts, chopped
2 tablespoons (30 ml) currants
2 tablespoons (30 ml) wheat germ
⅔ cup (150 ml) yogurt
1 tablespoon (15 ml) sesame tahini (optional)

Toast the sunflower seeds over low heat in a heavy skillet without oil. Stir to prevent scorching. Combine with remaining ingredients in a large bowl. If sesame tahini is used, combine with the yogurt before pouring over the fruit.

Variation: Try persimmons, pineapple, melons, figs, raisins, strawberries, grapes, apricots, peaches, tangerines or other fruit.

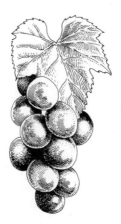

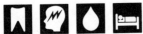

Chicken-Grape-Walnut Salad

Makes two servings

1 cup (250 ml) skinned, cubed chicken breast
½ cup (125 ml) seedless grapes, halved
½ cup (125 ml) chopped celery
¼ cup (60 ml) walnuts, broken
Tofu Mayonnaise
lettuce or spinach leaves

Combine the chicken, grapes, celery and walnuts in a serving bowl, toss with *Tofu Mayonnaise,* and chill. Serve on lettuce or spinach leaves as a luncheon salad.

Variation: Try the chicken salad with bean sprouts, water chestnuts or chopped cucumbers in place of celery, or try pineapple and sunflower seeds in place of grapes and walnuts.

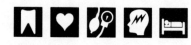

Makes six servings
2½ cups (625 ml) cooked
      brown rice, chilled
½ cup (125 ml) walnuts,
      chopped
1 cup (250 ml) diced
      pineapple
¾ cup (175 ml) pitted cherries
      with juice
¼ cup (60 ml) sunflower seeds
1 cup (250 ml) yogurt
½ teaspoon (2 ml) cinnamon

Rice 'n' Fruit Jubilee

Looking for a fast salad to go with a main dish that already has green veggies in it? Try this one.

Combine ingredients in a large bowl and serve.

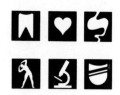

Makes four servings
4 cups (1 l) loosely packed
      spinach leaves
½ cup (125 ml) *Mushrooms
      Italian-Style*
½ cup (125 ml) chopped
      broccoli florets
1 carrot, sliced
¼ cup (60 ml) sliced *Blanched
      Almonds*
1 cup (250 ml) alfalfa sprouts
1 large tomato, cut into 8
      pieces
2 scallions, chopped

Herbed Mushroom Salad

Place spinach leaves in a salad bowl and decorate with concentric rings of the other ingredients. Make the mushrooms the center of attention.

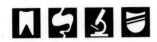

Pepper Cabbage

Makes six servings
2½ cups (625 ml) shredded
    cabbage
1 carrot, shredded
1 green pepper, finely
    chopped
1 stalk celery, finely chopped
¼ cup (60 ml) *Tarragon
    Vinegar*
¼ cup (60 ml) water
1 tablespoon (15 ml) honey

    Combine shredded and chopped vegetables in a large serving bowl. Mix *Tarragon Vinegar,* water and honey together in a jar or small bowl. Pour over cabbage mixture and toss. Refrigerate until the flavors blend, stirring occasionally. Makes about 3½ cups (875 ml).

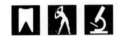

Cauliflower Salad

Makes four servings
½ medium head cauliflower
2 tablespoons (30 ml) *Tarragon
    Vinegar*
2 teaspoons (10 ml) sesame oil
1 teaspoon (5 ml) basil
2 scallions, chopped
2 tablespoons (30 ml) yogurt
1 tablespoon (15 ml)
    watercress, minced

    Break cauliflower into florets. Steam very lightly, only three to four minutes, so cauliflower retains some crispness. Combine steamed cauliflower with remaining ingredients in a large bowl while hot; allow to cool, then chill before serving.

BREADS

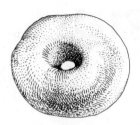

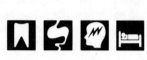

Reformed Bagels

Makes about 16 bagels
1 medium unpeeled potato,
     cubed
1½ cups (375 ml) water
2 tablespoons (30 ml) active
     dry yeast
1 teaspoon (5 ml) blackstrap
     molasses
1 egg
1 cup (250 ml) wheat germ
4 cups (1 l) whole wheat flour
     whole grain cornmeal
     Yogurt Cream Cheese

Love bagels but feel guilty eating white flour? Sink your teeth into these chewy, healthier bagels and enjoy with an easy conscience.

In a small saucepan boil the potato in 1½ cups (375 ml) water until tender. Process cooked potato plus water in a blender on low speed. You should have 2 cups (500 ml) of potato-water mixture; add water, if necessary. While the potato-water mixture is still warm, place in a large mixing bowl and add yeast and molasses. When yeast has dissolved, beat in egg and wheat germ.

Add flour ½ cup (125 ml) at a time, beating batter until smooth after each addition. Knead in remaining flour as dough becomes too firm to beat. Sprinkle flour on kneading surface, and work dough for 5 to 10 minutes.

Let rise in a lightly oiled bowl in a warm place until doubled in bulk. Punch down, knead briefly, and return covered dough to warm place until it has doubled again. Turn dough onto lightly floured surface. Knead and divide dough into 16 pieces. Roll each piece into a "rope" about five to six inches (13 to 15 cm) long, with tapered ends overlapped to make a circle.

Allow bagels to rest while a large kettle of water is brought to the boil. Drop bagels five or six at a time into the boiling liquid. After the bagels have come to the surface, allow them to boil a minute or two, then turn them over and boil two or three minutes longer. Remove the bagels with a slotted spoon and allow to drain on a cake rack which has been covered with a paper towel.

Place bagels on a lightly oiled cookie sheet that has been dusted with whole grain cornmeal and bake at 400° F. (200° C.) for 40 minutes, or until golden brown.

Spread with *Yogurt Cream Cheese,* maybe adding a little crushed garlic.

Whole Wheat Popovers

Makes one dozen
1 cup (250 ml) whole wheat
    flour
1 teaspoon (5 ml) honey
1¼ cups (300 ml) skim milk
1 teaspoon (5 ml) soy or corn
    oil
3 eggs

A delicious accompaniment to vegetarian stews, fish chowder and soup and salad meals.

Combine the flour, honey, milk and oil by beating with a spoon in a large bowl or processing in a blender on low speed. Beat the eggs with an electric mixer or by hand and fold into the flour mixture. (Air must be incorporated into the eggs for rising of the popover, so they must not be processed in a blender.)

When ready to bake, divide the batter between 12 muffin cups which have been lightly oiled. Place the popovers in a cold oven, turn the heat to 425° F. (220° C.), and bake for 45 to 50 minutes. If the popovers become too dark, turn the oven down to 350° F. (175° C.) after 30 minutes. (You should have a glass window for determining this, because opening the oven door before the end of the baking time will cause the popovers to fall.)

Serve the popovers immediately. To prevent them from becoming soggy, cut a small gash in the top of each, and pull slightly open to allow the steam to escape.

Crackling Brown Rolls

Makes 16 rolls
3 cups (750 ml) whole wheat
    flour
1 tablespoon (15 ml) active dry
    yeast
½ cup (125 ml) bran
2 tablespoons (30 ml) wheat
    germ
2 tablespoons (30 ml) lecithin
    granules
1 teaspoon (5 ml) bone meal
2 cups (500 ml) cottage cheese
¼ cup (60 ml) safflower oil
¼ cup (60 ml) water
1 teaspoon (5 ml) honey
1 egg, beaten
    whole grain cornmeal
    skim milk
    sesame seeds

Stir together one cup (250 ml) of flour with yeast, bran, wheat germ, lecithin granules and bone meal in a large mixing bowl. Combine cottage cheese, oil, water and honey in a medium saucepan. Place over moderate heat, and stir until mixture is lukewarm. Add to the dry ingredients and add egg. Beat on low speed with an electric mixer, scraping sides of bowl, until ingredients are thoroughly combined. Then beat on high speed for three minutes. Stir in the remaining two cups (500 ml) of flour by hand. Turn dough onto a lightly floured surface, cover with inverted mixing bowl, and allow to rest for 10 minutes. Shape into 16 balls and place 1½ to 2 inches (4 to 5 cm) apart on a cookie sheet that has been liberally sprinkled with cornmeal. Brush rolls with milk and sprinkle with sesame seeds. Cover and let rise in a warm place until double in bulk, about 30 to 45 minutes. Bake the rolls at 350° F. (175° C.) for about 20 minutes, until brown.

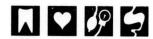

Pita Bread

Makes one dozen
1 tablespoon (300 ml) active dry yeast
1¼ cups lukewarm water
1 tablespoon (15 ml) corn oil
3–3½ cups (750–875 ml) whole wheat flour

While they are baking, these breads puff up, forming a pocket into which you can stuff your favorite sandwich combinations.

Dissolve the yeast in lukewarm water. Add oil and two cups (500 ml) of the flour. Beat until the dough is smooth. Add the remaining flour as you knead the bread in the bowl. Place dough on a well-floured surface and knead in some additional flour until the dough is firm. Rub the mixing bowl with some oil and return the dough to the bowl, turning to coat the dough with oil on all sides.

Let dough rise in a warm place until double in bulk. Punch down the dough and divide it into 12 equal pieces. Form the dough into balls and allow these to rest for at least 10 minutes. Cover with waxed paper or a tea towel to prevent them from drying out.

Roll out the balls until they are about ⅛ to ¼ inch (3 to 6 mm) thick and about 4½ inches (11 cm) in diameter. If rolled to a larger diameter, the rounds may not puff all the way to the edges.

For the pitas to bake properly, the heat source must be directly beneath the bread. If you have an electric oven, this might mean removing the top heating element. These are usually removable for cleaning. Bake the bread on the lowest rack. In a gas oven, raise the racks and place the baking sheet directly on the oven floor.

Bake in the bottom of a preheated 450° F. (230° C.) oven for five minutes, then open oven, place breads on a higher rack, and leave in the open oven for three to five minutes until the breads have puffed and begin to brown.

As they emerge from the oven, wrap the loaves in a slightly damp tea towel, cool, then store in the refrigerator. Do not allow the breads to become soggy.

Pitas can be reheated by sprinkling the loaves lightly with water, and placing them wrapped in aluminum foil in a 400° F. (200° C.) oven for a couple of minutes.

MAIN DISHES

Salmon Quiche

Makes six servings
½ cup (125 ml) low-fat
  cottage cheese
½ cup (125 ml) ricotta cheese
¼ cup (60 ml) buttermilk
2 scallions, finely chopped
2 eggs, beaten
15½ ounces (439 g) red salmon,
  with bones, drained
dash freshly grated nutmeg
9-inch (23-cm) unbaked
  *Whole Wheat Pastry
  Crust*

Enjoy the subtle flavor of salmon and get a double bonus of calcium in this low-fat quiche.

Combine the cheeses and buttermilk in a blender and process on low speed until combined. Place in a large bowl and add scallions and eggs. Flake salmon meat and crush the bones; add to the cheese mixture with a dash of nutmeg.

Pour salmon mixture into the pie crust and place in a preheated 400° F. (200° C.) oven. Bake for 20 minutes, then turn down the heat to 350° F. (175° C.) and bake 10 to 15 minutes longer, until quiche is puffed and golden brown. Serve hot or at room temperature.

Note: If desired, use one cup (250 ml) of cottage cheese or one cup (250 ml) of ricotta rather than the combination above.

Whole Wheat Pastry Crust

*Makes one 9-inch (23-cm)
  pie crust*
⅓ cup (80 ml) buttermilk
2 tablespoons (30 ml) corn oil
2 teaspoons (10 ml) active dry
  yeast
½ teaspoon (2 ml) honey
1 tablespoon (15 ml) lukewarm
  water
1 cup (250 ml) whole wheat
  pastry flour

Place the buttermilk and oil in a small saucepan and scald. Set aside to cool. In a large bowl, combine yeast with the honey and water. When yeast is dissolved and buttermilk mixture is lukewarm, add the buttermilk to the yeast mixture. Add ½ cup (125 ml) of the flour to the yeast mixture and stir briskly with a wooden spoon. Add remaining flour and knead by hand on a countertop until smooth. Place the dough in a lightly oiled bowl and set aside in a warm place to rise.

When the dough has doubled in bulk, punch down. Dust a pastry board with flour and roll the dough to fit a 9-inch (23-cm) pie plate. Fold round of dough in half, and lift carefully into the plate. Press into place. Handle dough gently.

Note: Double the amount above for a two-crust pie.

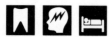

Mushrooms Stroganoff-Style with Toasted Cashews

Makes four servings

1 cup (250 ml) chopped
   onions
1 clove garlic, minced
1 tablespoon (15 ml)
   sunflower oil
3½ cups (875 ml) quartered
   mushrooms (about ¾
   pound [340 g])
1 cup (250 ml) cottage cheese
1 cup (250 ml) *Chicken Stock*
   or *Turkey Stock*
½ cup (125 ml) cashews,
   toasted
1 tablespoon (15 ml) chopped
   fresh parsley
2 teaspoons (10 ml) tamari
   dash freshly grated nutmeg

A hearty and flavorful dish with terrific texture. Makes a good introduction to meatless main dishes.

In a large skillet, saute the onions and garlic in the oil until tender. Add mushrooms and cook about 15 minutes, until they are tender.

In a blender, combine the cottage cheese and stock and process on medium speed until smooth.

Add blended sauce to the mushroom mixture, and add the cashews, parsley, tamari and nutmeg. Over low heat, stir ingredients until hot. Do not boil, as this may cause the mixture to curdle.

Serve over hot, steamed brown rice.

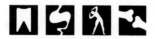

Classic Open-Face Sandwich

Makes one serving

1 slice Jarlsburg or Swiss cheese
1 slice whole wheat bread
1 large slice of tomato
¼ cup (60 ml) alfalfa sprouts

Turn oven on to broil or use counter-top broiler. Lay cheese on bread and heat until cheese bubbles and begins to brown. Do not let it get too brown. Remove from oven, add tomato and top with sprouts. If desired, add the tomato earlier so that it cooks with the cheese.

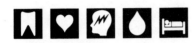

Cashew Chicken with Brown Rice

Makes four servings
- 1 cup (250 ml) chopped onions
- 1 clove garlic, minced
- 1 tablespoon (15 ml) soy oil
- 1½ cups (375 ml) cottage cheese
- ¾ cup (175 ml) *Chicken Stock* or *Turkey Stock*
- 2 cups (500 ml) cooked, cubed chicken breast
- ½ cup (125 ml) cashews, toasted
- dash freshly grated nutmeg
- 2 teaspoons (10 ml) tamari
- 1 tablespoon (15 ml) chopped fresh parsley
- 4 cups (1 l) cooked brown rice
- 1 tablespoon (15 ml) soy oil

In a large skillet, saute onions and garlic in oil until tender. In a blender combine cottage cheese and stock. Process on medium speed until smooth.

Add blended sauce to the vegetables, and stir in chicken breast, cashews, nutmeg to taste, tamari and parsley. Over low heat, stir constantly until ingredients are hot, but do not boil, or the cheese sauce may curdle.

Serve over hot, cooked brown rice.

MISCELLANEOUS

Seasoned Popcorn

Almost everyone is surprised at how good this tastes.

Makes four servings
- 2 teaspoons (10 ml) corn oil
- 3 tablespoons (45 ml) popcorn
- 1 tablespoon (15 ml) brewer's yeast

In a heavy pan over high heat, shake a covered pan containing the oil and popcorn. When most of the kernels have popped, remove from heat and serve the popped corn dusted with brewer's yeast.

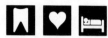

Stuffed Mushrooms

Makes three servings

6 large mushrooms
2 teaspoons (10 ml) corn oil
¾ cup (175 ml) soft whole
    grain bread crumbs
1 clove garlic, minced
2 tablespoons (30 ml)
    chopped walnuts
2 teaspoons (10 ml) minced
    fresh basil or tarragon
1 tablespoon (15 ml) cottage
    cheese
1–2 teaspoons (5–10 ml)
    buttermilk
dash paprika
grated Parmesan cheese

Can be served on a small slice of toasted whole wheat bread, accompanied by sprigs of parsley or cherry tomatoes. Delicious!

Clean mushrooms with a damp towel, but do not peel. Remove and chop stems, setting aside the mushroom caps. Saute stems in one teaspoon (5 ml) of oil for a minute or two in a medium skillet. Add the bread crumbs, garlic, nuts, herb and cottage cheese. Add a little buttermilk to moisten stuffing, and flavor with paprika. Divide stuffing between mushroom caps, and sprinkle with a little grated Parmesan. With a pastry brush, baste mushroom caps with the remaining oil and place under a broiler for five minutes, until sizzling hot.

Variation: Very large mushroom caps can also be stuffed with pureed lentils or pureed peas.

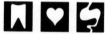

Sesame Crackers

Makes eight dozen

¾ cup (175 ml) warm water
2 teaspoons (10 ml) active dry
    yeast
2 teaspoons (10 ml) honey
2 tablespoons (30 ml) sesame
    tahini
1½ cups (375 ml) whole wheat
    pastry flour
sesame seeds

Combine water, yeast and honey in a small bowl, allowing yeast to dissolve. Add tahini. In a large mixing bowl, place flour and stir in yeast mixture. Combine ingredients, kneading briefly by hand, if needed. Allow dough to rise in a warm, draft-free place about a half hour, or until nearly doubled in bulk. Punch down, and knead dough briefly on a floured board. Divide dough into four pieces, and roll each quite thin, sprinkling with a thin layer of sesame seeds while rolling. Cut dough with a round cookie cutter. Place cutouts on a lightly greased cookie sheet and bake in a 350° F. (175° C.) oven until crisp and browned, 10 to 15 minutes. Turning crackers near the end of baking will help insure crispness.

Variation: For *Onion-Sesame Crackers,* while rolling dough, sprinkle with minced scallions, shallots, or onions. Roll with sesame seeds, as above.

Whole Wheat Croutons

Makes two cups (500 ml)

1 tablespoon (15 ml) corn or
    soy oil
1 teaspoon (5 ml) grated
    Parmesan cheese
¼ teaspoon (1 ml) thyme
    (optional)
1 clove garlic, crushed
    (optional)
2 cups (500 ml) dry whole
    wheat bread cubes

A great use for stale bread: use to garnish soups and salads.

Combine the oil, cheese and thyme and garlic, if desired, in a large, shallow ovenproof dish. Toss the bread cubes with the seasoning mixture. Place in a preheated 250° F. (120° C.) oven until crisp, about 30 to 45 minutes.

Chapter 9

Other Health Problems

ARTHRITIS

Most doctors would probably say that worthwhile treatments for arthritis include drugs, rest, physical therapy and, if need be, surgery. Some doctors, drawing on recent developments in psychology and holistic medicine, would add that the patient's *attitude* is also crucial. The arthritis sufferer who passively accepts his condition and believes he is stuck with it for the rest of his life might well be insuring that outcome by his belief. The person who makes up his mind to fight arthritis, who actively cooperates with his physician in seeking relief, and who refuses to become depressed and give up hope, is much more likely to get better.

Your decision to seriously try a dietary approach to arthritis (complementing whatever medical regimen you and your doctor have worked out) is a logical part of that positive, optimistic approach. And despite what the arthritis party line may tell you, nutrition *can* have a very beneficial effect on arthritis.

One dietary facet of arthritis which even the most conservative physicians accept is that any extra weight you are carrying around can only make your condition worse. When your cartilage or bone has become damaged, the less stress it has to put up with, the better. Banging your arthritic knee into a table leg will obviously hurt, but if you're carrying 40 extra pounds of fat on you, the weight of all that fat is, in a sense, banging down on your poor joint with every step you take—unless, of course, you're walking in a swimming pool, which happens to be a very good exercise for arthritis. So, if you are overweight, be sure to read the chapter Slenderizing Naturally.

Several other nutritional aspects are what might be called only *slightly* controversial, because they aren't concerned with treating the arthritis so much as they are with mopping up some of the brush fires caused by the condition or the drugs taken to treat it. Aspirin, for instance, which so many arthritics take, can actually triple the amount of vitamin C excreted by the body. Since vitamin C is so important to the connective tissues, as well as your health in general, it's only common sense that anyone taking aspirin should make sure they get extra amounts of vitamin C from fruits, juices and raw vegetables. (For a list of the best dietary sources of vitamin C, see the *Index.*) Aspirin aside, doctors at Trinity College in Ireland found that patients with rheumatoid arthritis had extremely low levels of vitamin C, indicating that the inflammatory disease process was somehow causing the body to lose this important vitamin.

Rheumatoid arthritis patients may also need more zinc, according to a report from the University of Washington Medical School. There a small group of patients given zinc supplements reported less joint swelling and morning stiffness than patients who were given inert placebo pills. "That doesn't mean that rheumatoid arthritis is caused by a zinc deficiency," Peter A. Simkin, M.D., told us. "There is no evidence of that. It *does* suggest that rheumatoid arthritis, like many other chronic illnesses, may be complicated by a zinc deficiency." A loss of zinc in the joints, in other words, may make arthritis worse, and replacement may make it better.

Extra zinc cannot be obtained as easily as extra vitamin C. Oysters and beef have high amounts, but we don't recommend oysters because of water pollution, and beef is too fatty and otherwise undesirable. Good sources of zinc include fish, green beans, lima beans, nuts, wheat germ and whole grain products. (For a complete list of recommended dietary zinc sources, see the *Index.*) If you can't seem to fit much zinc into your diet through food, consider a supplement in the range of 10 to 30 milligrams a day.

If your doctor has put you on cortisone for your arthritis, or has suggested it to you, you should know that this drug can cause an amazing number of side effects, ranging from ulcers to mental derangement, with many equally unpleasant stops in between. That is not to say you ought never to take cortisone; only that your doctor or pharmacist should alert you to the early signs of these side effects. On the nutritional front, your doctor should be checking you to see if you are retaining water or developing high blood pressure, because these drugs may cause you to hold sodium and excrete large amounts of potassium. If that is the case, you should be on a sodium-restricted diet and eating foods rich in potassium. (For a list of these foods, see the *Index*.)

Responsible physicians will not continue to prescribe cortisone-type drugs for a long period of time unless absolutely necessary. Nevertheless, that is done in quite a few cases, with potentially devastating effects on the body's very foundation. Taken over a period of several years, even small doses of cortisone can cause a large amount of calcium to be drawn out of the bones and contribute to the development of osteoporosis. The first symptom is usually a nagging, chronic pain in the low back, the kind of pain that always seems to be there. Seldom, in our own experience, are patients warned of this possibility or told to eat extra calcium. Their first inkling that something is wrong may be an unexplained fracture resulting from that bone loss.

Cortisone aside, it's possible that many people with osteoarthritis, the most common form of arthritis, could do themselves a lot of good by substantially boosting their calcium intake. When there is arthritic inflammation at a joint, there is often a localized loss of calcium, and it's possible, just possible, that pain can be reduced with extra calcium. We don't say that because there is any scientific or medical evidence to back it up, but because we have heard that story from literally *thousands* of people. What these people did was not just drink an extra glass or two of milk a day, but take about six or eight calcium tablets a day, in the form of bone meal, dolomite, calcium gluconate or calcium carbonate. If you have read our section "Building a Stronger Foundation" in the chapter Getting Stronger Every Day, you know why we consider supplemental forms of calcium to be food, rather than just "pills."

But before we share some of these stories with you, we want to emphasize that they are just that—personal accounts—and should not be confused with scientific studies. On the other hand, there is every good reason to consider these anecdotes seriously, albeit cautiously. Don't for one minute suppose that these nutritional ideas are dangerous or illogical while the medical approach is safe and logical. First of all, doctors do not know what causes arthritis. They do not know why it sometimes goes away and never comes back. They do not understand why some people with all the physical signs of arthritis feel no pain, while others with minimal joint damage suffer constantly. There is not a single drug ordinarily given for arthritis that is completely safe. A list of their possible side effects could fill several pages of this book. What's more, doctors don't understand why these drugs seem to help some people and make other people feel worse. Nor do they understand how these drugs work (when they do). It is believed, for example, that some drugs given for very severe forms of arthritis work by suppressing the immune system. That action ties in with the theory that arthritis is a so-called autoimmune condition in which, for unknown reasons, antibodies that are supposed to attack only invading germs turn against the lining of the joints and try to destroy them. Curiously, however, a drug that *stimulates* the body's immune system has also shown apparent benefit in certain arthritic conditions. The punch line is that it is not necessary to feel foolish or guilty when trying something on your own, so long as it's safe and not very expensive.

In 1977 and 1978, *Prevention* magazine conducted an informal survey of its readers concerning their use of calcium. When the staff was done tabulating approximately 3,000 responses, we were astonished to discover that nearly half of all the respondents—1,379 to be exact—said that bone pain had been either relieved or abolished after taking calcium. But numbers don't even begin to tell the real story. Here, for instance, is what we heard from Mrs. T. L. (all respondents were promised anonymity):

"My health was always good, except for arthritis of the hip of five years' duration, with agonizing, gnawing pain. Much of that time I had to walk with a cane, could not carry anything heavy, and literally crawled up stairs, holding onto the banisters with both hands. I was told by the M.D.'s that I'd have to learn to 'live with it.'

"After six months of calcium, the pain vanished completely, and has not returned. My health is excellent—my back straight and very strong, and I can *run* up stairs."

Now, we're sure there are many people who find a story like that just about unbelievable. In fact, Mrs. T. L. herself considered the possibility that her recovery may have had nothing to do with her self-prescribed regimen of 1,200 to 1,500 milligrams of calcium a day in the form of bone meal and dolomite, plus some vitamin D. "I have often wondered if I'd simply had a 'spontaneous remission' of arthritis," she said, "but I'm very, very strongly of the opinion that it has been due to the calcium I've taken religiously for the past eight years."

Mrs. E. M., 56, of Carmel Valley, California, confessed, "Two years ago I was literally crippled. My trouble started at 53, with pain in my back, neck, elbows and shoulders. I went to one of our leading orthopedic doctors and x-rays revealed arthritis and osteoporosis. My left arm and hand were completely numb. The doctor injected me with cortisone on several visits. Finally I was referred to a neurologist who ordered more x-rays, a brain scan and a complete skull series, as he had found diminished sensation on the entire left side. All tests were normal, though, except the arthritis. They fitted me with an orthopedic back brace, my right arm was put in a sling, and I was given a Philadelphia collar for my neck. I was forced to quit work and go on Disability Social Security.

"We were fortunate to have a young orthopedic surgeon come to this area. As I felt things could not get much worse, I went to see him. More x-rays. Three days later, he called me to his office and—now what I call the 'miracle'—he ordered 750 milligrams of calcium three times daily, plus 500 milligrams of vitamin C, and 500 milligrams of niacinamide, plus at least a quart of milk daily with a high-calcium diet. I was advised how to position myself for sleep (the hardest part as I had been a stomach sleeper). The first month I discarded the back brace and sling and used the soft collar another month. The only pain I have now is occasionally in my left elbow. I exercise and can do anything from turning cartwheels to using the trapeze bar. I have also returned to full duty work."

Those are only a few of the many stories we received in response to the survey. But they say a lot. Our high-calcium recipes appear in the section on osteoporosis and in the chapter Healthier Teeth and Gums.

It's also possible that some cases of arthritis—we have no idea how many—may be aggravated, or even caused by food allergy. Professor Norman F. Childers of Rutgers University has a theory that arthritis in some people is caused by an allergy or intolerance to plants in the nightshade family. Those include tomatoes, potatoes, peppers, eggplant and tobacco. It isn't easy to stick with a diet that eliminates all those foods. But if you're interested in giving it a try for several months to see if it helps, it can't hurt. At this time, Professor Childers' theory is a kind of university-born folk remedy.

Moving on to folk remedies pure and simple, the one we've heard most about is alfalfa—sprouts, tablets or tea. Cherries, sweet or sour, also a folk remedy for gout, are believed by some to help with arthritis as well. Herbalists frequently mention lemon, parsley and watercress as being helpful for arthritis, or rheumatism as it used to be called. Nutritional folk remedies focus on fish liver oil, vitamin C and high-potency B vitamins.

ATHLETIC STRESS

Chances are, your introduction to organized athletics came during the not-so-ancient era when the word "marathon" was more likely to conjure up images of dancers shuffling around a ballroom at four o'clock in the morning than of 10,000 half-naked people charging across the Verrazano Narrows Bridge on the opening spurt of an incredible 26-mile foot race. If that's the case, it's likely that you didn't learn very much at all about diet and exercise when you were in school. And that what you did learn—like what *we* learned—was probably wrong.

What most of us came away from school believing about nutrition and athletics went something like this:

If you sweat a lot, you should take salt tablets to replace your losses. If you get leg cramps, you can stop them with those same salt tablets. And, if you're trying to become strong and powerful, like a football player or a weight lifter, you should be eating huge amounts of protein to build big strong muscles.

There is now wide agreement in sports medicine circles that those beliefs are fallacious in about 98 percent of all cases. Instead, the experts are now talking about the importance of eating the kind of diet which, when summed up, amounts pretty much to the kind of fare we present in this book. Let's see just why.

First of all, what about salt? How is it possible that an athlete doesn't need more salt, when all that salty perspiration is being lost? And how can a dietary approach such as ours, which is very low in salt, be adequate for a person who, let's say, jogs or plays tennis for two hours every day?

The answer is that when you begin to perspire, the relative concentration of salt in your blood actually goes *up.* That happens because sweating causes you to lose relatively more water than salt. So while in fact you are losing salt, the proportionately greater loss of body water increases the *percentage* of salt in the fluids that bathe your muscles and organs. The real problem with sweating, then, is water replacement, not salt replacement.

Now, it's possible that after a very long period of exertion in an uncomfortably hot environment—an August marathon in Florida, for instance—you may need some extra salt. But only *after* you had replaced several quarts of water would a need for extra salt arise. And even then, the requirement would be far from certain. (Actually, a person who cares about his or her health has no business running long distances in such heat to begin with.)

Taking a few salt tablets probably isn't going to do you any great harm unless you have high blood pressure. Still, it could do you *some* harm. Because while slightly higher than normal salt intake causes you to retain water, a great excess of salt in the body increases the amount of water passing into the bladder, possibly contributing to dehydration or even heat stroke. Too much salt can also decrease your potassium, and the importance of keeping your levels of potassium up during exercise is, in almost every case, more critical than maintaining the sodium level. More about that in a minute.

If you feel that perhaps you *do* need some extra salt, you would be better off eating foods that naturally contain some useful sodium, rather than taking salt tablets. Good bets would be spinach, carrots, or turnip greens, because they not only contain some sodium, but are very high in potassium. A tuna salad made with the usual kind of canned tuna (which contains added salt) and lots of celery (naturally high in sodium) would also be a good choice. Canned sardines are another basically nutritious food that contains very substantial amounts of salt. Dairy products such as yogurt, milk and cheese also have useful sodium, as do fish, chicken, liver and meat.

Actually, most athletes would probably be better off *restricting* their salt intake, as we recommend in this book, rather than worrying about getting more salt. When you have been on a low-sodium diet for an extended period of time, several months at least, your body learns how to *conserve* salt. You will lose very little sodium indeed while exercising. In fact, both medical and anecdotal evidence suggest that the athlete who has been on a long-term, salt-restricted diet will actually perform *better* during hot weather than people who have been eating salt freely—or taking salt tablets.

But let's return for a minute to the need for water. Many people avoid drinking water before or during exercise because they think it will give them cramps. Today, that's considered extremely unwise. The need for more water is the single most immediate and important nutritional requirement for exercise. It *won't* give you cramps unless you drink it ice cold or consume extremely large amounts at one time. Sports medicine doctors are now recommending that you drink about two glasses of water 15 minutes or so before and several times during a long period of exercise in a warm environment.

PROTEIN AND ENERGY FOR ATHLETES

What about protein? Well, strange as it may seem, even vigorous exercise does not create a need for more protein than what is ordinarily required to keep your body in good running order. Connected with the old-fashioned idea of loading up on protein is the notion that the best protein of all is from great big juicy steaks. That idea is wrong for two reasons. First, most cuts of steak contain very unhealthful amounts of fat. Second, from the point of view of actual performance, protein is simply the wrong food to be packing in when you're in training for competition. The food element that the body can burn most quickly and efficiently is *carbohydrate.*

Enlightened trainers in every sport involving any kind of endurance, from bicycling to football, are setting the precontest table with our good friends, the complex carbohydrates—pasta, noodles, bread, potatoes and vegetables. Beans, cabbage, apples and other "carbs" that are not quite as readily digested and absorbed are avoided to minimize any problems with gas on the playing field. Derek Clayton, who at this writing has held the world record in the marathon for many years, ate great quantities of potatoes while training for his historic run. A number of outstanding athletes are vegetarians, and many who aren't eat large quantities of fruits and vegetables.

The carbohydrate-energy trend is not just another fad. There's a lot of very solid evidence that it *works.* A classic study was carried out by Swedish scientists who gave nine athletes the same endurance tests on a bicycle after they had followed a particular diet for three days. One diet was especially high in meat (and therefore, protein and fat). Another diet was a mixed diet of protein and carbohydrates. The third diet was especially high in vegetables and grains, and therefore carbohydrates.

After the athletes were on the high-meat diet, their average endurance on the bicycle was 57 minutes. After the mixed diet, it was 114 minutes. But after the high-carbohydrate diet, it was 167 minutes. Further analysis showed this very impressive difference could be related to the varying amount of glycogen contained in the muscles of these athletes. Glycogen is a carbohydrate which is the most readily available fuel used by muscles. On the high-meat diet, the percentage of glycogen in the muscle was only 0.63 percent. On the mixed diet, it was 1.75 percent. On the high-carbohydrate diet, 3.51 percent.

The body can, if pressed, use either fat or protein for fuel (after converting it to glycogen). But biochemically, it's kind of an awkward process—something like a ship refueling in stormy seas. Carbohydrates are taken on board by the muscles much more smoothly. In simple terms, the story seems to be: high carbohydrate, high glycogen, high endurance. But if you want the best results, use *complex* carbohydrates: natural food, not plain sugar, which is a kind of pharmaceutical version of carbohydrate that can wind up short-circuiting your whole energy system.

The superiority of the complex carbohydrates over protein for body fuel is expressed succinctly by Julian Whitaker, M.D., director of the California Heart Medical Clinic in San Clemente. "Fat and proteins clog the system. A person who is seriously into running should be eating vegetable foods almost exclusively," the physician advises. "A large protein intake puts enormous stress on the body and causes increased losses of water, calcium and minerals." The kinds of foods he recommends are whole wheat cereals, potatoes, fruits, vegetables, nonfat milk and big green salads eaten without added oil.

There is a certain amount of debate currently going on about consuming sweet drinks during extended periods of exercise, such as long races. The most informed opinions at present suggest that while eating sugar at this time can theoretically provide quick energy, that same sugar actually slows down the absorption of water. So in an attempt to boost your energy, you could be running the risk of overheating and dehydration. Something on the order of fruit juice, probably diluted to less than its usual strength, combines the best of both worlds—a little bit of natural sugar and a lot of water.

POTASSIUM AND OTHER VITAL NUTRIENTS

Fruit juice is also a rich source of potassium, an essential body mineral that deserves serious attention by anyone indulging in long periods of exercise. Gabe Mirkin, M.D., in *The Sports Medicine Book* (Little, Brown & Co., 1978) says that early in his own career as a runner, there was a time when he felt so weak he could barely get out of bed. He felt so terrible, he thought he was seriously ill. But tests showed that the trouble was nothing more than a deficiency of potassium. "Downing massive amounts of fruit juices," he reports, "rejuvenated me." The reason athletes require so much potassium, Dr. Mirkin explains, is that "even in frigid temperatures, every muscle that is being exercised produces heat. To keep from overheating, the muscle releases potassium into the bloodstream. This widens the blood vessels, increases blood flow, and carries heat away from the muscle. The potassium is excreted from the body via sweat and urine. Thus an athlete must constantly be on guard to replenish his potassium supply."

The feeling of total exhaustion that can be brought on by potassium deficiency is apparently a result of the fact that potassium deficiency can prevent formation of glycogen in muscle. Without glycogen, of course, the muscle has no ready fuel.

Probably the most convenient source of potassium, as Dr. Mirkin suggests, is fruit juice. When you're not actually exercising, however, eating the whole fruit is even better. Other very good sources of potassium include bananas, brewer's yeast, broccoli, carrots, peanuts, potatoes, raisins, sunflower seeds, tuna fish and wheat germ.

Magnesium is another mineral that may be in short supply in endurance athletes, although the need for it is usually not as great as for potassium. Magnesium is especially important in controlling the tone of muscles. When muscles are short of magnesium, they can become spastic, even convulsive. If you suffer from muscle tightness and cramps, it's likely that a good deal of your problem comes from not doing enough stretching exercises. But a shortage of magnesium (and possibly potassium and calcium as well) could very well be involved. Magnesium is not as easy to get in your normal diet as potassium. Especially good sources include blackstrap molasses, nuts, peas, brown rice, soybeans, dark green leafy vegetables and whole grain products. Dolomite is a mineral supplement that combines magnesium and calcium.

Because athletic individuals must eat more in order to get the calories they need for energy, they are ordinarily at much less risk of developing nutritional deficiencies than sedentary people. But it's not safe to assume that such deficiencies in athletes *never* arise. Researchers in the nutrition department at Syracuse University reported in 1978 that when they analyzed the diets of many athletes at that school, they found the women tended to have a deficiency of iron, while *both* sexes "could probably use more thiamine for carbohydrate metabolism." Women, of course, need more iron because of their menstrual losses, and unless they are eating a good deal of liver or other meat, it may be difficult for them to get all they need. But what about thiamine—also called vitamin B_1? Well, the latest evidence suggests that how much thiamine we need for the best health depends on how many carbohydrates we are taking in. Thiamine, it seems, is necessary for carbohydrates to be metabolized. And since athletes with big appetites usually eat a good deal of carbohydrates, they need large amounts of thiamine. Now, if they were eating especially good diets, their food would almost automatically provide the thiamine necessary to take care of the extra carbohydrates. But the Syracuse study found that was not necessarily the case. And that's worth worrying about: if a thiamine deficiency becomes a problem, the results could be jumpy nerves or pain sensitivity among other things—something no athlete wants to be plagued with. Good sources of thiamine include brewer's yeast, nuts, liver, sunflower seeds, dark green leafy vegetables, wheat germ and whole grain products.

The Syracuse study also found that many of the young athletes were getting 40 to 50 percent of their daily caloric intake from fat, regarded as definitely too high for good health. The football players were consuming 225 grams of fat a day, the equivalent of half-a-pound of butter.

PRE-RACE CARBOHYDRATE LOADING

In an attempt to gain every conceivable competitive advantage, some distance runners will prepare for a major event by going through a process popularly known as carbohydrate loading. Very simply, what this involves is purposely depleting their bodies of carbohydrate stores (glycogen), beginning about a week before the big event. The depletion is done by long periods of exercise. At one time, it was thought that you should also avoid carbohydrate foods during this time in order to hasten their removal from muscles, but apparently that may not be necessary. According to Dr. Whitaker, whom we mentioned before, continuous high-intensity exercise would deplete glycogen stores regardless of what you're eating, because it takes muscles "several days to recover from strenuous exercise." Then, about three or four days before the big event, exercise is stopped completely and the runners load up on carbohydrates: grains, noodles, potatoes and vegetables. It seems that after the depletion phase, the body soaks up carbohydrates like a sponge and stores larger-than-usual amounts of glycogen in the muscles and liver, where they can be put to quick use during the long race.

Another technique that is said to improve performance in endurance events is drinking a large cup or two of coffee the morning of the race.

Having said all that, it is now time to point out that we don't approve of carbohydrate loading. For one thing, it can be used only for special occasions, and can do nothing for the person who is running or playing tennis or swimming several times a week. Second, there is something unnatural about the whole process of carbohydrate loading, and anything that is unnatural can be potentially dangerous. As for drinking coffee before a long run, that, too, is just another gimmick. Coffee affects the system like a drug, so if you are taking coffee for the specific purpose of improving your performance, you are, in a way, drugging yourself. It seems to us that athletics should be natural, spontaneous and enjoyable, and not the occasion to resort to bizarre programs calculated to boost performance by any means possible.

In summary, the athletic person should avoid consuming a lot of salt unless told to by a doctor, avoid large amounts of protein and fat, but pay a lot of attention to drinking plenty of good fresh water, and getting plenty of potassium, magnesium and complex carbohydrates. A diet high in fruits, grains and vegetables will take care of those last three requirements very nicely.

BENIGN BREAST LUMPS

Breast lumps are, of course, something you should always get checked out medically without delay. In most cases, as all women know, the lumps are not malignant. But although they're called "benign," they can be very distressing—and difficult to get rid of.

Most people, we imagine, would find it hard to believe that diet could have anything to do with breast lumps. But often, it's been recently discovered, the problem will completely clear up with some simple changes in what you eat and drink.

Some years ago, John Peter Minton, M.D., Ph.D., of the department of surgery at the Ohio State University College of Medicine, discovered that substances called cyclic nucleotides—which are known to stimulate the growth and division of cells—were found in especially high amounts in women suffering from growth of abnormal fibrous breast tissue. There is an enzyme in the body that ordinarily keeps cyclic nucleotides in check. But that enzyme can be crippled by certain chemicals, called methylxanthines, which occur naturally in certain foods. After further research, Dr. Minton set up a clinical trial to see if the elimination of these enzyme-crippling substances from the diet could bring about an improvement in women with a history of benign breast lumps.

The methylxanthines, suspected of doing the dirty work, are found in coffee, tea, chocolate and cola. So Dr. Minton instructed a group of 47 women—all of whom had undergone breast biopsy to rule out cancer—to remove these items from their diet.

As you might guess, many of the women failed to follow his advice. Of the 27 women who didn't fully comply, only 1 recovered from the breast disease in the ensuing months.

But of the 20 women who did cut those four items out of their diet, 13 became completely free of the problem within two to six months. That's a 65 percent recovery rate. Actually, the results were a little better than that, because 3 more women got better after 18 months of sticking to the diet and also giving up cigarette smoking.

After their breast nodules cleared up, some women went back to their old dietary habits, and in most cases the lumps returned.

Obviously, the majority of women who drink coffee and eat chocolate do not get breast lumps, but some women are apparently supersensitive to methylxanthines—a clear-cut example of what is called biochemical individuality, and a dramatic illustration of why foods that cause no apparent ill effects in some people may literally deform the bodies of others.

Another interesting note is that the four foods involved—coffee, tea, chocolate and cola—have been incriminated in countless other health problems ranging from severe anxiety to galloping tooth decay.

Is it possible that people who are sensitive to methylxanthines may develop problems other than benign breast lumps? Or, looking at it another way, is it possible that people who are not acutely sensitive to them may nevertheless be harmed by substances that can stimulate abnormal cell growth and division? No one can answer that question right now, but there's no law against using common sense. "I tell women who have a family history of breast cancer," says Dr. Minton, "to cut out methylxanthines completely" (*Journal of the American Medical Association,* March 23, 1979).

BODY ODOR

There are two kinds of body odor that this brief discussion doesn't include. The first kind is a very unusual or strong odor in infants. Such odors can be markers of serious metabolic disease and should always be carefully evaluated by a pediatrician. (Although one kind of body odor we discuss here is a result of metabolic impairment, it is not dangerous or life-threatening.) The other kind of body odor we are not talking about here is the normal, everyday odor which is generally no big problem and can usually be prevented or cleared up completely by normal bathing and dusting appropriate areas of the body with baking soda or cornstarch.

Some people, though, have an odor problem that no deodorant can touch. They bathe morning, noon and night, change their clothes two, three times a day. Nothing works. The answer, in at least some cases, seems to be extra amounts of dietary zinc. That finding was accidentally discovered by a number of people who were taking zinc supplements for other reasons, and found to their incredulous delight that long-standing problems with odor cleared up in just a few days. But at least one doctor has also seen zinc at work. Morton D. Scribner, M.D., of Arcadia, California, wrote in the *Archives of Dermatology* (September, 1977) that a patient who had been taking 50 milligrams of zinc three times a day as part of the management of recurrent leg ulcers noted that "while he was taking zinc there was a marked reduction in axillary [armpit] perspiration odor. This problem, which had been most distressing to him for most of his adult life, returned within days after the zinc was discontinued. When he again started taking the capsules, the odor markedly diminished (confirmed by his wife)." Subsequently, said Dr. Scribner, he has seen five other persons with a severe body odor problem respond very well to zinc—sometimes with doses as low as 20 milligrams a day. And all, he points out, "had tried a wide variety of deodorants and antiperspirants without success."

Currently, no one seems to understand this particular action of zinc. But, since zinc is involved in a great number of enzyme reactions, and since unusual body odors are often created by enzyme failures, we can reasonably suspect that some individuals need extra zinc to fuel the required enzyme reactions.

It's likely that the required amount of zinc to do the job is somewhere, on the average, between 25 and 50 milligrams of zinc a day, although it might be more or less for some individuals. It is quite difficult to get much more than about 15 milligrams of zinc a day into your diet unless you eat oysters or large amounts of meat, so the person with this kind of problem might have to boost his zinc intake with supplements. Meanwhile, zinc could be increased in the diet by eating more liver, dark turkey meat, wheat germ, nuts and sunflower seeds. (For a list of the zinc value of various foods, see the *Index.*)

If the kind of body odor problem we described above seems trying, imagine the plight of a 13-year-old boy with a body odor so unbelievably bad that his family actually took him to a hospital clinic a dozen times to see what could be done for his problem. Imagine, if you can, a body odor problem so severe that when his family tried to sell their house, they couldn't because potential buyers were practically knocked off their feet by the smell of "dead fish" which seemed to linger in every room of the home. Imagine the doctors at the clinic telling the family over and over again that there's "nothing that can be done" except to have the boy practice good hygiene and use deodorants—none of which worked. Imagine what it must feel like to be in that boy's place—depressed, guilty, ridiculed, fighting, getting thrown out of school. . . . And now, imagine all those problems being cleared up almost overnight by a simple change in diet.

Well, it happened. Warren A. Todd, M.D., reported that when he examined the boy the "putrid fish odor" immediately suggested "a possible defect in trimethylamine metabolism." For some reason, the boy's body built up abnormal amounts of this substance, which circulated through the body and caused the odor.

The boy was then put on a diet excluding those foods whose metabolic breakdown can give rise to trimethylamine. These happen to be foods that are high in choline —eggs, fish, liver, kidney and legumes such as beans, lentils and chick-peas. By no small coincidence, these happened to be among the boy's favorite foods. After just one week, there was barely a trace of trimethylamine to be found in his body. "A follow-up one year after the diet was begun," Dr. Todd reported, "revealed no problem with the odor. The young man also had a near straight-A average in the ninth grade, was dating, and had made many friends. No further signs or symptoms of depression were noted by the parents" (*Journal of Pediatrics,* June, 1979).

COLDS

Just yesterday a friend of ours told us he'd been suffering for five days with the worst cold (or *something*) he'd had in 10 years. It was so bad, he said, he went to the doctor, who gave him a prescription for tetracycline. He'd been taking his prescription for three days but the cold was as bad as ever. He was congested from his eyes to his chest and his voice was so basso profundo it would have been humorous if he hadn't been so miserable. Was there any kind of vitamin we knew of, he asked, or even a drugstore remedy, that would help end his misery? And how come the tetracycline wasn't working, anyway?

The first mistake our friend made wasn't really his, but his doctor's. Some five years before this whole story took place, a review of half-a-dozen controlled studies published in the medical literature concluded that antibiotics do *not* reduce the number of disease-producing organisms in the nose or throat, do *not* shorten the duration of upper respiratory infections, and do *not* prevent complications or secondary infections (*Pediatrics for the Clinician,* April, 1975). Just in case it's your sinuses that bother you, we should also point out that another study showed that sinusitis patients who took antibiotics didn't recover any faster than patients not taking the drugs (*Modern Medicine,* January 21, 1974).

Antibiotics, you see, are effective against many bacteria, but Nature in her wisdom has chosen to equip viruses with antibiotic-proof vests, so there's very little our drugs can do to intimidate the organisms responsible for the common cold.

Okay. But what about aspirin? Aspirin must help, because the TV ads always say that doctors recommend taking two aspirin and getting bed rest. They couldn't say that if it weren't true, could they? Well, finish reading this paragraph and then *you* be the judge. Edith D. Stanley, M.D., and colleagues of the Infectious Diseases Section of the Abraham Lincoln School of Medicine, University of Illinois College of Medicine, Chicago, found in a study that not only did aspirin fail to significantly reduce symptoms of the common cold, but it actually seemed to *enhance* the reproduction of the infecting viruses! Volunteers treated with aspirin discharged through their coughing and sneezing and running noses some 17 to 36 percent more live viruses than the volunteers who took a placebo or dummy pill. Writing in the *Journal of the American Medical Association* (March 24, 1975), Dr. Stanley and her colleagues suggest that whatever temporary relief aspirin may give, it does so at the price of interfering with the body's defensive response to infection. So while it may ease your distress, aspirin could actually be making it easier for the germs to multiply and migrate through your body—and also increasing the chances that you're going to spread live viruses to other people.

Well, so much for antibiotics and aspirin. What about the decongestants we hear so much about? Unless you're absolutely gasping for breath and your doctor prescribes them, decongestants could very well do more harm than good. That's because they temporarily shrink the mucosal lining of your nose, but if used repeatedly, they tend to chemically irritate that same tender lining. The result is that the lining swells up again later, becoming *more* swollen than before. Not only that, the decongestant lowers the amount of a natural antibiotic secreted by the mucosa, and partially cripples the cilia, those tiny hairs in your nose and windpipe that help expel germs.

Wow—this is beginning to sound really negative! But let's stop for a moment and think about the significance of all that negativity. Is it possible, just possible, that the underlying purpose of a cold—if you believe in such things—is to take us out of circulation for a couple of days, force us to get a good rest and just sort of pamper ourselves? Personal experience, if nothing else, suggests that obeying the impulse to lie down, cover up, and sip hot tea makes more sense than taking all those drugs and patent medications we mentioned. But while you're lying there on the sofa, what do you *eat?* And what do you *drink?*

"Take vitamin C!" we can hear a lot of people saying. We've no big argument with that, except that vitamin C will probably do you more good before, or in the very earliest stages of a cold, than after the virus has you roped and tied.

As for what to eat, one good bit of advice, which again seems to agree with experience and common sense, is not to eat much of anything, particularly if your appetite isn't there. The evidence isn't all in, but some research, at least, shows that when there's a knock-down drag-out battle going on in your system, the immune system can get in more licks against the enemy when the body doesn't have to devote any energy to digesting food. Eventually, of course, if you don't eat for a long enough period of time, you're going to become run-down and your immunity will suffer. But during a brief crisis, such as an acute infection, forcing yourself to eat big meals is probably an unwise tactic.

Drinking is a different story. A fever, especially, can dehydrate you, so you want to take plenty of fluids into your system to keep things balanced. Probably, you already know that because your mother told you all about the need for fluids—especially chicken soup. Well, it turns out that mom was right on both scores. You not only need fluids, but chicken soup really is special. If you need scientific proof for that statement, consider this. A team of doctors at Mount Sinai Medical Center in Miami Beach, Florida, asked

15 volunteers to drink hot chicken soup. Before the volunteers drank the soup, the researchers measured their nasal mucus velocity—how fast the top layer of mucus moved out of the nose—and then measured it again after they drank the soup. They found that hot chicken soup increased nasal mucus velocity by 33 percent. When the volunteers drank cold water, nasal mucus velocity *decreased* by 28 percent (*Chest,* October, 1978).

To make that chicken soup even more potent, spice it up with some garlic. Garlic and herbs and spices such as chili peppers and horseradish, writes Irvin Ziment, M.D., are natural expectorants—substances that thin mucus and clear it out of the system. In fact, Dr. Ziment feels you're better off using such spices to clear you out than most popular over-the-counter products, which he says have been found "relatively ineffective" (*Journal of the American Medical Association,* July 12, 1976).

Herbalists have long had a bagful of tricks to use for colds and congestion. You can make a tea out of any or all of them by steeping a teaspoonful of the herbal material in a cup of boiling water, straining, and sipping. To help the flavor—and the helpful effect —add plenty of fresh lemon juice, or even some fresh orange juice. Don't drink more than one or two cups of any one kind of herb tea in a day, to prevent any possible stomach upset. Herbs that have traditionally been used to help colds include, among others, coltsfoot, mullein, anise, fenugreek and sage.

CYSTIC FIBROSIS

Until recently, it was generally believed that the nutritional program for children with cystic fibrosis (CF) should be designed merely to compensate for the serious derangements in absorption that afflict these children. Today, though, there is increased hope that a more aggressive nutritional approach—even though it might not get to the unknown cause of this disease—may bring about considerable improvement in a CF child's overall health.

The new approach emphasizes the importance of giving children supplements with polyunsaturated fats, rich in linoleic acid. Although most of the trials in this approach involved direct infusion of oils into the bloodstream, taking them by mouth is also effective, even though the oil will not be absorbed as efficiently.

In 1974, Robert B. Elliott, M.D., of the department of pediatrics at Auckland University Medical School in Australia, reported that several young children who were diagnosed as having CF shortly after birth responded very well to intravenous infusions of an emulsion of soy oil. There was, in fact, gradual reversal of many symptoms, and these children did not seem to develop the characteristic chest disease that accompanies CF. One of the children, after 19 months, appeared to be completely well. But another youngster, whose treatment did not begin until she was eight, showed considerably less improvement.

Within a few years, two other studies of linoleic acid supplementation, where the oil was simply swallowed, reported that there was notable improvement in the children, including significant weight gains and a decrease in a number of problems, such as elevated white blood cell count.

In 1979, Dr. Elliott, in cooperation with two American physicians, published another study that was designed to rule out any possible psychological or placebo factors in response to linoleic acid supplementation. After one year, they reported, the children who received the supplements "gained significantly more in height and weight during their previous year and on cumulative data analysis showed greater improvement" than another group of children who were given additional medical attention but without linoleic acid (*Pediatrics,* August, 1979). While additional research is being carried out, these authors recommend that all children with CF have the levels of linoleic acid in their blood plasma measured at least once a year. If levels are low, one tablespoon of safflower oil should be taken by mouth once or twice a day along with pancreatic enzymes. Needless to say, this or any other change in the diet of a CF child should first be discussed with a physician.

There are other nutritional factors involved in CF which you may also want to discuss with your physician. The Medical Advisory Council of the Cystic Fibrosis Foundation notes that "patients having cystic fibrosis may have a number of nutritional problems secondary to their disease." Many, if not all, of these problems may result from the fact that 80 to 85 percent of children with CF develop a deficiency of pancreatic enzymes, which are needed to properly absorb nutrients. Consequently, many CF children develop vitamin and other deficiencies and fail to grow normally.

A physician will probably recommend pancreatic enzyme supplements to improve digestion and supplements of fat-soluble vitamins—A, E, K and possibly D as well. These vitamins should be taken in water-dispersed form, so that they can be utilized by a CF child, who may not be able to absorb vitamins dispersed in oil. Deficiency of vitamin E may be the biggest problem of all. Current opinion is that infants should be getting 25 to 50 international units of vitamin E a day, while older children and adults should receive 100 to 200 international units. Of course, vitamin supplements may not be necessary in every case of CF. But, if they are *not* being given, it ought to be because specific tests have clearly ruled out any need.

In addition to vitamins, the CF child or adult may have a problem simply getting enough calories for energy because of poor absorption. As the disease involves the lungs, breathing becomes labored, which burns up still more calories. These calories should ideally come from healthful foods rather than sugars, but in any case, they must obviously come from foods that the CF child or adult can digest and absorb without suffering indigestion. That is something that must be learned by each individual through trial and error. If chopped nuts, seeds and moistened dried fruits cannot be handled, natural sugars such as honey, and even better, blackstrap or medium unsulfured molasses, which can be added to other foods or drinks, are preferable to plain sugar, which is bereft of all vitamins, minerals and trace elements.

DIABETES

WARNING: *If you are a diabetic who is taking insulin, you should know that the diet described herein can be expected to reduce the amount of insulin you require to keep your blood sugar level under control. If you should continue to take your usual amount of insulin while your body is moving toward normalization of sugar metabolism, you might well be risking an overdose of insulin, which can drive your blood sugar level dangerously low. Therefore, before embarking on this dietary plan, you should discuss it carefully with your physician and make arrangements to have your blood sugar level and insulin dosage monitored as your body becomes able to control its sugar level with less outside assistance.*

Everyone "knows" that diabetics have to avoid carbohydrates. But do they really?

Twenty years ago or so, we wouldn't have had to put quotation marks around the word "knows." Very few people questioned that belief, or the practice of advising diabetics to get most of their nourishment from high-protein, high-fat foods such as meat and dairy products, along with a few green vegetables, while strictly limiting their intake of sugar, sweets, bread, potatoes, beans, noodles and other "carbohydrate foods."

Today, there are probably still many thousands of diabetics who accept that advice, and probably a good many physicians that have not told their diabetic patients any differently. But in fact, there is now growing agreement among scientists and doctors who specialize in diabetes and related subjects that the advice about carbohydrates given almost uniformly a generation ago is wrong. And that's putting it mildly. It's very possible that the "standard" diabetic diet is responsible for many of the complications associated with the disease. After all, the fact is that diabetics in Africa and Japan, who eat far more carbohydrates than Western diabetics, are much less likely to die from circulatory problems. Japanese diabetics, for instance, have a cardiovascular mortality rate only one-tenth of those in the West!

We're continuing to learn more about diabetes all the time. But as far as carbohydrates go, the big error that was made years ago was the assumption that the diabetic's system treats all carbohydrates the same, whether they're from sugar, white bread or whole wheat bread. It turns out that's not the case at all. All carbohydrates are not created equal. To find out more about different kinds of carbohydrates, and what it all means to the diabetic, we talked with James Anderson, M.D., who has published some exciting medical reports on his work with diabetic patients at the Lexington, Kentucky, Veterans Medical Center.

"We sent our greatest success home last Thursday," Dr. Anderson said to us on the day we visited. "He came into the hospital taking 38 units of insulin, and went home taking zero. This fellow had to spend a month in the hospital, but he had been insulin-dependent for eight years."

Dr. Anderson's treatment was a high-carbohydrate, low-fat, high-fiber diet, similar in many ways to the diet *everyone* ate before the advent of industrial food processing, and similar to the great majority of recipes used throughout this book. "We've been treating diabetics with this diet for about five years," he told us. "We've treated some 50 insulin-taking diabetics and about half of them have been able to discontinue insulin completely."

There is also ample evidence that the same diet could go a very long way toward *preventing* diabetes in many people who may be vulnerable to its development. That is a very important prospect, because 1 out of 20 Americans currently suffers from diabetes and the percentage has been rising steadily since the middle of the last century. People with diabetes not only get complications such as heart disease, which we mentioned before, but kidney failure, recurring infections and even blindness.

Scientists don't know what causes diabetes, but they have a pretty good idea of what goes on in people who have it. The healthy body maintains a constant level of sugar in the blood. It accomplishes that through a number of mechanisms that raise and lower the sugar level as needed. But the most important factor in lowering blood sugar is the hormone insulin, secreted by the pancreas. Insulin causes sugar to shift out of the circulating blood and into tissues. When there's not enough insulin in the blood or when, for some reason, the insulin is unable to hold down the amount of sugar, you have diabetes. Many diabetics require insulin shots to keep their blood sugar levels in check.

The popular notion that carbohydrates are bad for diabetics was tested by Dr. Anderson and his colleagues in one study in which 20 men dependent on insulin shots were fed the standard diabetic diet for a week. During that time, their insulin doses averaged 26 units a day. Then they were switched to a diet high in carbohydrates *but also high in fiber.* In other words, not carbohydrates from cake and soda, but from grains and vegetables. "On a high-carbohydrate, high-fiber diet, there was a rapid drop in insulin requirements," Dr. Anderson reported to a scientific forum. "Insulin doses had to be lowered to avoid dangerously low blood sugars. Insulin shots could be completely discontinued in eight patients. At the completion of the high-carbohydrate, high-fiber diets, insulin doses, which averaged 11 units per day, were less than half of those required on a standard diabetic diet. Despite lower insulin doses, blood sugars were about 20 points lower. Yet these diets lowered insulin requirements and led to improvement in the blood sugar."

When Dr. Anderson used the high-fiber diet to treat diabetics at the Veterans Medical Center, the results were much the same. Twelve patients treated were not taking insulin, but drugs that stimulate the pancreas to produce more insulin. Ten of the 12 were taken off the drugs completely, and 2 were able to substantially reduce the doses they were taking. Of the 18 patients who were taking low doses of insulin (between 14 and 20 units a day), 16 were able to quit insulin completely. Five of the 12 patients receiving moderate doses of insulin were also able to abandon their shots.

Now, here is something of critical importance. All those patients suffered from "adult" diabetes, named for the time of life when it often appears, and by far the more common variation of the disease. People with adult diabetes do not seem to be suffering from a lack of insulin. In fact, the levels of insulin in their blood are often *higher* than they are in healthy people. For some unknown reason, these people cannot keep the levels of sugar in their blood down even when they are producing plenty of insulin. They have what is often referred to as "insulin resistance." Dr. Anderson's diet has proved most effective with adult diabetics. Six patients he treated, though, were suffering from the other major type of diabetes, "juvenile" diabetes. Juvenile diabetics have a genuine lack of insulin, and more severe symptoms in general. The juvenile diabetics Dr. Anderson treated were receiving over 40 units of insulin a day. While none of them were able to discontinue their insulin shots when they switched to the high-fiber diet, all of them required less insulin than before.

Just how does a natural diet rich in carbohydrates and fiber help diabetics? No one knows for sure, but Dr. Anderson says it's quite clear that "the diet slows carbohydrate absorption. After you eat a meal, there is a big pulse of carbohydrate entering the system. Fiber slows the absorption of that carbohydrate, so there is a gradual release of it into the body. Further, by some mechanism that we don't really understand, the high-carbohydrate, low-fat content of the diet sensitizes the body to a burning of sugar. We hear a lot of talk these days about alternative fuels. On the standard diabetic diet, the body is usually geared to burning more fat for fuel. This diet switches the body to a sugar-burning system, and as a result, even juvenile diabetics, who are totally dependent on outside insulin, have been able to reduce their intake by 25 percent. The insulin goes farther on this diet than it did before."

Once Dr. Anderson has weaned his patients from insulin, he is generally able to keep them off it at home by prescribing a diet that is a little less strict than the hospital diet. Made up of foods readily available in any supermarket, the diet still delivers a high-fiber punch. "The fiber in the common diabetic diet averages 15 grams a day," Dr. Anderson says. "The average American takes in 12 to 20 grams of fiber a day. Our therapeutic diet averages 45 to 60 grams of fiber. That's three to four times as much as the standard diabetic diet." Of 20 diabetics taken off insulin and monitored for periods up to 48 months, none had to return to their insulin shots.

While some scientists who are using a similar approach are concentrating on adding supplements of fiber to a regular diet, Dr. Anderson told us, "We've found that if you eat a regular diet and supplement that with fiber, the effects on insulin intake are relatively small. We see reductions of 60 percent in the use of insulin when we change the entire diet, but only 20 percent if we just supplement an ordinary diet with fiber."

If you were brought up with the notion that diabetes is something you *inherit,* and the further idea that the discovery of insulin more or less took care of the whole problem, you may have a hard time accepting Dr. Anderson's perspective. If that's the case, consider this: historically, figures for New York City indicate an enormous jump in the number of diabetes deaths from 1875 to 1895, the same period that the United States switched from fiber-rich, stone-ground wheat flour to the more refined, roller-milled flour containing less fiber. During World War II and in the years of scarcity immediately following the war, Great Britain switched to a flour that used more of the wheat grain, and consequently contained more fiber. During that period, the death rate from diabetes fell an astonishing 55 percent in men and 54 percent in women. At the end of that period, in fact, the diabetes death rate for women was at its lowest level in the entire 20th century! If vulnerability to diabetes is inherited, clearly its effect on health is dependent on diet.

You may also be wondering about the emphasis Dr. Anderson placed on the desirability of diabetics lowering their requirement for insulin. Ironically, even though the body naturally produces insulin, there's good reason to believe that insulin shots are quite different, and that the more insulin the diabetic must take, the more he may be inviting complications, such as impaired vision.

The results achieved by Dr. Anderson are being duplicated by doctors around the world. In Israel, Dr. Yoram Kanter and colleagues in Haifa gave additional fiber to 22 people, including 11 diabetics, 6 overweight people, and 5 healthy people. After just three days, they noted that following a meal, blood sugar levels increased significantly less than they had prior to the fiber regimen. Interestingly, the effect was greatest in those subjects with outright diabetes—who, of course, stand to benefit the most from controlling blood sugar. But there was another beneficial effect as well. Insulin levels were also decreased. Here, the group that benefited most was the overweight folks. That's important, because high circulating levels of insulin are often a forerunner of diabetes. But in addition, it seems that high levels of insulin may also be a forerunner of heart disease. A Finnish researcher, Kalevi Pyorala, examined 1,040 men between the ages of 35 and 64. High insulin levels were associated with a two- to threefold increase in the incidence of heart attacks (*Family Practice News,* June 1, 1979).

"We conclude," said the Israelis, "that supplementing the diet with certain fibers can be regarded as an important therapeutic measure in the treatment of diabetic and obese patients" (*Israel Journal of Medical Sciences,* January, 1980).

In England, a group of doctors and nutritionists affiliated with Oxford University fed a diet high in carbohydrates and fiber (largely in the form of whole wheat bread) to

14 patients with adult diabetes and also concluded that "it is no longer justifiable to prescribe a low-carbohydrate diet for maturity-onset [adult] diabetes" (*British Medical Journal,* June 30, 1979).

Thomas and Powell in the *Journal of Human Nutrition* mention another important fact in diabetes control which is too often overlooked. And that is that the sheer *amount* of food—in terms of calories—is extremely important. It's been known for some time that losing excess weight is the first thing a diabetic should do as far as dietary change goes, and it's often been observed that normalization of weight can obviate the need for taking insulin by a maturity-onset diabetic. What's involved here is an improvement in insulin sensitivity—the readiness of the body to respond to insulin in the normal way. But we are reminded in this report that within just a few days of lowering calorie intake, there is a decrease in blood sugar levels, and this beneficial effect occurs whether the food reduction comes from carbohydrates, protein or fat. Overeating, in other words, is one of the worst dietary habits for a diabetic or someone who may be headed in that direction. Eating less (assuming you're overweight) will begin to have beneficial effects on your health almost instantly. (It's interesting that modern weight control emphasizes the desirability of eating complex carbohydrates to fill you up.)

One physician who believes in the new high-carbohydrate, high-fiber approach is Stephen Podolsky, M.D., of the Veterans Administration Outpatient Clinic in Boston. Dr. Podolsky told a meeting of the American Aging Association in Washington late in 1979 that he was particularly concerned about diabetic patients falling for "hidden sugar traps" in processed foods. "There is nothing more crucial than controlling the plasma glucose level," said the physician. "If it can be maintained within normal levels, the patient will reduce his risks and the disease process can often be slowed. The kind of patient who can be helped most is the middle-aged, overweight person." But, he complained, the job of getting the patient to those normal levels may be complicated by sugar hidden in processed foods—foods we don't even think of as sugared.

Some examples he cited included ketchup, which has more sugar than chocolate ice cream (29 percent vs. 21 percent) and Wishbone Russian Dressing, which has more sugar than Coca Cola (30 percent vs. 10 percent). Some other foods with very high sugar content, according to Dr. Podolsky, include: Coffee-mate nondairy creamer, 65 percent sugar; Hershey bar, 51 percent; Shake'n Bake, 51 percent; Quaker Oats 100 Percent Natural Cereal, 24 percent; and Ritz crackers, 12 percent. Except for the Hershey bar, most people wouldn't associate these foods with high sugar content, Dr. Podolsky said, so the patient must be made aware of the thousands of hidden food traps out there waiting to boost his blood glucose level (*Internal Medicine News,* December 1, 1979).

On the positive side of things, there are several specific nutrients believed to be especially important to diabetics. Probably the most interest has been stirred in scientific circles by the trace mineral chromium. "We're just at the beginning of extremely encouraging data," Walter Mertz, M.D., said in the keynote address at a major scientific conference on chromium held in Quebec in 1979. It was Dr. Mertz, chairman of the U.S. Department of Agriculture Nutrition Institute in Beltsville, Maryland, and Klaus Schwarz, M.D., whose early work first suggested a link between chromium and diabetes. They found that laboratory animals fed a diet of torula yeast (which is low in chromium) developed impaired glucose tolerance—their ability to utilize sugar and turn it into energy went astray. None of the usual dietary changes made any difference, but adding chromium to their diet corrected the problem. A new dietary agent was born, which Drs. Mertz and Schwarz dubbed the glucose tolerance factor, whose active ingredient was chromium.

Exactly how chromium does its work is not fully understood. What Dr. Mertz and others believe is that the mineral is a potentiator of insulin. In other words, it enables the body to use insulin in a more efficient and effective manner. It may help people with low blood sugar—hypoglycemics—and those with too much blood sugar—diabetics— to handle glucose adequately with less insulin.

According to Richard J. Doisy, Ph.D., who was associated with the State University of New York Upstate Medical Center in Syracuse, blood sugar problems due to inadequate intake of chromium may be quite common. In one of his experiments, Dr. Doisy and his colleagues worked with a group of 31 elderly people living in public housing units in Syracuse. All seemed active and in good health. Nearly half of them, though, were found to have impaired glucose tolerance. After taking brewer's yeast (one of the best sources of chromium) for only one to two months, 50 percent improved their glucose tolerance to within normal limits. Insulin-requiring diabetics were also studied by Dr. Doisy and found to be able to reduce their insulin requirements while taking chromium-rich brewer's yeast.

Rebecca Riales, Ph.D., a West Virginia nutritionist who has studied chromium told us that "people can get enough chromium in their diet if they're careful. We should try to get people to eat lots and lots of whole foods—a basic natural diet offering a variety of foods, especially ones rich in complex carbohydrates and fiber." In other words, plenty of whole grains, beans and fresh fruits and vegetables, instead of processed foods. Whole wheat bread, for instance, contains almost four times as much chromium as white bread. Brewer's yeast, as we mentioned before, is an especially rich source of chromium, although it's not easy to eat brewer's yeast in tremendous quantities. Other foods particularly rich in chromium include cheese, spices, mushrooms and liver.

Luckily, brewer's yeast and liver are also good sources of vitamin B_6, which diabetics also need. According to Australian research, diabetics have lower concentrations of vitamin B_6 in their blood than healthy people. Diabetics suffering with nerve problems also apparently have lower levels of B_6 than diabetics in general (*Australian and New Zealand Journal of Medicine,* December, 1977). Some research points to the fact that myoinositol, a compound related to the B vitamins, may also be involved in

Dietary Sources of Chromium

Food	Portion Size	Micrograms
Beef round	4 ounces	65
Calf liver	4 ounces	62
Potato	1 medium	32
Chicken dark meat	4 ounces	20
Banana	1 medium	18
Green pepper raw, chopped	½ cup	14
Thyme	1 teaspoon	14
Chicken breast	4 ounces	12
Whole wheat bread	1 slice	10
Parsnips cooked, diced	½ cup	10
Orange	1 medium	9
Brewer's yeast	1 tablespoon	9
Rye bread	1 slice	8
Haddock	4 ounces	8
Cornmeal white	½ cup	7
Carrots cooked	½ cup	7
Wheat germ	4 tablespoons	6
Cornmeal yellow	½ cup	6
Spinach raw, chopped	1 cup	6

SOURCE: *"Chromium in Foods in Relation to Biological Activity,"* Journal of Agricultural and Food Chemistry, *vol. 21, no. 1, 1973.*

preventing the nerve damage that often causes pain, numbness and impotence in diabetics. After clinical trials of 20 patients, Rex S. Clements, Jr., M.D., director of the Clinical Research Center of the University of Alabama Hospitals, reported a statistically significant improvement in nerve function in the high-myoinositol diet. Sources of this compound are not hard to find—particularly among our high-fiber, high-carbohydrate natural foods. They include cantaloupe, citrus fruits, peanuts and whole grains.

One last nutrient we'll mention here is another mineral, magnesium. According to Scandinavian researchers reporting in *Diabetes* (November, 1978), low levels of magnesium in the blood may be an important risk factor in the development of the major complication of diabetes. The complication, called diabetic retinopathy, involves tiny hemorrhages in the retina of the eye, which can lead to total blindness. When a team of doctors in Denmark examined a group of diabetics who had had the disease for at least 10 years, they found a "definite lowering" of blood magnesium levels. And those patients with the most advanced and severe retinopathy had the lowest magnesium levels of all.

Look for dietary magnesium in blackstrap molasses, nuts, peas, brown rice, soybeans, dark green leafy vegetables and whole grain products.

FATIGUE

Fatigue may be caused by almost anything and everything, including diet. But even when we narrow the causes down to diet, there are a multitude of nutrients that may be involved in any particular case of chronic tiredness. But don't be discouraged, because a sensible course of action is not at all difficult to plot.

First of all, before you begin reshaping your diet for the sake of combating fatigue, ask yourself if there has been a notable change in your life-style recently. Do you have a new job? A new hobby? Are you taking medication? There is no sense, you see, hoping to extirpate fatigue by a change of diet if 90 percent of the problem is coming from somewhere else. Here's another important point: If you have been unusually fatigued lately, and that represents a sudden change for you, you should definitely get a medical evaluation. Perhaps the problem is nothing more than an unwise crash diet you've been following, but in any case, get your problem medically checked out.

Now, assuming there is no physical cause that can be pinpointed for your fatigue, you can put your mind to designing a diet that contains the best pattern of nutrients to produce a steady flow of energy.

First, think about calories. Either too many or too few can wipe out your energy. We all know what a heavy meal makes us feel like—like going to sleep. Doctors call it postprandial stupor and all it means is a feeling of lightheadedness that comes upon us after a heavy meal. What's going on is that some of the blood that would normally be gurgling around inside your brain has deserted that organ to help digest the mighty supper you just ate, and the result is a desperate desire to lie down.

But beyond the acute effects of a big meal, just carrying around a lot of extra weight can drain your energy. If you're 50 pounds overweight, it's as if you are carrying around 50 pounds of bricks strapped to your body—all day long. And you've been sleeping with them, too. So our first bit of advice to those of you who are overweight is . . . *slenderize* and *energize.*

It can work the other way though, too. While some people are able to diet away many pounds and never really feel fatigued, other people, particularly if they're on a strict diet, may feel terribly tired. Our belief is that one pound a week is a fine rate to be losing, while more than two per week is likely to get you into trouble. Aside from the sheer number of calories you're taking in during a diet, the food you're cutting back on can make a big difference in how you feel. If you cut out foods that are particularly important to energy production, you're much more likely to wind up feeling that losing weight isn't worthwhile.

That brings us to a consideration of exactly which nutrients *are* the most important in preventing fatigue. A logical place to start is with the mineral magnesium. According to Ray Wunderlich, M.D., a nutrition-minded physician in St. Petersburg, Florida, "a deficiency of magnesium is a common cause of fatigue." That assertion is backed up by a number of studies. In one, 200 men and women who were tired during the day were given extra magnesium and in all but two cases, fatigue disappeared (Second International Symposium on Magnesium, University of Montreal, June, 1976). The richest sources of magnesium include blackstrap molasses, nuts, peas, brown rice, soybeans, dark green leafy vegetables, whole grain products and wheat germ. It's easy to see why so many people can be deficient in magnesium, especially if they're on a diet and are cutting out "starches."

While fatigue or tiredness may be hard to define, sometimes it's as simple as muscles that feel like they just can't do any work. The lack of magnesium, which helps muscles contract, can cause that tiredness. But so can a lack of potassium. Potassium deficiency is a well-known hazard among long-distance runners and professional athletes. The mineral helps cool muscles, and hours of exertion use it up. If it's not replaced, the result is chronic fatigue—even for a highly trained athlete.

But a potassium deficiency and the weakness that goes with it aren't limited to athletes. In one study, researchers randomly selected a group of people and measured their potassium intake. Those people with a deficient intake of potassium—60 percent of the men and 40 percent of the women in the study—had a weaker grip than those with a normal intake. As potassium intake decreased, so did muscular strength (*Journal of the American Medical Association,* October 6, 1969).

You could probably put up with a few days of weakness. But after a few *months* you'd feel terrible. "In chronic potassium deficit," wrote a researcher who studied the mineral, "muscular weakness may persist for many months and be interpreted as being due to emotional instability" (*Minnesota Medicine,* June, 1965).

Potassium is one mineral that anyone on a natural foods diet should have no trouble getting plenty of, as evidenced by this partial list of foods containing ample amounts: apples, apricots, bananas, brewer's yeast, broccoli, carrots, oranges, peanut butter, potatoes, sunflower seeds, tomatoes and wheat germ.

Lack of iron is another cause of fatigue that makes life seem burdensome to many, particularly women. Women lose iron during periods and pregnancy and while on reducing diets. One nutritional survey shows that over eight percent of American women have outright iron deficiency anemia. But even if your blood tests show adequate levels of hemoglobin, your energy levels still may be compromised by inadequate iron, a phenomenon discussed in more detail in our section on "Energizing Your Blood." Dr. Wunderlich, mentioned before, maintains that "this syndrome of iron deficiency without anemia is an exceedingly important cause of fatigue."

Liver, as you probably know, is the best source of iron, but any kind of meat, fish or fowl offers a goodly amount. In the vegetable world, turn to legumes such as peas and beans, potatoes, dark green leafy vegetables, or whole grain products. When fruit rich in vitamin C is eaten along with vegetable sources of iron, the amount of iron you can actually absorb is greatly increased. However, in cases of real anemia, we urge liver or other animal foods, because of the greater amount of iron and the greater rate of absorption.

Iron deficiency is, of course, caused by a lack of iron. But anemia—which means too little hemoglobin, the pigment in red blood cells that carries oxygen through our bodies—has other nutritional causes as well. "The commonest cause [of anemia] is iron deficiency, but folate deficiency . . . can also be a cause," says a report in *Lancet* (February 21, 1976). The report goes on to cite a study in which women received either iron alone, folate alone, or iron and folate together. Only 26 percent of those who received a single nutrient had a rise in hemoglobin, while 96 percent of those who received iron *and* folate had a rise.

Folate, a B complex vitamin, is a must for the creation of normal red blood cells. Without enough of this nutrient, red blood cells are too large, strangely shaped and have a shortened life span. The result is lethargy, weakness, fatigue. One psychiatrist, in fact, found that four of his patients with "easy fatigability" and other symptoms had low levels of folate. He supplemented their diet with the nutrient, and as their folate levels rose, their fatigue disappeared (*Clinical Psychiatry News,* April, 1976).

If you want foods that contain iron *and* folate in helpful amounts, turn to liver, peas, beans and other legumes, dark green leafy vegetables and whole grain products. Brewer's yeast also contains both of these important blood-builders.

Years ago, it was thought that vitamin B_{12} was a kind of miracle energizer, but like all medical infatuations, that one passed, too. Still, B_{12} remains an important vitamin, although many of today's physicians are excessively cynical about it. We believe that many people, particularly older folks, do better when their B_{12} levels are boosted. Here again, liver is your best choice, but almost any animal source of food, such as meat or fish, or even yogurt, has B_{12}.

We mentioned in the beginning that many things can cause fatigue, but one dietary cause we haven't mentioned is an intolerance to sugar. Call it low blood sugar or hypoglycemia or reactive hypoglycemia or what you will, what it means is that your body is overreacting to the sugar you eat, producing so much insulin that your blood levels of glucose drop to the point where you suddenly become profoundly tired. That is a different kind of fatigue than we have been talking about here, and we refer you to our discussion in the section "Low Blood Sugar (Hypoglycemia)." Usually, people with low blood sugar have satisfactory energy levels at certain times of the day but feel extremely tired at other times. If that seems to be your problem, by all means read the discussion of low blood sugar. You will find out in that discussion why the worse thing you could do to get more energy is to take the advice of TV ads that tell you to eat "energy foods" loaded with sugar to carry you through a period of fatigue. We look at it this way: if we human beings really needed cakes, candy and soda for energy, the Good Lord would have provided us with junk food trees instead of fruit.

GALLSTONES

Gallbladder disease is uncomfortably common in the developed nations, particularly among women. In the United States alone, the pain (and danger) of gallstones pushes an estimated half million people onto the operating table each year. Yet, the disease is found much less often in Africa and the Orient, the same areas of the world that also have a very low rate of heart and bowel problems. That observation, plus the fact that four out of five gallstones are composed mainly of cholesterol, seems to suggest that the same Western diet that encourages so many other problems may also be responsible for gallstones.

The latest research shows, however, that while the typical low-fiber Western diet does indeed encourage gallstones, the co-conspirator is not fat, but sugar. That seems a little illogical, because it's the cholesterol in the bile secreted by the liver that precipitates into stones. Nevertheless, experiments with animals seem to indicate that the sugar bowl may do more damage than the butter dish.

Sugar, of course, is a carbohydrate minus its natural fiber. What would happen if you turned the tables, and took away the sugar but kept the fiber? When a Canadian doctor fed generous amounts of wheat bran to his patients with gallstones, he found that the amount of cholesterol in their bile decreased significantly. Whether or not the bran regimen would actually cause gallstones that are already formed to dissolve is not yet known. Apparently, though, a high-bran diet *may* be useful in *preventing* gallstones (*Family Practice News,* April 15, 1979).

If you are a gallstone patient, you may have heard of a new experimental drug called chenodeoxycholic acid—or "cheno" for short. Cheno is a natural bile acid which increases the cholesterol-dissolving capacity of the bile. Experiments at a number of centers suggest that it may help prevent gallstones, but there remain certain questions about its safety. The good news is that it may be possible for you to actually increase the amount of cheno in your body *naturally*—by taking bran. English doctors have reported that in the patients they tested, bran caused an average 27 percent increase in the amount of cheno available in the bile.

Soybeans are also a good bet for helping to prevent gallstones. In fact, in hamsters, a diet high in soybeans has been shown to actually *dissolve* a significant portion of gallstones.

A wise diet for helping to prevent further problems with gallstones would seem to be very low in refined sugars such as sucrose, high in bran, and with plentiful amounts of soybeans. It's likely that most of the staple items in our dietary approach, including beans and whole grains, are also helpful in fighting a problem estimated to cost Americans more than $2 billion a year and an enormous amount of suffering.

GOUT

Gout is a good example of a disease that is inherited—but doesn't have to be. In other words, you may be born with a tendency to develop gout, just as you may inherit a tendency to develop heart disease or gallstones. But depending upon your diet and life-style, you can either prevent that vulnerability from ever bothering you, or you can invite it to lay you low with pain and drug dependency.

The metabolic flaw in gout, put simply, involves a disorder of uric acid metabolism. Uric acid is derived from substances called purines, which occur in certain foods and which are also manufactured by the body. The real trouble is not the purines themselves. It's just that, for unknown reasons, people with gout overproduce uric acid from them, which they then have trouble excreting. When the system becomes supersaturated with uric acid, crystals form in the small joints—notably the big toe, but sometimes the knee or ankle or other joints—causing extremely painful inflammation.

A high level of uric acid in the blood is not in *itself* considered a dangerous condition. But it is a warning that worse things may come. In other words, even though you have inherited the tendency to develop high levels of uric acid, you may well be able to prevent it from progressing to the point where crystals are deposited in your joints and true gout flares up. That may not be true in every case, but it is in many.

How do people invite gout into their lives? One way is by eating large amounts of rich, animal-source foods such as sweetbreads, mincemeat, goose, partridge, mussels, kidneys and herring. (Note that those foods are among the favorites of the wealthier 18th and 19th century Englishmen who were famous for their painful gout attacks.) All are high in purines—as are every type of organ meat, any kind of meat concentrate or extract (such as bouillon), anchovies, sardines, scallops, and yeast, both bakers' and brewer's. Yeast, by the way, is the only nonanimal food with a really high concentration of purines.

Fat contains no purines, yet may be very harmful to the gout patient when eaten in large amounts. That's because fats are believed to prevent the normal excretion of uric acid.

Drinking a lot of alcohol is also a good way to get into trouble, because it has the same effect on uric acid that fat does.

Finally, permitting yourself to be overweight is another open invitation to a gout attack. Putting all these factors together, we see that a diet high in animal products, fat, alcohol and excessive calories all conspire to ignite the wicked flames of gout—just as they do so many other chronic diseases.

To alleviate or prevent gout, one obvious step is to avoid all those high-purine foods we mentioned earlier. In addition, you will want to go light on *all* meat, poultry and fish. Don't eat those foods more than a few times a week and limit your portions to about three ounces. Do the same for the legume family—beans, lentils and peas—as well as mushrooms, spinach and asparagus. During a gouty crisis, your doctor may want you to stay away from those foods altogether, but when no trouble is evident, moderate amounts shouldn't cause any problem.

There is a wide variety of nourishing foods that are practically free of purines and can be eaten freely. Wheat, corn, rice, grain products such as spaghetti, and dairy products such as milk, yogurt and cheese all fall into that category. So do fruits, nuts and vegetables not mentioned above. You should have no trouble getting enough protein in your diet by emphasizing recipes that combine grains with dairy products or nuts.

Be sure to drink plenty of water and eat a goodly amount of fruits and fruit juices. They will help flush excess uric acid out of your body.

You should also lose weight, but the last thing you want to do is to go on a crash diet. The rapid loss of weight, particularly when your gout is flaring up, can actually make your condition worse. By concentrating on whole, natural and unprocessed foods, you will lose weight both naturally and gradually, probably not more than a pound or so a week. And by drinking a lot of water, several quarts a day, you will not only help to flush uric acid out of your system, but also sharply reduce your desire for snacks.

In the realm of folk remedies, strawberries and cherries are both valued for their supposed antigout properties. When these fruits are in season, you can try eating a lot of them for a few days and see what happens. If the cherries bring relief, the anecdotes we've heard indicate that canned or frozen are just about as effective as fresh. A tea made from the flowers of the broom plant is mentioned in the works of traditional herbalists as being beneficial for gout, too.

HEADACHES

A lot of tests and drugs can go by before the doctor ever mentions diet in connection with your headache—if he mentions it at all. But that does not necessarily mean that only the rare headache is caused by diet. While there is still an astonishing amount of controversy concerning the causes of the common headache and migraine, enough has been reported by reputable doctors for us to be able to give you more than an inkling of the many connections between what you eat and what you suffer.

First, consider coffee. We look upon it as the most widely used drug in modern society. That's not to say a cup or two will turn you into a degenerate. But if you're a regular coffee drinker, *not* having that cup or two you're so accustomed to can set your blood vessels gnawing at your brain with caffeine hunger. It's called a caffeine withdrawal headache. And it hits you when you haven't had your caffeine fix for about 18 hours or so, according to John F. Greden, M.D., of the University of Michigan Medical Center at Ann Arbor (*Family Practice News,* July 15, 1979). If you're the kind of coffee lover, then, who drinks only during the day, when you wake up in the morning you've already been without caffeine for 12 to 14 hours. That doesn't give you much time to get coffeed up again, and chances are you feed your habit with great regularity. But once in a while, probably on the weekend, or on a day when your schedule changes for some reason, you don't drink your cup of coffee in time and—wham, you've got it. People have been known to get coffee withdrawal headaches just by staying in bed too long on a Sunday morning.

But why is this happening? Is coffee really like heroin? Well, it is in the sense that our bodies become addicted to it. Precisely what is going on, even the *British Medical Journal* (July 30, 1977) can't be sure, but in an editorial, they suggest it has something to do with the fact that coffee causes blood vessels in the brain to constrict. When the supply of caffeine is withdrawn, the blood vessels may simply expand in some kind of perverse reaction, triggering a headache. Usually these headaches respond to caffeine, whether in drug form or simply a cup of coffee.

From all this, you can draw one of two different morals. The first is, never miss your daily coffee fix. The second is, *gradually* reduce the amount of coffee you drink to such a small amount—if not absolute zero—that it no longer has control over your nerves. And a devilish master it is, too. As the *British Medical Journal* notes: "Too much coffee produces symptoms indistinguishable from those of anxiety neuroses: recurrent headaches, mental irritability, cardiac arrhythmias and gastrointestinal disturbances."

Coffee is, in fact, so disturbing a force in modern life that its story has even managed to involve the Almighty. Yom Kippur, the highest of all holy days for Jews, you see, is set aside as a day of fasting. But while going without food is not usually a cause of great suffering for adults, going without *coffee* for 24 hours can be extremely painful for those sensitive to caffeine withdrawal headaches. According to an article in a medical journal written jointly by a doctor and a rabbi, that poses a serious religious problem. If a headache interferes with devotion, it destroys one of the main purposes of the fast (*New York State Journal of Medicine,* February, 1977). To observing Jews who are addicted to coffee—or any other people who plan to go on a short fast—the authors give two choices. First, wean yourself off coffee, as we mentioned before. Second, the authors suggest, take caffeine on the morning of the fast in suppository form. While nothing except water should pass the lips on the day of the holy fast, there is apparently nothing wrong with a suppository. It is a sad commentary on our enslavement to caffeine, however, that anyone should have to confront his Maker on the highest of holy days with the chemical equivalent of a cup of coffee stuck up his rear end.

HEADACHES FROM FOOD AND ADDITIVES

Ever hear of the "Chinese Restaurant Syndrome"? In a mild case there would only be pressure and tightness in the face, burning over the trunk, neck and shoulders, and a pressing pain in the chest. But if a headache comes, it usually takes the form of pressure throbbing over the temples and a bandlike sensation around the forehead. The culprit isn't actually the Chinese food but the monosodium glutamate or MSG which is often used quite heavily to "enhance" flavor.

Since MSG is used in so many processed foods—especially soups, stews, and lunchmeat preparations—by manufacturers who want to give you the flavor of meat without actually using more than a smidgen of the real thing, you don't have to eat "Chinese" to get the headache. Nearly 20,000 tons of MSG are manufactured in the United States every year. Usually, though, it's most troublesome in Chinese restaurants simply because of the amount used.

Hot dogs are probably the last thing in the world you'd ever find being sold in a Chinese restaurant, but franks can give you a headache every bit as nasty as a big plateful of chop suey. Again, it's not the food per se but the additives—in this case, the sodium nitrate and nitrite. Actually, if you're sensitive to chemicals, you should also avoid other cured meats such as bacon, ham, sausage and salami, all of which will probably contain nitrates.

It's possible that some cases of migraine may be triggered by the excessive amounts of salt that nearly everyone eats today. When John B. Brainard, M.D., put 12 migraine patients on a diet that prohibited all salted snack foods, he noticed a definite improvement after six months. In three cases, the headaches disappeared completely (*Minnesota Medicine,* April, 1976). Dr. Brainard feels that salty snacks are particularly likely to cause migraine in susceptible people if they are eaten on an empty stomach.

Back in 1975, a question from a doctor about dietary allergies was published in the *Journal of the American Medical Association* (April 28). The answer included a series of cautions by Donald J. Dalessio, M.D., of the Scripps Clinic and Research

Foundation in La Jolla, California. Besides some of those items we already mentioned, Dr. Dalessio warns the migraine-sensitive person against

- all kinds of alcohol, particularly red wines and champagne
- strong aged cheese, particularly cheddar
- chicken livers, pickled herring, canned figs, broad bean pods, and chocolate
- skipping meals, fasting and eating an excessive amount of carbohydrates (such as cake) at any one time.

That last caution raises another point. It may not be *what* you eat that's causing your migraine, but *when* you eat. Dr. Dalessio mentions that hypoglycemia, or low blood sugar, can definitely trigger a headache in a susceptible person. That's something many of us know on our own, even if we don't get headaches all that often. The hypoglycemia headache comes when we skip a meal. Or when we eat too much sugar or other refined carbohydrates, triggering a flood of insulin from the pancreas, which drives the blood sugar so low that our brain starves for fuel and a headache results. In some people, alcohol can also induce hypoglycemia.

James D. Dexter, M.D., and two colleagues in the departments of psychiatry and neurology at the University of Missouri-Columbia School of Medicine decided to test the hypoglycemia theory of headache in a group of 74 patients. Giving them a five-hour glucose tolerance test, they found 56 patients had a blood sugar curve indicative of what is called reactive hypoglycemia, meaning that after eating a large dose of sugar, their blood sugar takes a dramatic nose dive. These 56 patients were put on a diet that eliminated table sugar and featured six small meals a day, which is pretty much a standard meal plan for hypoglycemics. The results of the diet were quite promising. Well over half the patients enjoyed better than 75 percent relief from their migraines, while many others experienced worthwhile improvement (*Headache,* May, 1978).

THE FOOD ALLERGY CONTROVERSY

In describing reactions people have to the foods we've been talking about, we have purposely not used the word *allergy.* We call it "sensitivity," because most allergists tell us that allergies to food, as compared to allergies to pollen, for instance, are remarkably rare. Some doctors argue that even food sensitivities are, in fact, largely psychological. So what we are basically talking about here are reactions whose nature is not quite understood. However, there are *some* physicians, mostly in the field known as clinical ecology, who maintain that allergies to food are extremely common. Most other doctors don't believe them, claiming that what they are seeing are psychological effects. Whatever the truth, Dr. Ellen C. G. Grant of the department of neurology, Charing Cross Hospital in London, has reported that in testing a group of 60 migraine patients, the most common foods found to cause suspicious symptoms were, in descending order, wheat, oranges, eggs, tea and coffee, chocolate, milk, beef, corn, cane sugar, yeast, mushrooms and peas. In fact, Dr. Grant said, "when these foods were avoided, all patients improved. . . . only nine (15 percent) still had headaches or occasional migraine attacks. An average of 115 tablets per month had been taken by each patient before the diet and afterwards only 0.5 tablets" (*Lancet,* May 5, 1979). Incidentally, Dr. Grant also reported that all those migraine patients who had high blood pressure experienced a drop of diastolic blood pressure to 90 or below when on the elimination diet. All of that sounds impressive, but most doctors would say, as did one medical critic, that what might be going on here is "faith healing." That same critic also expressed the opinion that the extensive elimination diet approach should be much more carefully tested and proven before "depriving anyone unnecessarily of the pleasures of the table" (*Lancet,* May 26, 1979). Our feeling is that eliminating foods from the diet is certainly worth a try, especially when other approaches are not productive.

HEARING

In your school days, you may have read stories about tribespeople of distant lands, whose hearing is remarkably sharp. The moral to be drawn was that living in quiet solitude is conducive to good hearing, while our own world of constant rumbling and grinding destroys the natural sensitivity of our ears. And no doubt, there is a good deal of truth to that interpretation. But is there something more involved here? Could diet, in fact, have anything to do with good hearing?

Some years ago, an international team of otolaryngologists, or ear and throat specialists, wondered about that question after testing the hearing of the primitive Mabaan Tribe of the Sudan. The scientists were particularly impressed with the exceptional hearing of the older folks who, they noted, also "seemed to age more slowly than we do." Could this have something to do with the fact that their diet was low in saturated fat, consisting mainly of millet seed, wild dates, nuts, corn and fish? Could their excellent hearing be related to the fact that they all had low cholesterol and that high blood pressure and heart disease were extremely rare?

To test that hypothesis, the scientists turned to a unique living laboratory, consisting of two mental hospitals in Finland. There Finnish doctors were conducting important trials of a low-fat diet. For the first five years of this study, the population at one hospital was fed the usual Finnish diet, which is high in saturated fat from animal products such as cheese, eggs and meat. Meanwhile, patients at the other hospital were fed a diet in which polyunsaturated fats from vegetable sources were used instead of saturated fats.

The doctors found that after five years, the patients eating the polyunsaturated fats not only had healthier hearts, but had significantly better hearing as well. At that point, the diets were reversed, and four years later, another test of hearing was performed. Results? Patients who previously had the best hearing now had the worst. More exciting, patients who previously had the worst hearing now had the best. In fact, the doctors said, it was "startling" that the effect of the aging process itself was "not only arrested—but even reversed" in those patients who avoided saturated fat for all those years (*Acta Oto-Laryngologica,* October, 1970).

Remarkably similar findings were reported by an American doctor, James T. Spencer, Jr., M.D., of West Virginia University School of Medicine. Many cases of inner ear disease, Dr. Spencer found, can be successfully treated by putting patients on a high-nutrition, low-fat diet similar to that generally prescribed for heart patients (and used throughout this book). Dr. Spencer examined 444 patients with hearing loss, ringing or fullness in the ears, vertigo and other symptoms of inner ear problems. Staggering, nausea, vomiting and headaches were also present in some cases. Laboratory analyses revealed that nearly half of the patients were suffering from elevated levels of cholesterol, triglycerides or similar fats in the blood. Abnormal glucose tolerance indicative of diabetes or a prediabetic condition was evident in 87 percent of the patients. And 80 percent of them were overweight to the point of obesity. Putting the emphasis on what he calls "good basic nutrition," Dr. Spencer altered the patients' diet to restrict saturated fats, refined sugars and starches, and concentrated sweets. He also urged all overweight patients to reduce their weight to an ideal level.

Among those who conscientiously followed his instructions, the majority reported significant improvement. "Phenomenal gain in hearing has resulted with as much as a 30-decibel improvement in an affected ear," Dr. Spencer reported (*West Virginia Medical Journal,* September, 1974). Ear discomfort, vertigo, headaches and other symptoms were also relieved as blood fat levels fell." In addition to these improvements," Dr. Spencer wrote, "these patients generally improve in appearance from weight loss, exhibit or admit to having more energy, and feel more youthful. They are very grateful patients."

It should be no surprise that Dr. Spencer believes that hearing loss and other inner ear symptoms may actually be early forerunners of heart and artery disease. That belief would find affirmation in the results of heart studies in the two Finnish hospitals we mentioned before.

For hearing, then, we would recommend particularly the dietary approach described in our section on the heart, although the great majority of recipes in this book would be perfectly appropriate for a low-fat approach.

The high vitamin A content found in many of our recipes, particularly those with dark green leafy vegetables, carrots, sweet red peppers and liver, may also be doing good things for your ears. Investigations carried out by Richard A. Chole, M.D., Ph.D., at the University of California at Davis, revealed that the inner ear, or cochlea, has a concentration of vitamin A 10 times higher than most other body tissues. Only the liver, which serves as vitamin A's storage depot, contains more. Further, animals deprived of vitamin

A were found to develop "very dramatic middle ear changes that I believe lead to a greater incidence of middle ear infections," Dr. Chole told us. These findings tie in nicely with work done more than a quarter of a century before, by M. Joseph Lobel, M.D., a New York City physician. Dr. Lobel reported dramatic improvement in hearing among patients given injections of vitamin A—alone or in conjunction with vitamin B complex. "Results in 300 patients on whom this therapy was used indicated an average hearing gain in the left ear of 18.9 percent and in the right ear 17.3 percent," Dr. Lobel wrote (*Archives of Otolaryngology,* May, 1951).

ITCHING

By "itching," what we really mean is rectal itching, a phrase one hesitates to bandy about too freely in a cookbook. The term is too blunt even for physicians, who prefer the Latinate *pruritus ani.* The reason we have to drag pruritus into this book at all is that it is probably the single most common complaint heard by proctologists. That, and the happier fact that this tormenting, embarrassing problem may sometimes be eradicated by a few simple changes of diet.

In certain cases of pruritus, there is a specific cause, such as a dermatological condition. But in about 90 percent of the cases, there is no obvious cause for the suffering —which may last for years. William G. Friend, M.D., a proctologist associated with medical centers in the Seattle area, has written in a professional journal that in many instances, what "no obvious cause" really means is sensitivity to certain foods or drinks (*Diseases of the Colon and Rectum,* January/February, 1977).

The six foods which he says most often cause pruritus are coffee, tea, cola, beer, chocolate and tomatoes (including ketchup). The most common cause of all, Dr. Friend told us in a telephone interview, is coffee, including the decaffeinated kind.

What to do, says the good doctor, is to quit consuming all the aforementioned products for two weeks. Assuming that the itching stops, you may then experiment to see if you can return to consuming small amounts of the offending foods without bringing your problem back again. Be warned, though, that the threshold of trouble is usually about two or three cups of coffee a day, although it may be as little as half a cup. If a food is going to cause you trouble, the itching should return between 24 and 48 hours after it is eaten.

Lester Tavel, M.D., D.O., a proctologist from Texas, told us that besides eliminating chocolate, coffee, tea and cola from your diet (they are all irritants, he explains), it is a good idea to *add* yogurt culture—*Lactobacillus acidophilus* or *Lactobacillus bulgaricus.* Making your own yogurt at home with viable bacteria makes this an easy job. Dr. Tavel's advice, by the way, is backed up by a study of 87 people who were given *Lactobacillus acidophilus.* For 84 percent, the itching completely or almost completely disappeared (*Diseases of the Colon and Rectum,* May/June, 1969). Dr. Tavel also recommends B vitamins, so taking your yogurt with some wheat germ would be a good idea.

KIDNEY STONES

What do kidney stones have in common with gallstones, diabetes, heart attacks and Monday Night Football? You guessed it, they're all diseases of civilization. In fact, kidney stones are not only associated with civilization, but affluence as well.

When British doctors took a long look at the incidence of kidney stones between 1958 and 1976, they found what they considered to be a fairly clear-cut pattern. From 1958 to 1969, there was a 45 percent increase in kidney stone cases in British hospitals. Why? Perhaps, the doctors suggest, because the rate of kidney stones is closely tied to eating *expensive* food: for every rise in food expenditure, there was a corresponding rise in kidney stone incidence two years later—a kind of delayed effect. However, they claim, when rampant inflation got going in the early 1970s, and people were buying less food and cheaper kinds of food, the rate of kidney stones suddenly leveled off, and even dropped in some regions.

But certainly, kidney stones aren't created by high price tags. The real culprit, according to this theory, is animal protein—basically, another word for meat. As meat consumption went up in England, so did the rate of kidney stones. And when it leveled off, the same thing happened to kidney stones. The figures show, the researchers report, that animal protein was the big factor involved in these changes—and not protein in general, nor sugar, phosphorus, magnesium, or even calcium or oxalate (*Journal of Chronic Diseases,* vol. 32, no. 6, 1979).

Those last two suspects—calcium and oxalate—are what the most common type of kidney stones are composed of, and it's important to realize that how much of these substances you eat has very little, if any, effect on kidney stone formation. Of course, if you cut back your calcium intake to practically nothing, you would theoretically be making it harder for your kidneys to form calcium stones. But in practice, putting people on diets restricted in calcium has proven to be a fairly useless way of dealing with the problem. If your body has the tendency to form stones, it may do so even on a diet very limited in calcium. A study reported in 1979 in the *British Journal of Urology* (vol. 51, no. 3) found that restricting calcium seemed to work over the long haul in just 12 of 74 patients. What the long-term consequences of such strict calcium denial might be on the bones after years of such a diet is another matter.

Other researchers second the idea that a diet high in meat predisposes people who are genetically vulnerable to kidney stones to actually form those stones. But another school of thought underlines the importance of refined carbohydrates in the diet as a cause of the problem. When naval doctors in England gave varying amounts of sugar to normal young men, they found that the more sugar in the diet, the more calcium was excreted in the urine, creating the possibility of stone formation. What's more, the greatest amounts of calcium that were passed were going through the urinary tract just as the highest amounts of oxalate were present, creating an obvious opportunity for mischief (*British Journal of Urology,* vol. 50, no. 7, 1978). By the way, it's likely that the reason animal protein could lead to kidney stones is similar: high amounts of protein cause body calcium to be moved through the kidneys and excreted from the body.

Which school of thought is closer to the truth—the animal protein theory or the sugar theory—we can't yet say. Some doctors, of course, would say that neither school is right, that the only thing to do is to take diuretic medicines, which cause more water to flow through the kidneys and lower the concentration of minerals. A doctor of the latter persuasion is ignoring the fact that people of primitive cultures who eat very little meat and very little sugar get very few kidney stones. But we must also admit there's really no strong evidence, no actual clinical trial, in which people who already have an established tendency to pass kidney stones were helped by avoiding either meat, sugar, or both. But do not despair, followers of dietary therapy, help is on the way.

Curiously, it turns out that the most efficacious natural approach to stopping kidney stones in people who are already getting them concentrates not on what you *don't* eat, but what you *do* eat. And the important thing to eat is magnesium. Vitamin B_6 can help too, but magnesium is the boss.

The pioneering work was done in the United States by doctors in the Boston area who eventually involved some 64 urologists in different parts of the country in their research. The punch line of the whole project was that on a daily regimen of 180 milligrams of magnesium and 10 milligrams of B_6, most people with a history of passing stones were absolutely symptom-free. And not just for a few weeks or months either, but for *years.* Oddly, or maybe not so oddly, although this study was carried out by researchers with impeccable credentials, and published in the *Journal of Urology* (October, 1974), it seems to have disappeared into some kind of black hole as far as the universe of medicine is concerned. Most doctors simply don't care. Yet, to our knowledge, the magnesium approach has never been disproven. In fact, research teams in both France and Sweden have *confirmed* that supplemental magnesium does in fact prevent many kidney stones.

All these studies cited above used magnesium supplements, such as magnesium oxide, as well as vitamin B_6 pills, rather than foods. Scientists doing vitamin research always take that approach, in order to isolate the effect of individual vitamins. Whether or not the same beneficial results could be achieved using magnesium naturally occurring in foods (which might not be absorbed quite so completely as magnesium in pills), we cannot say. But it's possible that it would. To that end, see the following table for a list of some of the practical magnesium sources we can turn to to get our 200 milligrams a day.

Selected Sources of Magnesium

Food	Portion Size	Milli-grams	Food	Portion Size	Milli-grams
Soy flour	½ cup	155	Peanuts roasted, chopped	¼ cup	63
Soybeans dried	¼ cup	138	Beet greens raw, chopped	1 cup	58
Tofu (soybean curd)	4 ounces	126	Banana	1 medium	58
Buckwheat flour	½ cup	112	Blackstrap molasses	1 tablespoon	52
Wheat germ	¼ cup	97	Potato	1 medium	51
Almonds	¼ cup	96	Oatmeal	1 cup	50
Cashews	¼ cup	94	Spinach raw, chopped	1 cup	48
Lima beans dried, large	¼ cup	81	Salmon sockeye	4 ounces	43
Brazil nuts	¼ cup	79	Milk skim	1 cup	34
Pecans halved	¼ cup	77	Brown rice	½ cup	28
Kidney beans dried	¼ cup	75	Ground beef lean	4 ounces	28
Whole wheat flour	½ cup	68	Peanut butter	1 tablespoon	28
Shredded wheat spoon size	1 cup	67			

SOURCE: Adapted from Composition of Foods, Agriculture Handbook No. 8, U.S. Department of Agriculture, 1975.

LOW BLOOD SUGAR (HYPOGLYCEMIA)

The symptoms of low blood sugar, or hypoglycemia, range from simple fatigue and inability to concentrate, to shaking, sweating and anxiety. A couple dozen other emotional states—such as depression, forgetfulness, suicidal tendencies, extreme sensitivity to slight noises—could be tossed in for good measure. When you get right down to it, almost any kind of emotional or behavioral problem can be theoretically caused by hypoglycemia.

The real question, however, is whether or not *your* problem is related in some way to sugar metabolism.

The conservative medical opinion is that very few people suffer from hypoglycemia and, in those rare cases, it is almost always associated with a specific physical condition, such as a history of stomach surgery or liver disease. There is another school of thought, though, that insists that hypoglycemia is extremely common in our society and that it is a major factor in many nervous disorders, as well as school problems, marital difficulties, alcoholism and outbursts of violence. But no matter how many dramatic case histories this side comes up with, showing astounding recoveries following a change of diet, the conservative medical camp dismisses all of them as mere anecdotes involving people who cannot get themselves to admit that they have an emotional problem.

The interesting thing is, the tortured question of which side is right is largely meaningless to you as a concerned individual. That's because it's possible for you to determine, entirely on your own, whether or not you have a condition that can be helped by diet. We're assuming, of course, that if your symptoms are serious and persistent, you have sought medical advice. We're also assuming your physician has told you your problems cannot be explained by any obvious problem which might be affecting your energy level or moods, such as diabetes.

One way to investigate hypoglycemia is to take a glucose tolerance test. However, the conditions under which that test are given are extremely artificial and may not have much relevance to your everyday experience. A more logical approach is to simply adopt for a specified length of time—10 days, for instance—the dietary plan that is now widely used in cases where hypoglycemia *is* diagnosed. If your symptoms improve dramatically, stick with it as long as the benefit lasts.

There are two fundamental rules that must be followed in any successful approach to controlling low blood sugar. First, eliminate all sugars and sugar-rich foods from your diet. Second, divide your food intake into about six small meals a day. To understand *why* these rules are fundamental to the control of hypoglycemia, we have to understand a little bit about the condition.

At the nub of the whole matter is the fact that the brain—more than any other organ in the body—demands a steady supply of blood sugar, or glucose, to function normally. While some parts of the body can store glucose, and burn reserves if the circulating supply drops below normal, or in a pinch use substances other than glucose for fuel, the brain is a finicky eater. *No glucose?* I'll show *you!* And what it might show you is any of those symptoms we mentioned before—or maybe a brand new one.

But if the brain needs glucose, a form of sugar, why don't hypoglycemics simply eat sugar and put an end to their problems? Sounds logical. But while that might indeed bring relief for a few moments, in the long run it would do more harm than good because it's the sugar that gets most hypoglycemics into trouble to begin with.

For one reason or another, a heavy sugar intake in some people may cause the pancreas to pump out excessive amounts of insulin, the hormone that keeps blood sugar under control. If there is too much insulin, too much glucose is swept out of the bloodstream and the result is low blood sugar.

By avoiding sugar, then, you avoid triggering an outburst of insulin which could bring your spirits as low as your blood sugar.

By eating six meals a day, you're protecting against another source of blood sugar problems—what's usually called *fasting* hypoglycemia. As the name implies, that form of hypoglycemia occurs when you haven't eaten for too long a time and your brain becomes starved for glucose—perhaps before your stomach does. By eating a number of small meals throughout the day, your system—which can synthesize glucose from carbohydrates, fat, or even protein—manufactures a steady stream of glucose, enough to keep the brain satisfied, but not enough to get the pancreas all riled up.

At one time, doctors who treated hypoglycemia emphasized the importance of a high-protein, low-carbohydrate diet, believing that carbohydrates in general, not just sugar, triggered excessive insulin release. Now, there is a whole new approach to hypoglycemia, based on the discovery made by many researchers that a diet high in complex carbohydrates—basically grains, beans and vegetables—triggers the smallest degree of insulin activity and therefore keeps blood sugar levels the most stable. There is also widespread agreement that the fiber content of these complex natural carbohydrates is of critical importance in this process.

A classic experiment in diet and blood sugar was carried out by researchers at the Royal Infirmary in Bristol, England. Dr. G. B. Haber and his colleagues wanted to see what would happen if they fed three different forms of the same basic food to a group of people. First, they fed apples, just as they come off the tree. Second, they fed the same amount of apple turned into applesauce—to which no sugar or anything else had been added. Finally, the same amount of apple was juiced and the juice fed to the people.

When the apple was eaten, blood sugar increased and gradually fell to a point just slightly below where it had been at the beginning, before leveling off at normal. When the applesauce was eaten, the falling side of the blood sugar curve went down considerably lower before rebounding to normal. With the juice, the effect was even more exaggerated, with blood sugar levels dropping quite markedly below the normal level before stabilizing. While all this was going on, insulin levels were also being monitored and, as might be expected, drinking the apple juice rather than eating the apple caused considerably greater production of insulin. And the more insulin, the greater the dip in blood sugar levels.

Apparently, when carbohydrates are eaten in their natural form—in this case, a whole apple—the fiber slows down the rate at which the carbohydrate portion of the food can be absorbed by the body, thereby moderating the insulin response. Interestingly, although you might think that turning an apple into applesauce isn't doing any more than your teeth do, you might be mistaken. It appears as if the particles that have been blended in the machine may be finer than mouth-processed fruit, and permit faster sugar absorption, leading to greater insulin reaction. And without any fiber at all—just the carbohydrate-rich juice—the insulin reaction is at its maximum (*Lancet,* October 1, 1977).

Now, what does all this mean to the average person? If you're the average person who isn't bothered by hypoglycemia, not a heck of a lot. But if you're the average hypoglycemia victim, the lesson is pretty clear: take in your carbohydrates surrounded by fiber and you're going to make life a lot easier for your sugar metabolism—which in turn will make *your* life a lot more pleasant.

Translated into dietary action, what we're talking about looks something like this:

For breakfast—which you should eat promptly and without fail every day—go for some oatmeal or other hot grain cereal, or a bowl of muesli. A couple of whole wheat muffins wouldn't be bad either. Watch out for pancakes, though, because if you can't eat them without some kind of syrup, you're probably better off avoiding them. (Later, after the test period, you can try some applesauce on them.) All the foods we've mentioned are high in fiber and the complex carbohydrates that you want. If you eat them with some yogurt, you're getting plenty of good protein, too.

What you *shouldn't* be eating for breakfast if you're hypoglycemic is white toast with butter and jam, which is not only low in fiber, but is high in sugar. Although eggs have in the past been recommended for hypoglycemics because of their protein, they contain no fiber at all. So you will probably be better off concentrating on a breakfast of grains and some whole fruits, such as sliced apples.

What about juices for breakfast? For you, no. At least, not at first. Many people with blood sugar problems find eventually they are able to eat a certain amount of natural sugar-rich foods and get away with it, but we don't recommend it at this point. Right now, the most important thing for you to do is to go on as "perfect" a diet as you can for a week or two so that you can find out whether or not the change is going to help you. So give the hypoglycemic diet an honest chance to work.

In the midmorning, you should by all means have a snack. And needless to say, the last thing in the world you want to snack on is a doughnut. Try one of our nice fruited muffins, or half a sandwich, or some sliced apple and cinnamon in a cup of yogurt. The important thing is, eat. Don't let the momentum of work carry you past 10:30 without eating.

When lunchtime comes around, you will probably have to eat less than you are accustomed to, but since you've got a fairly substantial amount of food in your system already, you shouldn't be all that hungry. Your choice of food here is very wide, because all you really have to do is avoid anything that's excessively sweet or a meal that contains no fiber. If you do have some fish or poultry, which contain no fiber in themselves, be sure that you have some vegetables or grain products with them, to give you the fiber you're looking for.

While the hypoglycemic really does not have to concentrate on eating special foods, it might be worth mentioning that rice, corn, apples and carrots may be especially valuable for an insulin-sparing effect. There are many recipes employing these foods throughout our book, but regardless of what you're eating, you could always have a raw carrot for an appetizer and a fresh apple for dessert.

Stick to this regimen, as we said, for at least a week or more. Take your first meal early in the morning and your sixth meal shortly before retiring. If it's going to help you, you will be the first to know, and it will be up to you to decide how strict a diet you will have to keep with to maintain your benefits.

It's possible, if your symptoms only bother you sporadically, that you will have to keep up your test diet for longer than a week to see if you improve. If you have been bothered by several migraines a month, for example, and no physical cause has been found, you'll need at least several weeks to determine the therapeutic effectiveness of your new eating regimen.

If migraine is your problem, by the way, it's worth knowing that hypoglycemia may indeed be at the root of your problem. Intrigued by the fact that early medical workers associated hypoglycemia with headache, but that the association had been largely ignored of late, James D. Dexter, M.D., and colleagues, mentioned previously, evaluated 74 patients who suffered from migraine typically during the midmorning or midafternoon, when they hadn't eaten for several hours. When these patients were given a glucose tolerance test, 6 of them were classified as diabetic, while 56 had various degrees of hypoglycemia—of the type we've been talking about. Following diet therapy (the kind of program we've already discussed), all the patients who demonstrated a diabetic glucose tolerance curve "showed an improvement of greater than 75 percent, and 3 have been headache free." Of the 56 patients who showed signs of reactive hypoglycemia—low blood sugar several hours after eating—48 returned for follow-up examination. Out of that 48, 27 (or 56 percent) said they enjoyed at least 75 percent or more relief from pain, while the others reported at least some significant degree of relief (*Headache,* May, 1978).

Oh, yes, we forgot one thing. If you believe you may be hypoglycemic, stay away from alcohol, which under certain conditions can cause a hypoglycemic episode. Particularly lethal, however, is gin and tonic. Why? Because, although few people know it, tonic contains a good bit of sugar, and the combination of sugar and alcohol can be a left-right combination to the head of a sugar-sensitive soul. Two English physicians have seriously suggested, in fact, that a significant number of traffic accidents may stem from attacks of hypoglycemia following alcohol ingestion. The alcohol itself, of course, can disrupt thinking, but these doctors showed that the effect of gin and tonic on the nervous system was much worse than the effect of gin and diet tonic (*Lancet,* June 18, 1977).

There's at least one other important dietary aspect to controlling blood sugar metabolism, and that is a little-known but very important trace mineral—chromium. We discuss this mineral in more detail under the heading of "Diabetes," but for now, let's just say there's overwhelming evidence that this mineral helps the body use insulin in a much more efficient manner. As a result, less insulin is needed to control blood sugar and there's less likelihood of extreme fluctuations of blood sugar in either direction. The best sources of dietary chromium are brewer's yeast, cheese, mushrooms and liver.

MULTIPLE SCLEROSIS

Multiple sclerosis (MS) is a puzzling disease notorious for its unpredictable ups and downs, or in scientific language, remissions and exacerbations. Remissions may last for weeks, months, even years, which while wonderful for the MS patient, makes it extremely difficult to describe with any certainty the effect of a dietary change. Or any other treatment, for that matter. There is always some question as to whether the improvement was due to the treatment or simply a spontaneous remission.

But when all is said and done, the important thing is that MS patients want an approach that is at least worth trying. And one approach they can turn to with considerable hope is the work of Roy L. Swank, M.D., Ph.D., Professor Emeritus in the department of neurology at the University of Oregon Health Sciences Center in Portland. For some 30 years, this respected neurologist has been treating MS patients with what seems to be remarkable success, relying largely on simple changes of diet.

In his book, *The Multiple Sclerosis Diet Book* (Doubleday, 1977), Dr. Swank discourages patients from eating animal fats while, at the same time, encouraging them to greatly increase their consumption of unsaturated oils, rich in essential fatty acids. Patients following the diet, Dr. Swank maintains, do remarkably well. He compares his own results with those of a large group of MS patients treated at a well-known health center who did not use his low-fat diet. Fifty percent of those people were completely disabled after 10 years. But after a similar span, only 25 percent of the patients on the Swank diet were unable to work or walk. While normally, Dr. Swank says, about 70 or 80 percent of MS victims are still alive 15 years after the onset of the disease, he has been able to increase that percentage to 94. And while ordinarily only 30 percent of MS patients survive for 35 years after the onset of the disease, some 79 percent of patients on the Swank diet lived that long or more. Perhaps most encouraging, Dr. Swank observes, is that "when treatment was started in the early stages of the disease with little or no evident disability, 90 to 95 percent of the cases remained unchanged or actually improved during the following 20 years."

Interestingly, Dr. Swank notes that the geographical distribution of multiple sclerosis is very similar to that of heart disease, with the highest occurrence in those parts of the world where there is high consumption of beef, butter, milk and other animal-fat foods. In low-fat areas—such as India, the Far East, Latin America—this disease claims far fewer victims.

Switzerland is an especially interesting case. The northern Swiss, who follow

Germanic eating patterns, high in animal fats, have one of the highest rates of MS in the world. Their countrymen in the south of Switzerland, whose diet is akin to Italian with much less animal-source food, very seldom get the disease.

Dr. Swank isn't sure of the exact mechanism by which his diet helps, but he says that excessive saturated fat in the diet triggers clumping of tiny blood components called platelets. Those clumps of tiny clots may get carried along the bloodstream to lodge in the small vessels of the brain, where they may cause the nerve fiber damage that occurs in MS. Unsaturated oils like cod-liver, safflower and sunflower on the other hand, tend to inhibit the platelet-clumping effect. (For precisely the same reasons, many doctors and scientists investigating diseases of blood circulation also recommend avoidance of animal fats and increased use of the unsaturated oils.)

In his book, which is certainly worth consulting for full details, Dr. Swank says his patients are strictly forbidden to eat such high-fat foods as whole milk, cream, butter, sour cream, ice cream, chocolate and frankfurters. Packaged cake mixes, cheeses, commercial sauces, pies, cookies and similar processed items are also forbidden because they contain hidden or unknown amounts of saturated fat. Margarine, although derived from vegetable sources, is forbidden because the hydrogenation or solidifying process increases saturation.

If you have read much of our book, you will instantly recognize that none of these items, with the exception of very small amounts of cheese and milk, are used in any recipes or recommended for any purpose.

To help boost unsaturated oils, patients are advised to take one teaspoon of cod-liver oil a day. Vegetable oils can be used liberally in salads and other dishes, and consumption of sunflower and pumpkin seeds, nuts, fish, and whole grain breads and cereals is encouraged. Wheat germ or wheat germ oil is suggested as a good source of vitamin E, necessary to keep the unsaturated oils from being oxidized inside the body. A daily high-potency multivitamin capsule with minerals is also suggested.

The vast majority of recipes in our book are appropriate for this dietary approach. Meat is not excluded entirely, but is limited to one four-ounce serving of lean beef or the equivalent a day. Stay away from any recipe calling for cheese, other than low-fat ricotta or cottage cheese. While in many recipes we have kept the amount of oil to a minimum, it might well be increased, in salads for instance, to obtain the required amount.

MUSCLE SPASMS

Some muscle spasms or cramps make sense. After a winter's indolence you dig your whole garden in one afternoon, and the next day it feels like someone has done a spading job on your backbone. Or maybe you just twist into a funny position and suddenly one of your muscles turns into a baseball of pain. But some cramps *don't* make sense. Their severity is way out of proportion to any physical abuse you may have given yourself. Or there may be no physical element involved at all. Just a spasm, over and over. What's going on?

Well, aside from everything else that could be happening in your mind and body at that moment, it's possible that you have a low blood level of calcium. William Rea, M.D., head of the Environmental Control Unit at Brookhaven Hospital in Dallas, Texas, told us in an interview in 1980 that a low blood level of calcium is something virtually all serious cramp patients have in common. "For muscle contraction to be normal, adequate levels of calcium must be present in the body," says Ralph Smiley, M.D., a colleague of Dr. Rea. "We make sure all our patients with cramps are getting enough calcium," he told us.

"Some patients with tetany [severe muscle spasms], in particular, may need calcium to relieve their cramp," says Dr. Rea. "Once you get them on a maintenance dose, calcium lessens the seizurelike activity of tetany and helps prevent it from occurring." For milder cases of cramps, the "maintenance dose" is 900 milligrams of calcium a day, says Dr. Smiley. But, he adds, not only cramp patients need this amount. "The average American is low in calcium, and it would be a prudent preventive measure for most people to supplement their diet with the mineral."

Don't think, though, that you have to be hospitalized in a state of tetany to benefit from adding calcium to your diet. Several years ago, the editors of *Prevention* magazine conducted an informal Calcium Research Project, asking readers to describe any noteworthy experiences with calcium: good, bad or indifferent. Almost 3,000 readers responded, and what surprised us most when we completed tabulating all the responses was that over half of the respondents said calcium relieved their muscle spasms or cramps. "I had a muscle spasm in my back, shoulder and down the left arm," wrote Mrs. J. S. of Indiana. "Calcium relieved all that in two weeks." A letter from Mrs. R. F. of Arizona told us "I had arm cramps sometimes going from my little finger up to my shoulder and all the way down my spine." After taking 1,800 milligrams of calcium daily in the form of bone meal, she wrote, "all the cramps were completely eliminated." Mrs. N. C. of Texas reported that calcium relieved cramping in her calves. At age 60, she said, she retired from nursing and went into selling. She had to stand on hard floors for long hours on end, causing a great deal of pain and cramping in her legs at night. She began taking one dolomite tablet (a good source of calcium) before each meal and another at bedtime. "It made a new woman out of me," is the way she put it.

Nearly 1 out of every 10 respondents to the survey reported improvement or total relief of menstrual cramping and distress. Mrs. A. G. of Phoenix, Arizona, remarked that "for 10 years I took birth control pills to avoid the terrible menstrual cramps that sent me to bed every month since I began menstruating. But I was afraid of the Pill, so I tried calcium. Now I have absolutely no incapacitating menstrual cramps."

A "Mailbag" letter published in *Prevention* in 1977 illustrates the fact that while low back pain is usually considered to be purely physical in origin, it may have a critically important nutritional component. Mrs. G. K. M. of Ohio wrote as follows: "We have two children, ages three and six. Although for both pregnancies I was seeing a reputable obstetrician/gynecologist—reputed by some to be the 'best' in the area— I still suffered from intense lower back pain. As years passed, my troubles continued. Sometimes I would bend over and could not straighten up. Many times I've crawled up our stairs on my hands and knees. When the trouble first started, I asked my doctor about it. This fine, reputable man gave me quite a lecture and said something like this: 'It happens to all women when they have children. It gets worse with each pregnancy. The 'glue' just goes out of your lower back and pelvis.' Being naive and ignorant of such things, I let his comments pass.

"Now I know differently. About eight months ago I was leafing through a nutrition book and came upon one statement that leaped out at me: 'When a body is deficient in calcium, the mineral is drawn first from the lower back and pelvis.' I was on my way! I read everything I could find about calcium, and stocked up on bone meal and dolomite. At the first sign of lower back pain, I take a 'calcium break' of three or four bone meal tablets and a glass of milk. In an hour the pain is gone. Although I am a 'yogurt freak' and I have always eaten lots of cheese and milk, I was apparently not getting enough calcium. Now I lead a healthy, active life building stone walls, shoveling dirt and toting firewood."

Letters such as that, whether part of a survey or not, do not pretend to be "scientific" in any way. So if you are reading this as a scientist, simply ignore it. But if you're reading it as a person with chronic muscle aches, use your common sense. If you are left wondering exactly *why* you may need more calcium or how it works, you're in the same boat as the doctor who, pondering the success of calcium in treating cramps, wrote to a medical journal asking, "Why does this therapy appear to work in many patients in whom there is no obvious calcium deficiency and in whom the results are too-long-lasting to be a placebo effect?" (*Postgraduate Medicine,* November, 1975).

While doctors are figuring out the answer, cramp sufferers can try to end their misery by increasing their calcium intake with yogurt, tofu, salmon with bones, or simply bone meal, a kind of cross between a food and a supplement.

Vitamin E has also been credited with alleviating certain kinds of cramps but, as usual, it's been employed in amounts far greater than can possibly be supplied by normal foods. Doses in the range of 400 international units per day are said by some doctors to relieve leg cramps that occur at night, such as during sleep. And combined with a program of progressive walking over a period of weeks, the same dose of vitamin E reportedly brings about notable improvement of intermittent claudication, which is a cramping of the calf that occurs during walking—generally afflicting people with poor circulation.

PREGNANCY AND BREASTFEEDING

Perhaps you never gave a thought to the relationship between nutrition and good health. Then, suddenly, you're pregnant, and it begins to dawn on you: whatever you put into your mouth will go toward building your baby. You don't want to give birth to a child with all the mental and physical stamina of a jelly-filled doughnut—so, it's time to think about good nutrition.

First, think about how big a project this is going to be. While in the past pregnant women were warned to keep their weight gain down to 15 or 18 pounds, current recommendations range between 20 and 30 pounds for women of normal height. Even if you are overweight, do not choose pregnancy as the time to lose. Dieting restricts nutrients essential to the child. Research has shown that dieting in the obese woman during pregnancy causes a metabolic derangement that creates an abnormal environment for the fetus which may impair brain and nerve development, particularly in the three months before birth.

Restriction of calorie intake can also result in infants of lower birth weight. In general, bigger babies are healthier babies, and there is a strong association between mother's weight gain and the birth weight of the infant. A "fetus may be more vulnerable to maternal dietary deficiencies and excesses than has often been assumed," Richard L. Naeye, M.D., concluded after studying the relationship between weight gain and outcome of pregnancy (*American Journal of Obstetrics and Gynecology,* September, 1979).

Like any good builder, you will want to find the best materials in laying a sound nutritional foundation for your child. One of the most important is protein, familiar as the "building block" of life. Protein forms the hard and soft tissues of the baby's body, the placenta and the expanding uterus. You also need your own share of protein for the constant repair of body tissues.

The Recommended Dietary Allowance of protein for a pregnant woman is about an additional 30 grams per day, the amount contained in a cup of uncreamed cottage cheese. A 128-pound woman over the age of 19, for example, ordinarily needs a recommended level of 46 grams of protein daily. During pregnancy, her Recommended Dietary Allowance would be 76 grams. The following foods contain about 15 grams of protein: one cup of yogurt, one cup of cooked dry beans or peas, one-half cup of sunflower seeds, one-quarter cup of peanut butter and about three ounces of fish or poultry.

Protein has also been found to have a function in preventing or curing toxemia of late pregnancy, a severe condition marked by high blood pressure, excessive protein in the urine and fluid retention.

Tom Brewer, M.D., an obstetrician who headed a toxemia-prevention project in Contra Costa County, California, from 1963 to 1976, concluded that toxemia can be prevented with a proper diet.

"Women, poor women, who eat junk food are lacking many nutrients," Dr. Brewer told us. His study emphasized that without the proper amount of good, nutritious food in a diet, protein will be burned for energy instead of being used for the building of maternal and fetal tissues. Dr. Brewer stressed the vital protective role of adequate nutrition in human reproduction.

A more recent study, this one at Tuskegee Institute in Alabama, links dietary fat intake to the possibility of toxemia in pregnancy. A research team, headed by Ronald Chung, Ph.D., studied the diets of 65 pregnant women in their final three months of pregnancy. They found that those women who ate "significantly greater amounts of cholesterol and fat-containing foods" developed some degree of toxemia, while the other women, who ingested significantly less fat, did not.

For this, and other reasons stated elsewhere in this book, we recommend mostly nonanimal sources of protein, along with low-fat fish and poultry, with only occasional use of red meat. Liver, because of its tremendous store of vitamins, minerals and protein, is also recommended.

What about occasional news reports about vegetarian or macrobiotic mothers who give birth to less than healthy offspring? Is it possible to avoid meat and still get the protein and other nutrients necessary to insure a baby's healthy growth?

The answer is yes; but some careful planning is necessary. First, any extremes in diet, such as relying heavily on only a few foods for all nutritional needs, must be avoided. A wide range of foods should be chosen, as much as possible in their whole and fresh state, to insure good health.

Second, it pays to understand combinations of vegetable foodstuffs that will increase protein intake. Complementary proteins might be compared to bricks and mortar: neither one is at its strongest standing alone, but together they make a solid foundation.

Amino acids, which make up protein, are comparable to bricks and mortar. There are eight amino acids that cannot be manufactured in the human body. For these, we must depend on our food intake. Meat and animal products, such as cheese, contain all of the necessary amino acids in a proportion best utilized by the body. These amino acids are also available from grains, beans and other vegetable sources, but in each source, the proportions vary.

Here is where the complementing comes in. Where one source, such as grain, is weak in a certain amino acid, another, such as beans, is strong. By combining the two foods at one meal, all of the essential amino acids, in the proper proportion, can be provided.

Rather than worry about each amino acid, keep a few rules in mind:

1. Serve whole grains with beans, tofu, peas or lentils.

2. Combine whole grains with milk products, such as cheese.

3. Combine beans, peas or lentils with seeds.

More information on complementing proteins is available in Frances Moore Lappe's book, *Diet for a Small Planet* (Ballantine Books, 1975).

Societies all over the world have traditionally relied on vegetarian combinations as a protein source: corn tortillas and beans in Mexico, Middle Eastern hummus made with chick-peas and sesame seed paste, and tofu (made from soybeans) and rice in the Orient.

Relying on nonmeat sources of protein can allow you to meet the high protein requirements of pregnancy without overspending on calories or loading up on saturated fats. Many chemical residues are deposited in animal fat, and reducing meat intake means that less of these chemicals will build up in your body. These chemicals can be transferred through the placenta and in breast milk to the child. The same thing is true of any hormones, antibiotics, tranquilizers or preservatives present in meats.

Vegans, those who eat no animal products, not even milk or eggs, must be even more careful in balancing protein sources. In addition, it is necessary to add vitamin B_{12} to the diet, a vitamin found in animal products. Nonanimal sources include specially grown nutritional yeasts and commercial supplements.

DON'T RISK IRON DEFICIENCY

Iron, too, is important for the baby, but in this case the fetus draws what it needs from the mother. Estimates of iron stores in newborns show little or no difference between groups of infants whose mothers had iron deficiency anemia and those mothers who were not anemic. So just when you are at your heaviest, you may find yourself dragging, unless you provide adequate iron coverage for your own nutritional insurance. The estimated need for iron in pregnant and lactating women is 18 milligrams daily. Three ounces of liver contain 7 to 12 milligrams of iron; one cup of prune juice contains about 10.5 milligrams. Other iron-rich foods are: whole grain products, dried beans, wheat germ, blackstrap molasses and apricots.

Extra iron is needed to build hemoglobin as your blood volume increases to nourish the baby through the placenta. Iron deficiency will make you less able to tolerate exercise, for one thing, and there is evidence that cellular immunity, intellectual function and intestinal nutrient absorption can all be affected.

There are some steps you can take to increase your intake of iron. One is to use the old-fashioned cast-iron cooking pots and skillets. With acid ingredients and long cooking times, an appreciable amount of iron will be imparted to foods. You can also enhance the absorption of iron from nonmeat sources by accompanying meals with some form of vitamin C, such as citrus fruit, orange juice or a salad with dressing made from fresh lemon juice. A small amount of meat, fish or poultry also enhances iron absorption from all sources in the diet. On the other hand, milk, tea and eggs all restrict the absorption of iron.

Often contributing to anemia is the lack of sufficient folic acid, or folate. Folate is also needed for a healthy nervous system and brain. A group of compounds in the B vitamin family, folate is found in leafy greens and whole foods such as soybeans and whole wheat. Nuts, broccoli, asparagus, liver, onions, wheat germ and legumes are other sources.

Relying on processed "enriched" grains (such as enriched white rice, white flour and breads) will mean missing some of the important B complex. Although 11 B vitamins, as well as trace minerals and other nutrients, are depleted in milling flour, only three B vitamins are eventually replaced. Some enrichment!

During the last three months of pregnancy, calcium becomes especially important in your diet. Again, the baby is not shy in making its needs known, and will take what it needs for teeth and bone formation, possibly to your detriment, if your diet is not adequate. Our recommendation for pregnancy is about twice the normal 800-milligram allowance for adults. A quart of milk contains just under 1,200 milligrams. Other good sources of calcium are almonds, broccoli, cheese, ground hulled sesame seeds, tofu, soybeans, canned salmon with the bones, and dark, leafy vegetables such as kale.

Adequate intake of vitamin D goes hand in hand with calcium because it helps the body to utilize the mineral most efficiently. The recommended amount of vitamin D during pregnancy is 400 units daily, about the amount added to one quart of fortified milk. Vitamin D is also found in canned salmon, liver and fish liver oil. Sunlight on the skin is another source of vitamin D, so spend some time each day enjoying this valuable free "supplement."

In the past, doctors often advised pregnant women to cut down drastically on salt intake because sodium was believed to cause preeclampsia. Preeclampsia can lead to toxemia of pregnancy. Modern obstetric research has shown that salt has little or no relationship to the development of preeclampsia. Now, however, doctors and researchers believe that adequate sodium intake (2,000 milligrams daily) is necessary to maintain fluid balance. A quart of skim milk has about 500 milligrams of sodium; a quart of buttermilk about 1,300; and seven ounces of regular tuna about 1,680.

Iodine is another important mineral, vital for the functioning of the thyroid gland. Kelp powder, used in some recipes in this book, contains both iodine and sodium. Saltwater fish and seaweed products also provide both sodium and iodine.

NUTRITION DURING BREASTFEEDING

Your nutritional responsibility to your growing child does not stop when the baby has left your womb. We will not go into all the advantages of breastfeeding here, both to mother and child, since entire books have been written on this subject. What we will point out is the continuing need for excellent nutrition throughout the period when you breastfeed.

In the four to six months following birth, the baby will double the weight it acquired throughout nine months in the womb. This is evidence of the heavy demands the breastfeeding infant makes on the mother.

If you have been observing good eating habits throughout pregnancy, you have a fine basis for breastfeeding. Your body will have built reserves of many nutrients, and some fat, to provide for lactation.

However, it is still important to continue good eating habits during this vital growing period of your baby. Save any efforts at losing weight (much will probably come off during this period, anyway) until the child is obtaining some foods other than breast milk.

An extra serving of complementary proteins, green and yellow fruits and vegetables, citrus fruit, two cups of milk and some additional calcium-rich foods above your normal (nonpregnant) daily diet will meet the requirements of lactation.

An extra 500 calories a day should be balanced to provide the nutrients you and your baby need for health. This should include 20 additional grams of protein (see *Index* for good sources of low-fat protein).

There are certain areas where special attention is needed for a healthy breastfeeding diet. Many women begin lactation with practically no folate reserves. Folate deficiency is the most prevalent nutritional problem during pregnancy. Because of this, it is a good idea to concentrate on foods high in folate during lactation. These include asparagus, broccoli, legumes, liver, nuts, onions, wheat germ, whole grains and dark green, leafy vegetables.

Calcium levels, again, should be about double those of a nonpregnant woman's diet. We earlier mentioned food sources high in calcium. In order for the calcium to be absorbed by the baby, vitamin D is necessary. Although human milk contains some vitamin D, careful exposure of the baby to sunlight will also protect against deficiency.

During lactation, there are several substances that should be avoided. One of these is caffeine. Newborns eliminate caffeine much more slowly than adults, and can develop high concentrations of caffeine if it is regularly transmitted through the breast milk. The half-life of caffeine in the newborn averages 80 hours, while for an adult, 3.5 hours is the average. Although the average half-life of caffeine for infants is unknown, if it is comparable with newborns, toxic concentrations might accumulate if nursing mothers have large caffeine intakes (*Archives of Disease in Childhood,* October, 1979).

Oral contraceptives can also affect a lactating mother's milk. Some hormones can be transferred to the child in physiologically active doses (*American Journal of Clinical Nutrition,* April, 1980).

Some children can show a sensitivity to foods ingested by the mother. Colic, for example, may be a symptom of intolerance to cow's milk. Studies with some mothers have shown that infants may be affected by cow's milk proteins transmitted through the breast milk. By eliminating cow's milk products, some mothers have found that they can make the colic disappear (*Lancet,* August, 1978). More information on allergies and breastfeeding is available in the book, *You Can Breastfeed Your Baby . . . Even in Special Situations,* by Dorothy Patricia Brewster (Rodale Press, 1979).

While we have outlined some of the most important building elements for you and your baby here, every vitamin, mineral, and trace element is important during this rapid time of change and growth. Following a few simple rules will help to make the period of pregnancy and breastfeeding a healthy and nutritious one:

1. Rely on whole foods, such as whole grain bread and pasta, and unrefined cereals.

2. Eat fresh fruits and vegetables whenever possible, since freezing and canning destroy some amount of important nutrients.

3. Avoid refined flours, sugar and highly processed foods, since these will be taking the place of healthier foods needed in your diet.

4. Keep fat intake to a minimum.

What you don't eat can have as important an effect on your unborn offspring as what you do eat. There is some concern among experts, for example, that any amount of alcohol can cause potential damage to the fetus at any time in pregnancy. There is also some evidence that heavy caffeine intake (from coffee, tea, cola drinks or cocoa) can lead to poor pregnancy outcomes. Smoking, too, should be eliminated to provide the healthiest uterine environment for the baby. Also, pregnancy is a time to be especially suspicious of any chemicals or additives added to foods, such as saccharin, nitrites and nitrates, BHA, BHT and artificial coloring.

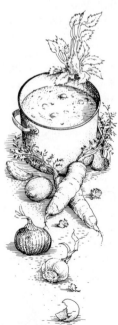

MAIN DISH

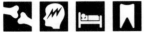

La Leche League Salmon Loaf

Makes four servings
15½ ounces (439 g) red salmon, with bones, drained
1 cup (250 ml) dry whole grain bread crumbs
2 stalks celery, chopped
2½ cups (625 ml) chopped mushrooms (about ½ pound [225 g])
¾ cup (175 ml) chopped scallions or 1 small onion, minced
1 clove garlic, minced
1 egg, beaten
2 egg whites, beaten
2 tablespoons (30 ml) lemon juice
½ cup (125 ml) cottage cheese
2 teaspoons (10 ml) minced fresh dillweed
½ teaspoon (2 ml) basil

We developed this recipe, high in calcium needed by pregnant women and nursing mothers, for the 1979 annual conference of the Pennsylvania La Leche League. Turned out to be delicious, too!

Crush salmon bones and toss together with the flaked salmon in a mixing bowl. Add bread crumbs to bowl. In a skillet, steam-stir celery, mushrooms and scallions, using a few drops of water to prevent scorching before vegetables begin releasing their juices. Add garlic, and steam until vegetables are tender and liquid has evaporated; then combine in a large mixing bowl with the salmon, crumbs and the remaining ingredients. Place mixture in a 9 × 5-inch (23 × 13-cm) loaf pan and bake in a preheated 350° F. (175° C.) oven for 30 to 45 minutes, until firm.

DESSERTS

Vanilla Pudding

Makes four servings
3 cups (750 ml) whole milk
3 tablespoons (45 ml) cornstarch
¼ cup (60 ml) medium unsulfured molasses or honey
1 teaspoon (5 ml) *Vanilla Extract*
1 egg, well beaten
4 strawberries

Gently heat 2½ cups (625 ml) of the milk in a heavy-bottom saucepan. Into the remaining ½ cup (125 ml) of milk, stir in the cornstarch until dissolved. When the milk in the pan is hot, but not boiling, stir in the cornstarch mixture. Add the molasses and *Vanilla Extract*. Lower the heat, and cook very gently about 8 to 10 minutes, until the pudding is thick. Remove from heat.

Stir ½ cup (125 ml) of the pudding into the egg. Return the egg and pudding mixture to the pan and heat a couple of minutes, stirring constantly.

Pour pudding into individual serving dishes and chill. To serve, wash and remove stems from strawberries. Cut berries in half and place in center of each pudding.

Almond Cheesecake

Makes 12 servings

Crust:

¼ cup (60 ml) sunflower seeds
½ cup (125 ml) wheat germ
1 tablespoon (15 ml) soy oil
1 teaspoon (5 ml) honey

Filling:

2 cups (500 ml) ricotta cheese
1 cup (250 ml) low-fat cottage cheese
3 eggs
2 egg whites
½ cup (125 ml) honey
1½ teaspoons (7 ml) *Vanilla Extract*
¼ cup (60 ml) *Blanched Almonds,* chopped
1 teaspoon (5 ml) finely grated lemon rind
1 tablespoon (15 ml) whole wheat flour

The flavor is so extraordinary you won't believe this is a "health" dish—with about one-half of the calories and one-third the fat of ordinary cheesecake.

To prepare crust, grind the sunflower seeds into meal in a blender with short bursts on high speed. In a small bowl, combine the sunflower seed meal and wheat germ. Add the oil and honey and stir with a fork until combined. Press into a lightly oiled 9-inch (23-cm) springform pan, covering the bottom and halfway up the sides.

For the filling, remove any lumps from the ricotta and cottage cheese by mashing them with a wooden spoon against the sides of a large mixing bowl. The cottage cheese can also be pressed through a sieve for smoothness.

Beat the eggs and the additional egg whites together in a medium bowl until light. Add to the cheese mixture along with the honey, *Vanilla Extract,* almonds, lemon rind and flour. Stir together until combined. For a light-textured cheesecake, beat the mixture for 5 to 10 minutes on high speed with an electric mixer.

Pour cheese mixture into the prepared crust and place the pan in a 350° F. (175° C.) preheated oven for 45 minutes to an hour. At the end of that time, turn off the heat and let the cheesecake cool in the oven with the door ajar for about one hour. Remove from the oven and allow to cool to room temperature before chilling. Allow to chill at least six hours before serving.

Variation: Substitute 3 cups (750 ml) ricotta cheese or 3 cups (750 ml) cottage cheese for the combination above. Substitute ¼ cup (60 ml) raw ground sunflower seeds for the *Blanched Almonds.*

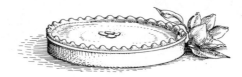

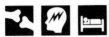

Rice Pudding

Makes six servings

½ cup (125 ml) brown rice
⅔ cup (150 ml) water
4 cups (1 l) whole milk
½ teaspoon (2 ml) finely grated
    lemon rind
3 tablespoons (45 ml) honey
1 egg yolk
½ teaspoon (2 ml) *Vanilla*
    Extract
2 egg whites
dash freshly grated nutmeg

Rinse the rice and place in a large enameled saucepan with the water. Bring to a boil, reduce heat, cover and simmer until water is absorbed.

Add the milk, lemon rind and honey. Simmer 20 to 25 minutes, until the rice is tender, stirring occasionally. Remove from heat.

When rice has cooled slightly, add a spoonful of rice to the egg yolk, then add yolk mixture and *Vanilla Extract* to remaining rice. Beat the egg whites with an eggbeater or on low, then medium speed with an electric mixer. Fold the egg whites gently into the rice mixture.

Pour the rice mixture into a lightly oiled, 8 × 8-inch (20 × 20-cm) shallow baking dish. Dust with a little freshly grated nutmeg. Place pudding in a preheated 300° F. (150° C.) oven for about an hour, until the surface is browned. Serve hot or cold.

Variation: Add ½ cup (125 ml) seedless raisins, chopped pitted dates or chopped figs to the pudding before baking.

PROSTATE PROBLEMS

Ask a doctor about a prostate gland that's been acting up and if you're a man over the age of 40, the reply will probably contain such phrases as "extremely common," "not much we can do about it except surgery," and "no one really knows what causes it." If you're over 60, you may even hear phrases like "at your age, it's perfectly natural."

Well, it's true that as men become older, the problem of an enlarged prostate —as well as other problems with the gland—become increasingly common. Some estimates put the figure of prostate sufferers at 12 million, nearly every one of them middle-aged or older men.

But while prostate problems may indeed be extremely common, does that mean they're "natural"? And because no one understands why prostate glands cause trouble, does that mean there is nothing a reasonable person can do to help avoid problems? Consider the following facts before framing an answer:

According to one prostate researcher, Erik Ask-Upmark, M.D., of the department of medicine at Sweden's University of Upsala, prostate disease "represents a relatively new pathologic entity. When I was studying medicine, one heard of its existence, but chiefly as a . . . curiosity" (*Grana Palynologica,* vol. 2, no. 2, 1960). Apparently, in our century some basic change has come about that has made what was once a rare disease all too common. And—no surprise—there is some good evidence suggesting that this basic change has something to do with the way we Westerners now eat.

For one thing, a high-fat diet may encourage the most common kind of prostate trouble—benign prostate hypertrophy, or BPH for short. In that condition, the gland is swollen (but not cancerous), and may pinch off the urethra, leading to burning pain, inability to void, and worse if left untreated. And all of this from a high-fat diet? That's the indication of studies by Carl P. Schaffner, Ph.D., professor of microbial chemistry at Rutgers University. Interested in the observation that dogs share man's propensity to develop prostate problems, Dr. Schaffner discovered that by reducing the cholesterol levels in aged dogs, he was also able to reduce the size of the animals' enlarged prostates (*Proceedings of the National Academy of Sciences,* August, 1968).

Another study, reported to the American Urological Association in 1976, using human prostates, corroborates the possibly harmful effect of high cholesterol levels on prostate disease. Camille Mallouh, M.D., chief of urology at Metropolitan Hospital, New York City, examined 100 prostates from men of all ages and found an 80 percent increase in cholesterol content of prostates with BPH.

There has been some indication that zinc may also play a protective role in the prostate story. Doctors in Chicago have found that patients with chronic prostatitis generally suffer from low levels of zinc in both prostate and semen. They have further reported that of 19 patients with BPH who were given zinc supplements, all reported an easing of painful symptoms and, on examination, all but 5 showed a decrease in prostate size. A larger number of patients who were given zinc for infectious prostatitis were also significantly helped, according to these reports. However, to our knowledge these good results have not been duplicated by other physicians. And those doctors who carried out the work admit that zinc therapy cannot replace conventional treatments of most prostate disorders.

The best bet, then, for helping the prostate gland through nutrition would be to follow the general tenor of eating in this book—the low-fat high-nutrition approach. Detailed dietary information about zinc is given in the section on "Sexuality."

SEXUALITY

Imagine a romantic dinner. What do you see? In the way of food and drink, we mean. Probably, what slips into your mind first is an image of wine. Champagne, perhaps. And then? How about a sweet dessert? Something really special. Followed, perhaps, by some freshly ground coffee, or an after-dinner cordial. In most of our minds, such are the essential ingredients that go along with candlelight and soft music for a romantic dinner. Yet, for some of us, the kind of dinner we just described might be a large part of the reason why the result of a night of romance is too often frustration instead of fulfillment.

Let's start with the wine, because that's the most direct cause of problems. Alcohol, to put it bluntly, is a downer—in more ways than one. The man who drinks four or five bottles of beer a night may think he's pretty manly when he's chugging the brew, but his manliness could abruptly end when sex begins. Tolerance varies, of course, and two bottles of beer may do to one person what it takes three double highballs to do to another. The important thing to be conscious of here is a daily pattern in which either partner chronically goes to bed with just enough of a load on to be sexually dulled. Keep in mind that the same amount of alcohol that had no effect on you 10 years ago may be doing you in today. Other people get in trouble because they become anxious about their sex life, and drink to "relax" before going to bed. Finally, we wonder how many men realize that alcohol tends to lower their testosterone level (*New England Journal of Medicine,* October 7, 1976). Any way you look at it, drinking significant amounts of alcohol on a regular basis constitutes nothing less than an antisex regimen.

Sweet things would seem to be an appropriate finish to a special meal, but to a person with potency problems, sugar may be the very thing that's souring his or her sex life. When a researcher gave glucose tolerance tests to impotent men and to women unable to have orgasms, he found that an unusual number, particularly the men, seemed to have trouble processing the sugar they ate. People with this kind of hypoglycemic tendency may become weak or confused or headachy after consuming large amounts of refined carbohydrates. And apparently, the syndrome doesn't do their sex life any good either. Hypoglycemia surely isn't the only thing that might be behind a sex problem, but it deserves to be looked at (*Journal of the American Medical Association,* August 25, 1975).

Clinical psychologist Barry Bricklin, Ph.D., affiliated with Hahnemann Hospital in Philadelphia, told us that "I have observed a relatively high proportion of sexual problems in patients who have been medically diagnosed as hypoglycemic. They tend to be bothered by all varieties of problems relating to sex. They may be too distracted, too irritable, too depressed or too argumentative with their spouse to enjoy relations. Or they simply fall asleep too fast because they are so exhausted." Looking at it the other way, when patients come to Dr. Bricklin complaining of impotence or another sexual problem, they are referred to a physician for a medical evaluation which includes a glucose tolerance test. It is often the case that the physician, in lieu of a glucose tolerance test, may suggest that the patients go on a strict hypoglycemic diet (described later) for a few weeks. If hypoglycemia is involved in their problem, then their symptoms should clearly improve during that time.

"Although I have found that a fair number of people with sex problems have hypoglycemia, and improve when they go on a proper diet," Dr. Bricklin says, "I can't say that I've ever seen a case where the entire sexual and behavioral problem cleared up simply with a change of diet. Two things could be happening in these cases. First, if a person has a tendency to hypoglycemia, he usually develops emotional problems as a result. These problems can create difficulties with spouses, damage relationships and otherwise become serious problems in themselves. Or, the initial problem could be basically psychological—but with anxiety, often comes hypoglycemia. In these cases, a dietary and physical dimension becomes a serious part of the psychological problem. So in most cases, we have to look at both aspects. Often, they coexist in the same person, creating a vicious cycle of anxiety, poor diet and impaired metabolism, leading to more anxiety, and so on.''

The management of a low blood sugar problem entails avoiding refined carbohydrates in all forms—including not only soda, cake and sweets, but also honey and even excessive amounts of fruit juice (whose natural sugars are absorbed by the body more rapidly than they would be from the whole fruit). It also means a regimen of six small meals a day, which helps keep blood sugar levels on an even keel. Each meal, from the first in the morning to the last at night, should contain something fairly substantial, whether it be meat, vegetables, whole grains, yogurt, cheese or nuts. Don't rely on fruits, which have very little protein and too much fruit sugar.

In recent years at least two new dimensions have been added to our understanding of how blood sugar problems may be improved. The first is by consuming a diet high in fiber-rich unrefined carbohydrates. These, of course, are foods such as whole grains, potatoes, beans—the kinds of foods that appear regularly throughout this book. The modulating effect of these unrefined, natural carbohydrates on blood sugar is so strong that high-fiber diets have proven effective in getting people with mild diabetes off insulin completely. For the hypoglycemic, it is likely that the high-fiber approach would also be very beneficial, probably because the rate at which food sugars can be absorbed is slowed down. Slower sugar uptake means that even a relatively impaired metabolism can handle them with less need for insulin.

In addition to a diet high in complex carbohydrates, the person with a tendency to develop unstable blood sugar levels would do well to pay attention to brewer's yeast. Brewer's yeast, an excellent source of so many nutrients, is also one of the richest natural sources of chromium, a trace element. Chromium is believed to play a very important part in the way our bodies use glucose or blood sugar. Supplements of this trace mineral have been shown to improve the ability of people with impaired metabolism to handle sugar. A leading expert on chromium, Dr. Richard Doisy, whom we mentioned previously, also told us that taking about a tablespoon of brewer's yeast every day might *prevent* glucose intolerance from developing in the first place.

What about that strong, freshly brewed cup of coffee in our imaginary, romantic meal? Generally speaking, one or two cups of strong coffee are not as likely to have detrimental effects on sexuality as the equivalent dose of alcohol or sugar upon individuals with vulnerable metabolisms. However, drinking significant amounts of coffee throughout the day—say, four or five cups or more—can very easily interfere with sexual relations for the simple reason that the amount of caffeine we're talking about affects the entire nervous system, which of course influences sexual behavior. In the words of one medical journal, the coffee habit can produce such symptoms as irritability and stomach upset which are "indistinguishable" from those of anxiety neurosis. That is not exactly a good frame of mind (or body) to be in at bedtime. The effect of coffee on nerves (tea is not much better) is discussed at great length in the chapter Take a Load Off Your Nerves. For now, let's just say that it is a good idea to be in a very relaxed state before entering into sexual relations, and drinking coffee will only make it more difficult for you to achieve relaxation.

The idea that specific foods may have a strongly positive effect on sex drive or performance is widely regarded as a myth. But it isn't. Not exactly.

True, there are no foods known to turn normal sex drive and potency into lust-on-the-loose. But what about people who *don't* have normal desires and abilities? For them, there is now real hope from better nutrition.

The breakthrough came several years ago, when researchers at the Veterans Administration Hospital in Washington, D.C., were studying four men with kidney disease, all of whom were impotent. They had trouble having erections and enjoyed sexual intercourse as rarely as once every six months. All four were on regular hemodialysis for their kidney disease. Their doctors wondered why the men were impotent since they were otherwise in "good condition" (*Lancet,* October 29, 1977).

Noting that the men had low levels of zinc in their blood, and knowing that zinc plays a major role in the health of the sexual organs, the researchers gave them zinc supplements. Three of the men soon reported an improvement in their sexual functioning. And when zinc was added to their "dialysis bath"—the solution in which their blood was purified—three of the men reported a "striking improvement" in potency after two weeks. The fourth noticed an improvement after four weeks. The men reported an increase in their ability to have erections and ejaculations, increased frequency of intercourse and a heightened sex drive. Not bad, huh?

"Zinc appears to be essential for the metabolism of testosterone, which is the primary male hormone," Lucy D. Antoniou, one of the researchers who conducted the study told us. Without enough testosterone, sex drive can't get in gear. And without enough zinc, testosterone levels are low.

Putting the whole picture of sex and nutrition together, we see that on the negative side are alcohol and sweets and on the positive side, small but regular meals, lots of complex carbohydrate foods, brewer's yeast (for its chromium) and zinc. For a complete list of zinc-rich foods, see the *Index.* For the time being, we'll mention liver, lamb, dark meat turkey, wheat germ, sunflower seeds, whole grain products, nuts and cheese. Oysters happen to be particularly good sources of zinc (which may be why folklore considers them aphrodisiacs) but we are too concerned about the possibility of pollution to recommend oysters as a source of zinc.

Reforming a diet along these lines is not going to transform anyone overnight. Common sense tells us not to expect much for a week, or a month, or possibly longer in some cases. But be patient, because these dietary changes will be doing so much good for you in so many ways that you will actually begin benefiting the very first day.

SMOKING

You could be eating the most healthful diet in the world, but if you are a smoker, you're still worse off than your neighbor who loves junk food—but doesn't smoke. Sure, sprouts are good for you, and sure, extra vitamins can help, but nutritionally, there's just nothing you can do to set right the harm done by those 75,000 puffs of smoke you take every year on your pack-a-day habit.

Interestingly, though, you don't see many people who *do* eat an excellent diet, high in natural foods, who also smoke. Why is that? Probably the most obvious answer is that people who are so interested in their health that they would eat natural foods can also be expected to have tried their best to kick the smoking habit. But there is another way to look at the situation: Is it possible there's something about natural foods that positively *discourages* smoking? That makes it easier to quit when you decide you've had enough? Could be, according to some doctors.

Here's one way it could work. Picture yourself having just put away a cheese omelet, home fries and a Danish. Now you're finishing it all off with a cup of coffee. How would a cigarette feel? Terrific, right? Or at least, logical. Now, picture yourself just having eaten a cup of hot vegetable soup, some whole grains, salad, and fresh fruit. *Now* how would a cigarette feel? At best, awkward.

We can think of at least three reasons why the natural, more healthful meal doesn't invite you to smoke. First, there is the matter of what psychologists call *cues*. Smokers have lit up so many times after having a cup of coffee that as soon as they smell it, or even think about it, they get an urge to light up again. But since precious few smokers actually developed the habit of smoking after a rice and fruit salad, eating one does not trigger that habitual response.

There is also the matter of taste. Even though taste is highly subjective, it does seem that *strong* flavors such as those in beef, pork, coffee, liquor and similar foods seem to serve as a good base for cigarette smoke, while the gentler, more subtle flavors of fish, rice, fruit and the like do not hanker to be topped off with tobacco smoke.

But there may well be another dimension in the relationship between food and smoking. Specifically, there is now this important news for all smokers: The possibility definitely exists that a diet consisting largely of vegetables and fruit may take a good deal of the pain and difficulty out of kicking the habit that is stealing life from you with every single puff.

The theory behind this diet is fairly simple. It's the result of speculation on the action of acids and bases in the body. And, according to A. James Fix, Ph.D., and David M. Daughten, a behaviorial research team at the University of Nebraska College of Medicine, nicotine is a strong base substance. "It has been shown that the more acid the body's chemical balance, the more readily nicotine is flushed out of the system," Dr. Fix told us. "Therefore, the more nicotine a smoker would need to take in to replace it." The opposite side of the coin is that the more basic or alkaline the body's chemical balance, the *less* nicotine is lost, and the less the smoker would need to take in from outside—*which just might reduce the urge to smoke enough to make the difference during a quitter's crisis.*

The man who pioneered work in this area is Stanley Schachter, Ph.D., professor of psychology at Columbia University. In January, 1977, Dr. Schachter and his colleagues published a series of five reports on the effects of acidity on smoking *(Journal of Experimental Psychology: General)*. Dr. Schachter was concerned with determining exactly what makes people smoke. He contended that the smoking habit is basically a nicotine addiction, not a psychological hang-up. To prove his contention, he first examined the effects of a highly acidic urine on smoking. "In the acid-condition" he found "there is an increase of roughly 17 percent in smoking (roughly seven or so cigarettes more per day for a two-pack-per-day smoker)."

Dr. Schachter then performed some tests which suggested why smokers may feel a greater need to indulge their habit when under stress, even slight stress: in such situations, he discovered, their urine becomes more acid.

When Dr. Fix heard about the research going on in New York, he decided to see what would happen if he gave participants in a stop-smoking program he was running either sodium bicarbonate—a base substance—or ascorbic acid, in addition to the usual therapy. The results?

"By the fifth week, the people taking sodium bicarbonate were virtually off cigarettes. Only one person in that group was smoking as much as two cigarettes a day. Everybody *except* the people taking bicarbonate was still smoking about eight cigarettes a day."

There were some statistical problems with the study, because some people forgot to take their pills. But while admitting these shortcomings, Dr. Fix is intrigued by the fact that "of those who had failed to reduce their smoking from one session to the next, 82 percent were in the acid group."

Are we going to ask smokers, then, to take sodium bicarbonate? No. Curiously, even Dr. Fix feels that an alkalizing *diet,* rather than a simple supplement, would produce much better results.

"In general, there are two problems that smokers face," according to Jack

Alkaline-Acid Effects of Some Common Foods

Food	Portion Size	Alkaline (+) or Acid (−) Effect	Food	Portion Size	Alkaline (+) or Acid (−) Effect
Molasses	2 teaspoons	+60.0	Onion	1	+1.5
Lima beans			Squash, summer		
dried	⅛ cup	+42.0	seeded	1 cup	+1.0
Raisins			Butter	2 pats	0.0
seedless	⅓ cup	+34.0	Honey	1 tablespoon	−1.1
Figs	1½	+33.0	Whole wheat		
Beet greens	1 cup	+27.0	bread	2 slices	−3.6
Spinach	1 cup	+27.0	Peanuts		
Dandelion greens	1 cup	+18.0	without skins	16	−3.9
Brewer's yeast	1 tablespoon	+17.1	Cottage cheese	⅛ cup	−4.5
Almonds	12	+12.0	Cheese, cheddar	1 cube	−5.0
Carrot	1 large	+11.0	Brown rice	3 tablespoons	−5.7
Soy flour	2 tablespoons	+9.5	Buckwheat flour	2 tablespoons	−7.1
Celery	2 stalks	+7.8	Walnuts		
Grapefruit juice	½ cup	+7.0	English	12	−7.8
Sweet potato	1	+6.7	Cod	4 ounces	−8.4
Tomato	1 small	+5.6	Lamb chops	2	−9.7
Strawberries	12	+5.5	Beef liver	4 ounces	−11.0
Peas			Beef loin	4 ounces	−11.0
dried	2 tablespoons	+5.0	Egg	1	−11.0
Mushrooms	7	+4.0	Chicken	4 ounces	−14.0
Apples	1 large	+3.7	Lentils		
Milk			dried	2 tablespoons	−16.0
whole	1 glass	+2.3	Wheat germ	2 tablespoons	−20.0
Buttermilk	1 glass	+2.2			

SOURCE: *Adapted from a chart appearing in* Hawk's Physiological Chemistry *(McGraw-Hill, 1965).*

NOTE: *All foods are calculated in the raw state and are meant as a guide for estimating average portions or servings.*

Smith, Ph.D., a nutritional biochemist who worked with Dr. Fix on the study. "One problem is that they want to lose their smoking habit, and the other is that they often find they are gaining weight when they stop smoking. If you consume a diet that mainly consists of vegetable foods, you produce a less acid urine and thus achieve the same thing as the sodium bicarbonate. Coincidentally, vegetables are foods that are not calorically dense. So vegetables not only make stopping smoking easier, but at the same time will not contribute to the weight problem. Fruits in general, excluding plums, prunes and cranberries—which acidify urine—are also good."

A quick look at the table will show that meat, fish, and poultry are all acid-forming foods. But aside from them, Dr. Fix says that "the other thing that's really a potent acidifier of the urine is alcohol. It is incredible how many people trying to quit fail when they take a drink, and suddenly get the urge to smoke. Alcohol also lowers willpower, which makes it even harder."

For those smokers who may be taking vitamin C supplements, the acidifying effects can be avoided by taking sodium ascorbate instead. Sodium ascorbate is alkaline and has been recommended by Linus Pauling, Ph.D., as a way to avoid any possible acid side effects of ascorbic acid in sensitive individuals.

Don't get the idea that there is something unhealthful about acid-forming foods, because there isn't. Or that you will have to avoid them forever, because you won't. All you are looking for is that little extra edge during the week or so that you're weaning yourself away from the worst health habit you could possibly have. During that period, eat generous helpings of spinach or beet greens and snack on raisins, figs, almonds, carrots and celery. Brewer's yeast in some juice would also be a help.

Vincent E. Gardener, M.D., director of the Better Living Center of Philadelphia, where a five-day stop-smoking program is run regularly by the Seventh-day Adventist Church, told us that on the first day of the plan, the diet consists of just fruits and fruit juices. That gives the smoker plenty of vitamin C "and has an alkalizing effect on the body, so that nicotine is excreted at a slower rate. On the second and following days, the diet consists of vegetables and whole grain cereal, also because of the alkalizing effect," Dr. Gardener told us. At the same time, he suggests avoiding sugar and junk foods, meat, coffee and tea. Even decaffeinated coffee should be avoided, according to Dr. Gardener, because of the association between coffee and smoking.

VARICOSE VEINS

There's nothing we know of a dietary nature that can make severe varicose veins disappear. However, we do know about something that may well be able to prevent varicose veins in people who are genetically disposed to their development, or halt their progress if the condition is still developing. That something is—believe it or not—fiber.

Fiber? That probably goes against everything you ever heard about varicose veins—probably against common sense as well. Yet, once you understand a few fascinating facts about anatomy, it all becomes perfectly reasonable. We learned this in an interview we conducted in London with the eminent British surgeon and medical researcher Dr. Denis Burkitt.

Q: *You say that varicose veins can be prevented by a high-fiber diet. Now surely the veins in the legs aren't directly connected to the colon. Many people must find it difficult to believe that a low-fiber diet can cause varicose veins.*

Dr. Burkitt: *Of course they would! And so would the average doctor. But there is no other hypothesis you can put to me that can hold any water. You see, we know by actual measurement that when we strain to pass constipated stools, we create pressures of between 200 and 400 millimeters of mercury in our abdominal cavity. We know also by actual measurement that all of those pressures are* transmitted down into the veins of the legs. *But they are blocked when they get to the first valve. If you keep putting these pressures in the veins every day for 30 or 40 years, the vein dilates. If the vein dilates, the cusps of the valves can't meet. And now we know by American work in Oregon that valves give way sequentially, one after another, down the leg. And we know that when the valves give way, abdominal straining plus gravity can put pressures in the veins of the ankle equal to or about that of arterial blood pressures [ordinarily much greater than the pressure in veins].*

Q: *That is a rather novel theory, isn't it?*

Dr. Burkitt: *Let me tell you a thing that your textbooks in America say on varicose veins. They say it is due to the fact that man isn't adapted to standing upright. Now, this is absolutely rubbish. People in native communities probably stand far more than the average person does in the West. Yet, varicose veins are extraordinarily rare in these communities. Secondly, they say it is due to pregnancy. But in fact, there is an inverse relationship, geographically, between pregnancies and varicose veins. The more pregnancies, the fewer cases of varicose veins.*

*A professor in an Indian university examined 1,000 pregnant women just before delivery and found 11 with varicose veins or 1.1 percent. When non-*pregnant *women of the same age group were examined in North America,* 30 percent had varicose veins. *So far, we've had several surveys of varicose veins done in India and in none of them did more than 3 percent of the people have varicose veins. And in every group, varicose veins were more common in men than women. And the men don't often get pregnant. Now, of course, if you have defective valves, then during the pregnancy they will become more noticeable. But they'll disappear again after the pregnancy.*

And there was a very extensive study done in the Pacific islands, and the only thing that related to the prevalence of varicose veins was the impact of Western culture. If we took age into account, the number of pregnancies made no difference at all. So these things which we are told to be the cause of varicose veins, they just don't stand up. And if you should say that heredity is a factor —well now, black Americans have just as many varicose veins as white Americans today, but the condition is rare in the parts of Africa where their ancestors came from.

Dr. Burkitt didn't mention it in his answer, but it's likely that the reason women have a greater incidence of varicose veins than men, at least in Western countries, is simply a reflection of the fact that they suffer more often from constipation. Or so it seems. And that would seem in turn to be a reflection of the fact that they simply eat less fiber than men: basically because they eat less *food* than men, but also perhaps because they tend to avoid bread, potatoes, beans and other high-fiber foods.

In our discussion, Dr. Burkitt also neglected to explain the mechanism by which pressure is transmitted from the colon down into the legs, which is actually what our first question was about. But later he referred us to an article he wrote in *Archives of Surgery* (December, 1976) that made it all quite clear. The pressure is not transmitted from the colon itself, but from the entire abdominal cavity. That's because when we strain at the stool, we squeeze our abdominal muscles, and in so doing compress *everything* inside, not just the colon. And one of the organs that is compressed is the large vena cava, which is carrying the blood being returned to the trunk from the legs. That pressure is transmitted down into the leg veins, distending them and weakening the valves whose job it is to prevent just such a back-up from occurring.

We want to make it clear that an advanced case of varicose veins, perhaps with complications, is not going to disappear just because you switch to a high-fiber diet. However, it seems to us that if you have reason to believe you are prone to develop varicose veins because of heredity, or if you now have a mild case, or maybe even if you want to prevent a fairly bad case from getting worse, making sure that you don't have to strain makes a lot of sense. We suggest turning to our chapter Better Digestion, Top to Bottom for more specifics about the prevention of constipation and plenty of recipes that are high in whole grains and bran. Drink some extra water, too.

VISION

The best-known connection between diet and sight involves vitamin A. The retina or back wall of the eye, which activates the optic nerve leading to the brain, is made up of light-sensitive cells called cones and rods. The cones are sensitive to color, while the rods are only able to detect different shadings of light. The rods contain a pigment called rhodopsin, which is a chemical cousin of vitamin A. When light strikes a rod, its rhodopsin is chemically broken down, and can only be restored to working order if vitamin A is present.

In this case, a vitamin is the very stuff from which vision is "made." If the body is lacking in vitamin A, the natural restoration of rhodopsin to working order does not take place, and the rods quit working. The first sign of the breakdown is a loss of night vision in the dim light where the eye can no longer distinguish colors and must rely totally on its black-and-white vision. Proper night vision is totally dependent on the rods, and vitamin A.

In severe cases of vitamin A deficiency, there is extensive damage to the cornea as well, but the center of vitamin A's action seems to be in the retina. Other nutrients have been shown to aid vitamin A there. Scientists working at the government's National Institutes of Health laboratories have demonstrated the close interaction of vitamin E with vitamin A in the retina (*Investigative Ophthalmology and Visual Science,* July, 1979).

Tests in rats revealed that vitamin E had an important effect on how much vitamin A was available for use in the eyes. But vitamin E was also shown to have a direct effect on the retina. Rats fed diets containing no vitamin E, but adequate amounts of vitamin A, developed significant retinal damage.

When the diets were deficient in vitamin A as well, the same damage occurred, plus an additional loss of light-sensitive rods and cones in the retina. "Rods and cones were involved equally," the scientists reported, "and their pattern of loss was not like that found in vitamin A deficiency." The lack of vitamin E seemed to compound the damage usually done by a lack of vitamin A.

Zinc is also closely tied to vitamin A in maintaining good vision. One of the highest concentrations of zinc in the body occurs in the retina of the eye. Zinc is necessary to keep blood levels of vitamin A at the proper level and to mobilize vitamin A for use from its storage place in the liver. Animal studies conducted at Harvard University have shown that "zinc deficiency can interfere with the metabolism of vitamin A, especially in the retina (*Journal of Nutrition,* November, 1975).

Revealing studies of zinc and vision were carried out by scientists at the University of Maryland. The researchers treated six patients suffering from cirrhosis of the liver and night blindness—a common complication of that disease and, as we have seen, of vitamin A deficiency. One patient, given both vitamin A and zinc from the start of the study, regained normal night vision within a week. Three patients treated with zinc alone also returned to normal.

But two patients fed vitamin A alone for a period of two weeks did not do so well. Though one improved, the other showed no response at all. Only when zinc was added to their treatment did their sight return to normal (*American Journal of Clinical Nutrition,* April, 1977).

Other nutrients are involved in good vision, in ways that have no apparent connection with the action of vitamin A on the retina. A study of some 900 schoolchildren in India revealed some interesting connections between the B vitamins and general good vision. The children were screened for signs of possible B vitamin deficiency and had their vision tested. One month later the tests were repeated.

"Of the 715 children with evidence of vitamin B complex deficiency, 126 (17 percent) had altered acuity of vision," the scientists reported, "whereas of 247 children without signs of vitamin B complex deficiency, only 6 (2 percent) had altered visual acuity. There was a significant association between different vitamin B complex deficiency signs on the one hand and visual defects on the other" (*British Journal of Nutrition,* January, 1979).

B VITAMINS CAN IMPROVE VISION

The clincher, however, came when the researchers tested the effects of B vitamin supplementation on the children's vision. When supplemented children were examined after one month, B vitamin intake was found to be closely associated with improvement in vision. "While 56 of 70 supplemented children had shown improvement, only 4 of the 26 unsupplemented children had improved."

Thiamine (vitamin B_1) has been used in other studies to correct disorders of the optic nerve interfering with normal vision. Here the problem was not with the sensitive cells receiving the image, but with the nerves that carry the image to the brain. Studies have shown that thiamine-deficient diets cause degeneration of the optic nerve in rats (*Medical Journal of Australia,* January 15, 1977). In more recent research, two ophthalmologists examined people on special diets who did not seem to be getting enough thiamine. In all four cases, the patients suffered similar losses of vision near the center of their visual field. And in all four cases, the problem was corrected when the patients were given thiamine supplements (*British Journal of Ophthalmology,* vol. 63, no. 3, 1979).

NUTRITION AND CATARACTS

Riboflavin (vitamin B_2) has been linked to the prevention of cataracts, another of the many disorders that can rob us of our vision. Cataracts are a clouding of the lens that focuses the image on the back of the eye. Researchers have produced this clouding in several kinds of fish by feeding them diets lacking riboflavin. When scientists at the University of Alabama tested cataract patients for riboflavin deficiency, they found 8 of 22 were not getting enough riboflavin. "Our data suggest that riboflavin deficiency may play a role in cataract development in man," the scientists concluded. "Exploration of this possibility is particularly attractive because . . . the administration of riboflavin [is] easily accomplished and might lead to either the prevention or regression of cataract formation" (*Lancet,* January 7, 1978).

Vitamin C might also be involved in preventing cataracts. Scientists at the University of Maryland recently found that vitamin C protects the lens against chemicals normally produced there by the action of light. That finding was particularly interesting given the high concentration of vitamin C naturally found in the lens of the eye and in the fluid directly in front of it, between the lens and the cornea. In fact, the concentration of vitamin C in that fluid, called the aqueous humor, is among the highest of any of the various fluids in the body.

"These findings," the University of Maryland scientists said, "further emphasize the concept of the importance of essential nutrients in prevention of certain forms of cataracts" (*Proceedings of the National Academy of Sciences USA,* July, 1979).

Vitamin E may also aid in the prevention of diabetic cataracts. Scientists in Canada reported last summer that experiments on rat lenses kept in a high-sugar solution indicated that vitamin E sharply reduced cataract formation. The scientists believe the action may have something to do with vitamin E's ability to protect tissue from oxidation reactions that occur naturally in the body.

If there is one food that a person concerned about a nutritional approach to better vision should be eating more often, it's liver. Liver is not only exceptionally high in vitamin A, it's also a rich source of riboflavin and all the other B vitamins, vitamin E and zinc. Liver is even a pretty decent source of vitamin C, if you don't let it sit around too long after it's been cooked. In other words, you will find in liver every nutrient we've discussed in this section. Wheat germ is also valuable, being both a good source of B vitamins and vitamin E. Almonds are good sources of riboflavin and vitamin E. Although many people fail to get enough vitamin A, if you have any appetite at all for natural foods, it shouldn't be much of a problem. If you don't go for liver, try apricots, broccoli, sweet potatoes, spinach or pumpkin.

Index of Recipes According to Problem

The recipes in this book are not prescriptive; only your doctor can prescribe a diet. Rather, our recipes are informational, which means they contain food elements our research indicates are believed to be generally helpful, or at least nonharmful, for various health problems.

Recipes given in chapters dealing with a certain subject, such as digestion or weight control, are designed especially for that area of concern.

However, because many recipes are appropriate for more than one health area, we use a system of cross-referenced symbols. This allows you to find recipes throughout the book that are considered appropriate for various dietary concerns. You may, for instance, find a recipe in the chapter on osteoporosis (Building a Stronger Foundation) that is marked as also appropriate for nerves and recuperation.

The index below permits you to locate recipes in every chapter which may be of interest to you.

 A HEALTHIER HEART CAN BEGIN TODAY

42; Steam-Stirred Red Onions—43; Baked Onions—43; Baked Stuffed Onions—43; Mushroom Stuffing—44; Onion-Apple Stuffing—44; Autumn Vegetable Puree—45; Mashed Potatoes with Green Beans—93; Potato Cakes—94; Corn on the Cob—94; Baked Butternut Squash—95; Fruited Baked Squash—95; Polenta—96; Basic Boiled Potatoes—136; Potato-Sauerkraut Casserole—136; New Potatoes in Garlic Broth—136; Mashed Potatoes with Yogurt—137; High-Protein Noodles—174; Baked Vegetable Rice—175; Toasted Brown Rice Stuffing—175; Italian Green Beans—204; Carrots Piquant—240; Kohlrabi and Carrots —240; Steamed Broccoli and Red Peppers—241; Steamed Mixed Vegetables—241; Hi-Pro Sprouts—244; Boiled Sweet Potato—267; Rice with Pears—269; Pennsylvania Dutch Baked Lima Beans—287.

Miscellaneous: Tofu Mayonnaise—45; Thick Onion-Tomato Sauce—45; Raw Marinated Mushrooms—46; Basic Tomato Sauce—46; Hot Taco Sauce—46; Stockpot Tomato Sauce—47; Black Magic Sauce—48; Soybean Tahini Dip—48; Hummus Tahini—49; White Lightning Cheese Dip—49; Eggplant Dip—49; Baked Garlic—50; Herbed Garlic Spread—50; Garlic Broth—50; One-Minute Cinnamon Applesauce—51; Strawberry Applesauce—51; Cinnamon-Apple Snack—51; Spiced Pear Spread—52; Baba Ghannouj—98; Hot Pepper Sauce —98; Pinto Bean Spread—138; Oven-Baked Chick-peas—139; Banana Hors d'Oeuvres— 176; Sesame Tofu Dip—176; Good Gravy—210; Whole-Wheat-Cornmeal Pie Crust—211; Apple Pancake Sauce—212; Cauliflower White Sauces—244; V-7 Juice—245; Garlic-Yogurt Spread—308; Garlic Dip—309; Onion Sauce—311; Stuffed Mushrooms—360; Sesame Crackers—360.

Beverage: Carob Yogurt Frosty—179.

Desserts: Banana Pound Cake—53; Frozen Banana Yogurt—104; Apple Delight—213; Sweet Potato Pie—245; Stovetop Rice Pudding—339.

 LET YOUR BLOOD PRESSURE GO DOWN

Breakfasts: Dutch Muesli—19; Apple Chunk Porridge—19; Raisins 'n' Spice Oatmeal—20; Porridge-Fruit Melange—20; Bulgur Breakfast—20; Choo-Choo Granola (Muesli)—80; Nutty Oatmeal—81; Date-Nut Porridge—81; Pear Porridge—81; Fruit-full Cereal Bowl—119; Orange-Cinnamon Cracked Wheat Cereal—120; Creamy Apple Porridge—120; Rice and Raisin Breakfast Cereal—163; Banana-Toasted Nut Cereal—164; Raisin Breakfast Rice— 189; Fruited Yogurt Muesli—190; Sweet Sugarless Muesli—299; Royal Elizabethan Breakfast —322; Apricot-Brown Rice Cereal—324; Mat's Himalayan Muesli—348; Hawaiian Punch —348.

Soups: Cream of Tomato Soup—82; Pureed Garden Soup—82; Peachy Plum Soup—83; Lentil Soup with Dill—123; Cream of Carrot Soup—258; Chilled Apricot Soup—300.

Salads: Simply Super Bean Salad—24; Orange-Date Salad—83; Molded Fruit Salad—83; Millet,

Fruit and Vegetable Salad—84; New Potato and Onion Salad—84; Chick-pea and Corn Salad—85; Basil Tomatoes—85; Cabbage-Grape Salad—86; Grape-Cucumber Salad—86; Sunshine Salad Dressing—86; Fabulous Fruited Salad—166; Cabbage-Apple-Date Salad—233; Orange and Grape Salad—259; Rice 'n' Fruit Jubilee—352.

Breads: Barley Bread—87; Quick Yeasted Date Bread—88; No-Knead Dill Bread—88; Quick Whole Wheat Bread—89; Pita Bread—356.

Main Dishes: Haddock with Mushroom and Bulgur Stuffing—35; Oven-Baked Lentils—38; Crunchy Chicken Tropicana—89; Poached Fish Fillets—90; Broiled Tuna Melt—90; Lentil Stew—90; Lentil-Tomato Sauce—91; Scalloped Cabbage—91; Zucchini Tortilla—129; Lentil Risotto—131; Soy Spaghetti Balls—237; Baked Vegetable Pie—239; Sweet Potato-Bean Pie—264; Savory Lentils—286; Mexican Lentils—286; Saucy Fish Fillets—331.

Side Dishes: Red Rice—41; Ratatouille—92; Zucchini Fiesta—93; "Grownup" Green Beans—93; Mashed Potatoes with Green Beans—93; Steamed New Potatoes—94; Potato Cakes—94; Corn on the Cob—94; Baked Butternut Squash—95; Fruited Baked Squash—95; Polenta—96; Carrots Piquant—240; Kohlrabi and Carrots—240; Steamed Broccoli and Red Peppers—241; Steamed Mixed Vegetables—241; Boiled Sweet Potatoes—267.

Miscellaneous: Thick Onion-Tomato Sauce—45; Basic Tomato Sauce—46; Hot Taco Sauce—46; Garlic Broth—50; One-Minute Cinnamon Applesauce—51; Vegetable Stock—96; Chicken Stock—97; Barbeque Sauce—97; Baba Ghannouj—98; Hot Pepper Sauce—98; Herbal Seasoning Mix—99; Season with Reason—99; Mediterranean Tomato Sauce—100; Curry Powder—100; Light Chicken Broth—101; Oven-Baked Chick-peas—139; Quick Pizza Sauce—210; V-7 Juice—245; Strawberry Topping—271; Turkey Broth—311; Tofu-Peanut-Banana Spread—334; Banana-Date-Nut Spread—334.

Desserts: Buckwheat Crepes—101; Fresh Strawberry Pie—102; Strawberry-Rhubarb Pie—102; Jeweled Raspberry Pie—103; Lemon Chiffon Pie—103; Frozen Banana Pop—103; Baked Currant-Pears—104; Frozen Banana Yogurt—104; Creamy Dessert Sauce—104; Tofu-Rice Pudding—105; Whole Wheat Bread Pudding—141; Banana-Rice Cream—180; Peaches 'n' Pear Sauce—212; Cantaloupe-Raisin Pie—290.

BETTER DIGESTION, TOP TO BOTTOM

Breakfasts: Dutch Muesli—19; Apple Chunk Porridge—19; Raisins 'n' Spice Oatmeal—20; Porridge-Fruit Melange—20; Bulgur Breakfast—20; Apple-Raisin Cracked Wheat Cereal—21; Molasses Pancakes—21; Wheat-Oatmeal Dollar Pancakes—21; Choo-Choo Granola (Muesli)—80; Pear Porridge—81; Powerhouse Pancakes—119; Fruit-full Cereal Bowl—119; Orange-Cinnamon Cracked Wheat Cereal—120; Sunshine Oatmeal—120; Creamy Apple Porridge—120; Banana Split Breakfast—162; Orange-Cinnamon Waffles—163; Whole Wheat Waffles—163; Rice and Raisin Breakfast Cereal—163; Wheat Pancakes—164; Raisin

TAKE A LOAD OFF YOUR NERVES

Rosy Tuna Salad—36; Hot Tuna Sauce—37; Chunky Chicken Tropicana—89; Poached Fish Fillets—90; Broiled Tuna Melt—90; Spaghetti with Herbed Cheese—130; Baked Fish Mediterranean—167; Super Second-Day Chowder—168; Chicken Liver Kebabs—168; Split Pea Vegetable Soup—169; Oriental Chicken Rolls—169; Split Pea Casserole—170; Pate Ring—170; Turkey with Vegetables—171; Red Flannel Tofu—171; Tuna Casserole—172; Spinach-Rice Casserole—173; Confetti Rice 'n' Beans—173; Fish Fillets Florida—198; Creamed Fish and *Pimiento*—199; Broiled Mushrooms on Toast—202; Macaroni with Ricotta—202; Broccoli-Cheese Quiche—237; Rainbow Rice—238; Liver Dressed for Dinner—262; Oven-Baked Chicken and Vegetables—263; Fettucini with Spinach and Mushrooms—264; Super Chili—281; Pate Meatloaf—282; Polynesian Liver—282; Chicken Livers, Mushrooms and Walnuts—283; Liver 'n' Onions—283; Liver Yucatan—284; Fish Fillets Florentine—304; Whole Wheat Crepes—305; Fancy Stuffed Macaroni Shells—306; Four-Star Beef Stew—327; Vegetable Meatloaf—328; Baked Chicken Breasts—328; Roast Turkey Breast—329; Saucy Fish Fillets—331; Mushroom-Walnut Sauce with Pasta—331; Salmon Quiche—357; Mushrooms Stroganoff-Style—358; Cashew Chicken—359; La Leche League Salmon Loaf —415.

Side Dishes: Red Rice—41; Baked Stuffed Onions—43; High-Protein Noodles—174; Baked Vegetable Rice—175; Toasted Brown Rice Stuffing—175; Thick Beef Spaghetti Sauce—285; Rice Waffles—332.

Miscellaneous: Tofu Mayonnaise—45; Pinto Bean Spread—138; High-Protein No-Roll Crust—139; Banana Hors d'Oeuvres—176; Sesame Tofu Dip—176; Mark's Trail Mix—176; Raisin Chews—177; Spinach Sauce—210; Yogurt Cream Cheese—308; Fabulous Date Bars—333; Seasoned Popcorn—359.

Beverages: Peanut Butter Toddy—177; Summer Drink on the Green—178; Banana-Strawberry Drink—178; Clove Tea—178; Hot Carob Drink—179; Warm Golden Milk—179; Carob Yogurt Frosty—179; Pineapple Punch—272; Hot Milk Unwinder—312.

Desserts: Lemon Chiffon Pie—103; Whipped Tofu Topping—140; Plum Kuchen—141; Sweet Potato Cheesecake—180; Banana-Rice Cream—180; Brown Rice Pie—181; Carrot Yogurt Cake—273; Body-Shaper Cheesecake—313; Peanut Butter Pie—337; Orange-Almond Cake—338; Stovetop Rice Pudding—339; Almond Cheesecake—416; Rice Pudding—417.

 SLENDERIZING NATURALLY

Breakfasts: Bulgur Breakfast—20; Creamy Apple Porridge—120; Raisin Breakfast Rice—189; French Toast—190; Fruited Yogurt Muesli—190.

Soups: French-Style Onion Soup—22; Green Pepper Soup—22; Gazpacho—23; Cream of Tomato Soup—82; Pureed Garden Soup—82; Peachy Plum Soup—83; Fresh Lima Chowder —121; Browned Potato and Cabbage Soup—121; Tomato-Lentil Soup—122; Minestrone —191; Oven Split Pea Soup—192; Thick Cream of Corn Soup—192; Chicken Soup Chi-

THE ANTI-CANCER DIET

Bread: Carrot Bread—261.

Main Dishes: Broccoli-Cheese Quiche—237; Mushroom-Tofu Delight—237; Soy Spaghetti Balls —238; Rainbow Rice—238; Baked Vegetable Pie—239; Mexican Vegetable Casserole— 263; Peanut Butter Tacos—265.

Side Dishes: Fruited Baked Squash—95; Potatoes and Broccoli—205; Carrots Piquant—240; Kohlrabi and Carrots—240; Steamed Broccoli and Green Peppers—241; Steamed Mixed Vegetables—241; Cauliflower Souffle—241; Capitol Dome Cauliflower—242; Broccoli Mousse—242; Oven-Braised Brussels Sprouts—243; Brussels Sprouts with *Lemon White Sauce*—243; Hi-Pro Sprouts—244; The Ugly Ducklings—267; Spicy Ginger Carrots—268; Curried Rice—288.

Miscellaneous: Cauliflower White Sauces—244; V-7 Juice—245.

Desserts: Sweet Potato Cheesecake—180; Sweet Potato Pie—245; Carrot Yogurt Cake—273.

 # INCREASING YOUR RESISTANCE

Soups: Peachy Plum Soup—83; Carrot-Apricot Soup—228; Green Zinger Soup—228; Sweet Potato Bisque—257; Chili-Pumpkin Soup—257; Cream of Carrot Soup—258; Chilled Peach Soup—258; Chilled Apricot Soup—300.

Salads: Tuna-Rice Salad—25; Green Bean Salad—27; Basil Tomatoes—85; Spinach-Orange Salad —165; Fabulous Fruited Salad—166; Minted Fruit Salad—194; Fresh Tomato Salad—196; Antipasto Alla Salute!—230; Very Orange Salad—232; Tossed Salad Vinaigrette—234; Spring Dandelion Salad—234; Mushroom-Cashew Salad—234; Cold Orange-Rice Salad— 236; Shredded Vegetable Salad—236; Spinach-Mushroom Salad—259; Orange and Grape Salad—259; Four Star Cabbage 'n' Fruit Salad—260; Zingy Spring Salad—260; Ruby Tofu Dressing—260; Creamy Vegetable Salad Dressing—261; Grapefruit and Prune Salad—280; Tossed Green Salad—349; Creamy Fruit Salad—351; Herbed Mushroom Salad—352; Pepper Cabbage—353.

Bread: Carrot Bread—261.

Main Dishes: Liver Dressed for Dinner—262; Kale Quiche—262; Mexican Vegetable Casserole —263; Oven-Baked Chicken and Vegetables—263; Fettucini with Spinach and Mushrooms —264; Sweet Potato-Bean Pie—264; Stuffed Butternut Squash—265; Peanut Butter Tacos —265; Super Chili—281; Polynesian Liver—282; Chicken Livers, Mushrooms and Walnuts —283.

Side Dishes: Baked Butternut Squash—95; Fruited Baked Squash—95; Carrots Piquant—240; Steamed Broccoli and Red Peppers—241; Cranberry-Stuffed Sweet Potatoes—266; Sweet Potato-Applesauce Souffle—266; Baked Sweet Potato and Pear—267; Boiled Sweet

ENERGIZING YOUR BLOOD

Miscellaneous: Mark's Trail Mix—176; Lentil Pate—289; Fig Bars—289; Prune Butter—290; Fabulous Date Bars—333; Date-Nut-Raisin "Jam"—335.

Beverage: Peanut Butter Toddy—177.

Desserts: Whole Wheat Bread Pudding—141; Carrot Yogurt Cake—273; Wet-Bottom Molasses Cake—290; Cantaloupe-Raisin Pie—290; Peanut Butter Pie—337; Orange-Almond Cake—338.

 # BUILDING A STRONGER FOUNDATION

Breakfasts: Dutch Muesli—19; Molasses Pancakes—21; Powerhouse Pancakes—119; Banana Split Breakfast—162; Brown Rice Pancakes—299; Broiled Cinnamon Pancake—299; Sweet Sugarless Muesli—299; Royal Elizabethan Breakfast—322.

Soups: Cream of Tomato Soup—82; Salmon Bisque—165; Green Zinger Soup—228; Chili-Pumpkin Soup—257; Broccoli Soup—300; Chilled Apricot Soup—300; Blueberry Soup with Yogurt—301.

Salads: Cucumber and Yogurt Salad—196; Coleslaw with Yogurt Dressing—235; Dairy and Fruit Salad—301; Garden Cottage Cheese Salad—301; Persian Cucumber Salad—302; Yogurt-Dill Dressing—302; Rosy Sesame Dressing—302; Sesame-Tofu Dressing—303; Cheese-Stuffed Pears—350.

Breads: Strawberry Muffins—29; Sunflower-Buckwheat Bread—128; Potato-Corn Muffins—128; Apricot-Corn Bread—303; Quick Date Bread—304.

Main Dishes: Sharon's Best Pizza—30; Skillet Turkey Dinner—33; Soy-Bulgur Casserole—39; Scalloped Cabbage—91; Spaghetti with Herbed Cheese—130; Autumn Cabbage Pie—133; Zucchini Pie—133; Potato Pizza—134; Split Pea Casserole—170; Eggplant Pizza—200; Macaroni with Ricotta—202; Broccoli-Cheese Quiche—237; Kale Quiche—262; Mexican Vegetable Casserole—263; Fish Fillets Florentine—304; Whole Wheat Crepes with Spinach-Ricotta Filling—305; Better-Than-Lox-and-Cream-Cheese Sandwich—305; Fancy Stuffed Macaroni Shells—306; Welsh Leek Tart—307; Salmon Quiche—357; Classic Open-Face Sandwich—358; La Leche League Salmon Loaf—415.

Side Dishes: Broccoli Mousse—241; Rice Waffles—332.

Miscellaneous: Tofu Mayonnaise—45; Pinto Bean Spread—138; Spinach Sauce—210; Cauliflower White Sauces—244; Fig Bars—289; Yogurt Cream Cheese—308; Garlic-Yogurt Spread—308; Herbed Cheese Ball—309; Garlic Dip—309; Whole Wheat White Sauce—310; Creamy Tofu Sauce—310; Zesty Lemon Sauce—310; Onion Sauce—310; Turkey Broth—310; Tofu-Banana-Peanut Spread—334.

Beverages: Peanut Butter Toddy—177; Banana-Strawberry Drink—178; Hot Carob Drink—179;

RECUPERATING FASTER

Roast Turkey Breast—329; Apple-Chicken Casserole—329; Savory Chicken Curry—330; Stuffed Haddock Fillets—331; Saucy Fish Fillets—331; Mushroom-Walnut Sauce with Pasta —331; Salmon Quiche—357; Mushrooms Stroganoff-Style—358; Cashew Chicken—359; La Leche League Salmon Loaf—415.

Side Dishes: Molasses Baked Soybeans—40; Creamy Succotash—42; Cranberry-Stuffed Sweet Potatoes—266; Sweet Potato-Applesauce Souffle—266; Oven-Baked Carrots—268; Curried Rice—288; Rice Waffles—332; Steamed Stuffed Potatoes—332.

Miscellaneous: Soybean Tahini Dip—48; Hummus Tahini—49; Sesame Tofu Dip—176; Mark's Trail Mix—176; Raisin Chews—177; Lentil Pate—289; Fig Bars—289; Prune Butter—290; Fabulous Date Bars—333; Peanut Sauce—334; Stuffed Prunes—334; Tofu-Banana-Peanut Spread—334; Banana-Date-Nut Spread—334; Date-Nut-Raisin "Jam"—335; Fresh Applebutter—335; Peanut Butter Cookies—335; Carob Syrup—336; Blanched Almonds— 336; Stuffed Mushrooms—360.

Beverages: Peanut Butter Toddy—177; Banana-Strawberry Drink—178; Banana Curd Shake— 312; Frosted Banana Whip—312; Sesame Milk—337.

Desserts: Banana Pound Cake—53; Lemon Chiffon Pie—103; Creamy Dessert Sauce—104; Tofu-Rice Pudding—105; Whole Wheat Bread Pudding—141; Sweet Potato Cheesecake— 180; Sweet Potato Pie—245; Pumpkin Pie—273; Wet-Bottom Molasses Cake—290; Body-Shaper Cheesecake—313; Peanut Butter Pie—337; Orange-Almond Cake—338; Baked Apple Custard—339; Stovetop Rice Pudding—339; Vanilla Pudding—415; Rice Pudding— 417.

◤ HEALTHIER TEETH AND GUMS

Breakfasts: Dutch Muesli—19; Broiled Cinnamon Pancake—299; Royal Elizabethan Breakfast— 322; Mat's Himalayan Muesli—348; Hawaiian Brunch—348.

Salads: Cabbage-Grape Salad—86; Autumn Roots Salad—195; Cabbage-Apple-Date Salad—233; Garden Cottage Cheese Salad—301; Tossed Green Salad—349; Stuffed Pears with Pineapple—349; Cheese-Stuffed Pears—350; Cottage Cheese Salad—350; Carrot-Raisin Salad— 350; Creamy Fruit Salad—351; Chicken-Grape-Walnut Salad—351; Rice 'n' Fruit Jubilee— 352; Herbed Mushroom Salad—352; Pepper Cabbage—353; Cauliflower Salad—353.

Breads: Crunchy Fruit Muffins—29; Strawberry Muffins—29; Pumpernickel Bread—127; Reformed Bagels—354; Whole Wheat Popovers—355; Crackling Brown Rolls—355; Pita Bread—356.

Main Dishes: Sharon's Best Pizza—30; Broccoli-Cheese Quiche—237; Mushroom-Walnut Sauce with Pasta—331; Salmon Quiche—357; Mushrooms Stroganoff-Style—358; Classic Open-Face Sandwich—358; Cashew Chicken—359; La Leche League Salmon Loaf—415.

Miscellaneous: Mark's Trail Mix—176; Fig Bars—289; Blanched Almonds—336; Seasoned Pop-corn—359; Stuffed Mushrooms—360; Sesame Crackers—360; Whole Wheat Croutons—361.

Dessert: Sweet Potato Cheesecake—180.

PREGNANCY AND BREASTFEEDING

Main Dish: La Leche League Salmon Loaf—415.

Desserts: Vanilla Pudding—415; Almond Cheesecake—416; Rice Pudding—417.

General Index